The Trauma-Informed Pediatric Practice

A Resilience-Based Roadmap to Foster Early Relational Health

R.J. Gillespie, MD, MHPE, FAAP

Amy King, PhD

With a Foreword by Andrew S. Garner, MD, PhD, FAAP

T0290986

American Academy of Pediatrics

DEDICATED TO THE HEALTH OF ALL CHILDREN®

American Academy of Pediatrics Publishing Staff

Mary Lou White, *Chief Product and Services Officer/SVP, Membership, Marketing, and Publishing*
Mark Grimes, *Vice President, Publishing*
Chris Wiberg, *Senior Editor, Professional/Clinical Publishing*
Theresa Wiener, *Production Manager, Clinical and Professional Publications*
Amanda Helmholz, *Medical Copy Editor*
Peg Mulcahy, *Manager, Art Direction and Production*
Soraya Alem, *Digital Production Specialist*
Sara Hoerdeman, *Marketing and Acquisitions Manager, Consumer Products*

Published by the American Academy of Pediatrics
345 Park Blvd
Itasca, IL 60143
Telephone: 630/626-6000
Facsimile: 847/434-8000
www.aap.org

The American Academy of Pediatrics is an organization of 67,000 primary care pediatricians, pediatric medical subspecialists, and pediatric surgical specialists dedicated to the health, safety, and well-being of all infants, children, adolescents, and young adults.

While every effort has been made to ensure the accuracy of this publication, the American Academy of Pediatrics does not guarantee that it is accurate, complete, or without error.

The recommendations in this publication do not indicate an exclusive course of treatment or serve as a standard of medical care. Variations, taking into account individual circumstances, may be appropriate.

Statements and opinions expressed are those of the authors and not necessarily those of the American Academy of Pediatrics.

Any websites, brand names, products, or manufacturers are mentioned for informational and identification purposes only and do not imply an endorsement by the American Academy of Pediatrics (AAP). The AAP is not responsible for the content of external resources. Information was current at the time of publication.

The publishers have made every effort to trace the copyright holders for borrowed materials. If they have inadvertently overlooked any, they will be pleased to make the necessary arrangements at the first opportunity.

This publication has been developed by the American Academy of Pediatrics. The contributors are expert authorities in the field of pediatrics. No commercial involvement of any kind has been solicited or accepted in the development of the content of this publication.

Every effort is made to keep *The Trauma-Informed Pediatric Practice* consistent with the most recent advice and information available from the American Academy of Pediatrics.

Please visit www.aap.org/errata for an up-to-date list of any applicable errata for this publication.

Special discounts are available for bulk purchases of this publication. Email Special Sales at nationalaccounts@aap.org for more information.

Printed in the United States of America

9-511/0624   1 2 3 4 5 6 7 8 9 10
MA1141
ISBN: 978-1-61002-740-3
eBook: 978-1-61002-741-0

Library of Congress Control Number: 2023947912

What People Are Saying About *The Trauma-Informed Pediatric Practice*

This book presents a down-to-earth path to becoming a trauma-responsive pediatric practice. Drs Gillespie and King give us a detailed, practical, and compassionate way forward, rooted squarely in relational health, the bedrock of resilience. Very actionable!

> M. Denise Dowd, MD, MPH, FAAP, editor of the Trauma Toolbox for Primary Care and professor of pediatrics at Children's Mercy Hospital

In this book, Dr King and Dr Gillespie recognize the pediatric advantage—and privilege—of longitudinal relationships with patients and their families. Pediatricians have regular opportunities to engage families as partners in care, taking the family's lead to discuss adversity, protective factors, and resilience. Their emphasis for the pediatrician's role is not to fix but to listen. I encourage practice teams to embrace this approach.

> Marian F. Earls, MD, MTS, FAAP, coauthor of "Mental Health Competencies for Pediatrics" and chair of the American Academy of Pediatrics Council on Healthy Mental and Emotional Development

The Trauma-Informed Pediatric Practice is a must-have for anyone looking to move beyond just summing the suffering to, practically and effectively, building the buffering. With tools and techniques drawn from the authors' combined years of experience, the authors move beyond the approximation of adversity to concrete strategies to build and restore relational health. In so doing, this roadmap charts a path for us all to follow.

> Heather Forkey, MD, FAAP, coauthor of *Childhood Trauma and Resilience: A Practical Guide* and professor of pediatrics at UMass Chan Medical School

We all know we *should* be implementing trauma-sensitive practices, but we get stuck in the *how*. This masterful book respectfully guides us how to support children, adolescents, and families in their journey toward healing. These authors are spot-on by focusing on relational health. We have special relationships with families, making us critical supports in their lives. Now, thanks to Drs Gillespie and King, we have a roadmap that recognizes our skills to listen wholeheartedly and then builds our capacity to sensitively support others in their path toward resilience.

> Kenneth R. Ginsburg, MD, MS Ed, FAAP, author of *Building Resilience in Children and Teens;* editor of *Reaching Teens: Strength-Based, Trauma-Sensitive, Resilience-Building Communication Strategies Rooted in Positive Youth Development;* and professor of pediatrics at Children's Hospital of Philadelphia

This book is essential reading for anyone who has thought that doing trauma-informed work is too hard or not worth the effort! Guided by clinical experiences and the evidence, the authors share their own personal and professional journey to developing a trauma-informed clinical environment and implementing trauma-informed care within the outpatient primary care setting. The book is full of practical tips that make trauma-informed care accessible to the masses and not just rewarding for the pediatric provider but frankly enjoyable to practice!

> Brooks Keeshin, MD, associate professor of pediatrics at the University of Utah

The Trauma-Informed Pediatric Practice is just the transformational book pediatricians need; it is full of practical, evidence-informed tips about identifying and ameliorating the effects of childhood adversity while promoting resilience and healing. This book reminds us all about why we became pediatricians and the joy of helping each and every child and family thrive. It is truly transformational.

> Moira Szilagyi, MD, PhD, FAAP, coauthor of *Childhood Trauma and Resilience: A Practical Guide* and past president of the American Academy of Pediatrics

Drs Gillespie and King, in partnership as pediatrician and child psychologist, have created this seminal work, *The Trauma-Informed Pediatric Practice,* that brings practical guidance and wisdom from years of integrated trauma-informed care (TIC) and early relational health (ERH) clinical practice. Together, often reflecting on each other's clinical experiences, they poignantly describe their research-to-practice journey in the development of new clinical skills from relational health history taking to empathic listening and guidance in support of family's growth, healing, and resilience. This must-read book, from nationally recognized TIC and ERH master clinicians, offers next-generation pediatricians the fundamentals and advanced practice tools, with the personal reflective processes, to become the needed innovative TIC/ERH clinicians of the future.

> David W. Willis, MD, FAAP, founder of Nurture Connection, the Movement to Promote Early Relational Health

American Academy of Pediatrics Reviewers

Committee on Psychosocial Aspects of Child and Family Health
Committee on Substance Use and Prevention
Council on Child Abuse and Neglect
Council on Foster Care, Adoption, and Kinship Care
Council on Healthy Mental and Emotional Development
Trauma Expert Leadership Team

Authors

R.J. Gillespie, MD, MHPE, FAAP
General Pediatrician
The Children's Clinic
Portland, OR

Amy King, PhD
Licensed Psychologist
Oregon Psychological Association
Amy King, PhD, LLC—CEO & Founder
Newberg, OR

Dedication

To you, my colleagues in the trenches…may this strengthen and support you as you give your hearts and souls to the care of your patients and families.

—R.J. Gillespie

To the children and families that have allowed me the honor of hearing their stories. Thank you for being the most amazing teachers. I hold your stories in my heart, especially yours, my sweet, freckle-faced friend whose only goal was to simply "get messy"; I hope you're thriving in the world—making messes and feeling loved.

—Amy King

Equity, Diversity, and Inclusion Statement

The American Academy of Pediatrics is committed to principles of equity, diversity, and inclusion in its publishing program. Editorial boards, author selections, and author transitions (publication succession plans) are designed to include diverse voices that reflect society as a whole. Editor and author teams are encouraged to actively seek out diverse authors and reviewers at all stages of the editorial process. Publishing staff are committed to promoting equity, diversity, and inclusion in all aspects of publication writing, review, and production.

Contents

Translation—and Transformation—Begin Here

It was the best of times, it was the worst of times...
A Tale of Two Cities, **Charles Dickens**

The phrase "bench to bedside" is often used to describe the lengthy process of translating advances in research into new diagnostic modalities, treatment guidelines, or clinical practices. Although estimates vary, the general consensus is that it frequently takes longer than a decade for the medical community to translate "what we know" into "what we do."

This translation gap is pervasive throughout medicine, and pediatrics is no exception. More than 25 years has passed since Felitti and Anda described the now well-established associations between adversities in childhood and poor outcomes in physical and mental health later in life. More than 25 has passed since the National Academy of Sciences used their report *From Neurons to Neighborhoods* to draw attention to the ecological, social, and developmental influences on child health and well-being. Thanks to *The Trauma-Informed Pediatric Practice* from Drs Gillespie and King, we now have a comprehensive roadmap to begin translating these and other advances in developmental science into clinical care that is squarely focused on the ability of early relationships to proactively nurture wellness...both in childhood and beyond.

The science is now clear: what happens in childhood does not stay in childhood. Recent advances in basic developmental sciences are revealing the molecular, cellular, and behavioral mechanisms that allow formative experiences in childhood, both adverse and affiliative, to drive outcomes in physical health and mental wellness decades later. Prepared with this more sophisticated understanding of how salient childhood experiences become biologically embedded, pediatricians are now poised to lead transformational changes in how medicine is taught, practiced, and funded.

If we assume—as has been done in the past—that most adults will lead healthy, productive lives regardless of their childhood experiences, pediatric care is perfunctory at best and superfluous at worst. But when we acknowledge that the foundations for both adult wellness and adult disease are being laid during childhood, then pediatric care becomes the linchpin of a reenvisioned, strengths-based health care system that is squarely focused on proactively building wellness and actually *preventing costly, seemingly intractable, adult-manifest, noncommunicable diseases*. From a "what we now know" perspective, it really is the best of times.

But change is hard, and there are significant barriers to change at multiple levels. At the societal level, discussions about relational health, listening with compassion, and expressing empathic curiosity seem downright countercultural in an era marked by division, distrust, and depersonalization.

At the systems level, the entire health care–insurance-pharmaco-industrial complex runs on 2 codes. A diagnosis code declares what is wrong with the patient, and a procedural code explains what was done to the patient. There is little room—or reimbursement—in such a deficits-based system for pediatric or other efforts to promote the safe, stable, and nurturing relationships that buffer adversity in childhood and build wellness in adulthood.

The reductionistic, deficits-based framework of traditional medicine continues to slant medical education toward the molecular, cellular, physiological origins of disease, while minimizing—if not ignoring—the significant ecological, social, and developmental forces that forge disease *and* wellness over time.

At the practice level, payment schedules continue to prioritize quantity over quality, and far too many quality metrics rely on dutifully clicking boxes in an electronic health record instead of focusing on the therapeutic relationships that are known to drive behavioral change and wellness in both children and their caregivers.

Finally, at the clinician level, pediatricians understand the developmental science, recognize the inherent value and power relationships, and yearn to build wellness in patients and their families, but *they feel thwarted at every turn.* From a "what we actually do" perspective, it really is the worst of times.

So how do pediatricians who feel distressed, beleaguered, and undervalued begin to bridge this discordant chasm between what we now know and what we actually do?

It all starts with this book. Drs Gillespie and King acknowledge that there are multiple barriers to implementing care that is trauma informed, grounded in developmental science, and centered on relationships. But in a clear, concise, and approachable manner, they outline the steps needed to transform pediatric practices into healing-centered medical homes for both children and their families. In doing so, they offer pediatric clinicians the knowledge, scripts, skills, resources, and, perhaps most importantly, the confidence to embrace a different kind of care. The care that Drs Gillespie and King endorse here is strengths based, longitudinal, and grounded in respectful, trusting, and therapeutic relationships.

Simply put, Drs Gillespie and King provide an accessible guide to begin bridging the chasm between what we now know and what we actually do at the clinician and practice levels. But the implications of this proactive, development-informed, strengths-based, relationally focused approach extend far beyond the walls of the pediatric clinic. Transforming how the rest of medicine is framed (strengths- vs deficits-based), taught (reductionistic vs holistic), practiced (quantity vs quality), and funded (procedures vs long-term value) will require the pediatric voice to be heard at all levels of leadership. Similarly, the system and policy changes needed to promote wellness—instead of waiting for disease to intervene—will require pediatric clinicians to lead interdisciplinary advocacy efforts.

Fortunately, that's what pediatricians have always done! From the introduction of child labor laws, to the use of immunizations, to the adoption of seat belts and car seats, pediatricians have always worked to translate what we now know into what we actually do.

But before pediatric clinicians transform the rest of medicine and tackle the complexities of public policy, we first need to set our own house in order. Thanks to Drs Gillespie and King, *we got this!*

Andrew S. Garner, MD, PhD, FAAP
Clinical Professor of Pediatrics
CWRU School of Medicine
Cleveland, OH
January 5, 2024

Preface

Listen.

You hear it, don't you? The rumblings are everywhere: Telling you that adverse childhood experiences (ACEs) are important. Telling you that responding to adversity, stress, and trauma may create a vital paradigm shift in how you treat patients. You've heard other clinicians talking about trauma; in fact, whole conferences have been dedicated to understanding the physiology and consequences of trauma. Public health officials declare it to be a chronic health crisis. Whole states are beginning to mandate screening for ACEs and reimbursing for completed question-naires. Schools are creating trauma-responsive practices in their transformation of education and in-school discipline. Even the media jumps in from time to time, lamenting the impacts of unresolved trauma on our communities. You have heard the science. You are well aware of the countless effects trauma has on your patients and families. You know in your gut that you're seeing these effects daily, and you feel you must do something.

But where do you start?

Doubts creep into the back of your mind. Questions come flooding out: *What can I do in my busy practice that would be meaningful to families and patients? Screening alone isn't enough to begin to heal people, is it? How do I create a meaningful response to patients or families that have experienced trauma? I'm not a mental health clinician; is this really something I can do? Is this in my scope of practicing medicine?* **How do I do this?**

You want to help…but you're also worried about doing it "wrong." You're worried that you may open a can of worms and not have adequate resources to meet the needs of your patients. No one has given you a roadmap for this, or any kind of plan. Since you're not quite sure what steps you need to take, you push it into the enormous to-do list on your desk, where it gets buried but not exactly forgotten. Someday you'll take the first step.

That day is today.

This book is a step-by-step guide to supporting families in building the relational skills they need to mitigate the effects of trauma. It's so much bigger than ACEs; it's about understanding early relational health (ERH) and the broadening definition of early trauma, figuring out barriers to relational health that caregivers are experiencing on a daily basis, and knowing how and when to help. And it's about providing hope and direction. As clinicians dedicated to the health and wellness of children, we hold prevention as one of our core values—so we're going to walk you through a better way than simply "screening" for trauma. We're going to walk you through how to prevent its effects and what to do when you see it.

By going upstream in the lives of infants, toddlers, and young children, and by supporting their caregivers in their parenting journeys, you'll be able to partner with families to create greater health and resilience. Then, these healthy and resilient families will be better able to thrive and withstand stressors when they happen, so they become tolerable stresses instead of toxic ones. We will walk you through the entire process—including how to prepare yourself and your prac-tice to embark on this journey, what tools and surveillance questions you'll need to implement, what to do with disclosures of trauma, and how to maintain your own wellness and equanimity in the process. Practical, evidence-based, and effective interventions for improving patient and family resilience will be a vital part of both your preventive efforts and your structured response to disclosures of trauma. We'll provide plenty of these interventions. Each chapter will conclude with some questions to consider based on quality improvement principles that, when answered, will help you personalize the workflow to best fit your needs and interests.

This text was written by practicing clinicians, in pediatric primary care and pediatric mental health, who have walked the walk and will guide you on an actionable path. We hope you find it relatable and practical, since our experience is based in the reality of navigating busy outpatient practices just like yours.

A few reflections from R.J.:

When I first decided to start asking about trauma in practice, I was pretty worried. What was I actually going to say if a patient disclosed trauma to me? What if they said something triggering… I mean, I have my own history to contend with. Would I actually have the words to help? Who were the allies that would help support me and my families?

The first time I intentionally asked a patient about ACEs was with a teenager I considered to be pretty troubled. You've probably seen a kid just like her, the one who "does everything wrong": skipping school so much that she was being expelled from a last-ditch high school, experimenting with drugs, having unprotected sex with a much older boyfriend, actually throwing furniture at her mother whenever they got in a fight. I think Mom had the police on speed dial, and the police could have probably driven to the house in their sleep. You get the picture: the kind of case where just hearing the kid's name makes your blood pressure go up.

So, when she came in for her 15-year checkup, I had a pretty long list of things to address. I'm her physician, so it's important for me to counsel her on how to get her life on track again, right? But at the same time, I wanted to back up and try to help her see the big picture. I started by asking her if she had any goals—for example, what she wanted to do when she finished school. She looked me straight in the eye and said, "You think I'm having unprotected sex because I don't have any goals? You're an < insert expletive here > !"

Yikes.

She had seen right through me. But at the same time, I knew there had to be more to her story, more to help me understand where she was coming from. After I caught my breath, I started to ask her about ACEs. I just listed them out and let her say yes or no. She had 5, and if you've read the research on ACEs, you know that's a lot. So, I let go of my agenda of needing to "fix everything" and let her drive the conversation while I just listened…

The conversation drifted to her interests, her dreams, and her passions—some of which she had probably forgotten, but they were still in there. It even turned out that we have a hobby in common, photography, so we talked about that for a few minutes.

I had her come back a month later for a follow-up, since we still had a lot to talk through. When she came in, she had quit drugs on her own and transferred to a Gateway program where she could earn a GED and an associate's degree at the same time. She had even dumped her boyfriend. I asked what had changed, and she said, "Those kids at my old school were losers; they didn't have any goals."

My heart still jumps a little bit when I think about that moment.

It defined how I would approach trauma histories in my office. There is something so well-known in mental health that we tend to undervalue in primary care: it's the magic of listening and of giving our undivided attention to our patients and families. This isn't master-level wizardry, but it is a practical, everyday kind of magic.

Obviously, there's a bit more to it than that—but not as much as you might think. A lot of it comes down to realizing the power of the skills you already have in your toolbox. It comes down to understanding what hurts our patients and families are carrying, recognizing when trauma is getting in the way of either child development or parenting, and then taking the day-to-day pieces of clinical care and turning them into dozens of ways to support our families.

To me, talking with a patient who has *already* experienced trauma feels woefully inadequate. From the moment I started learning about trauma and toxic stress, I was desperate to get upstream, to see what I could do to possibly prevent toxic stress from happening in the first place. One of my partners and I decided to embark on a precarious journey—asking parents about their histories of adversity—and that seemingly straightforward decision set me on the journey of learning how to support relational health of caregivers and their very young children. This book is the result of where that journey has taken us—thanks in no small part to the partnership I've had with Amy, which added some of the form and structure to the clinical process that is now part of our day-to-day practice.

A few reflections from Amy:

I'll never forget the feeling I had when I paused while speaking to a group of pediatricians about responding to childhood adversity. As I encouraged them to respond by listening to the messages behind behaviors; to bring more of themselves into the room; to celebrate character strengths in children and connection within families; and to begin to talk about feelings and fears with caregivers, many of them had blank stares. Some leaned forward. Some nodded with trepidatious agreement. I held my breath. Were they finding this cheesy? Too much? Were they terrified, interested, or ready to send me packing? Like many of you reading this book, they had heard about ACEs, watched Nadine Burke Harris' TED Talk, and felt compelled to take action in their clinics. They wanted something practical, strength based, and efficacious. I stepped into this meeting and, with their encouragement, proposed teaching resilience interventions at every well-child (health supervision) checkup, starting with newborn checkups. I encouraged small doses of education, guidance, and support that would enhance ERH, respond to infant and toddler mental health needs, and create more feelings of competence and confidence in my colleagues. One of the pediatricians suggested an array of interventions they could use throughout a child's development. I began to talk to them about trauma-informed practices, feeling states, family strengths, and proven interventions I had used for years as a psychologist specializing in complex trauma. And over dinners, coffee, and a slew of emails, I received feedback from practicing physicians on what felt meaningful, what inspired them, and what reassured them. They asked questions, requested scripts, dug deep into their own fears, and began to try out these conversations with their patients.

And they told me this work was *everything*. It was completely transforming how they interacted with children and families. They excitedly told me it felt like there was *finally* practical guidance to implement trauma-informed practices with resilience-building strategies that are meaningful, reassuring, compelling, and, more than anything, inspiring. Having started out compelled but nervous, these physicians became champions at their clinics. R.J., an early adopter, dived right in. Thanks to him and other pediatricians who were ready to be champions in the lives of children and families, this work has flourished.

A month or so after providing the first round of training on resilience interventions to pediatricians, I reached out to one of them to consult about a patient. It was a follow-up discussion about a first trial of stimulant medication, but he had also recently taken part in training around resilience building as a way to mitigate the effects of stress and trauma in children and families.

> **Amy:** Hey there, I was checking in about "Joey" and how things are going with the Ritalin trial?
> **Pediatrician:** Yeah, going great, but we need to talk...

Amy: *(Gulp. Had I messed up? Did I not send over notes? What call did I overlook?)* Sure, what's up?

Pediatrician: We need to talk about Yolky Feelings. *(For context, Yolky Feelings is a resilience strategy you'll learn about later, meant to build emotional intelligence and build resilience through increasing coping tools and communication.)*

Amy: OK, talk to me...

Pediatrician: This has completely changed how I'm talking to kids and families. I mean, I've always talked to them about behavior, but now I have a tool, a connection piece. I'm going to implement this strategy in every single 6-year-old well-child exam. What else do I have to talk about? I've covered immunizations, bicycle safety, but this—*this* is what I needed to connect with parents. This is how I can help them decrease anger in their house and respond to questions they have about tough feelings.

Amy: I'm so glad it feels helpful.

Pediatrician: This is everything. Thank you.

Over the course of the next several months, this pediatrician taught every clinician in his clinic about Yolky Feelings, his nurse made handouts, and he continued to call me and gush over successes he was having and his increased connection with parents and children.

As R.J. mentioned, this isn't unicorn magic, but it is a shift that *feels* magical. And you're already doing so much of this! If we do our job well in following this blueprint, practices that you've been engaging in for years will feel more meaningful and well-rounded. And those that need shoring up will feel accessible and actionable.

In other words, you can do this. We're here to walk you through everything you need to know—even if you are starting out feeling terrified, worried, nervous, or burned out. We've been there. We wrote this book to help.

Acknowledgments

R.J. Gillespie: First, I'd like to thank my colleagues at The Children's Clinic—the most dedicated and innovative group of clinicians I've ever met. When we first approached them with the idea of asking caregivers about their trauma histories—an outrageous idea at the time—they thought it through and enthusiastically said "Yes, we can do that." This book wouldn't exist without their compassion and love for the families that walk through our doors.

I've had many professional mentors who have influenced and shaped my professional career—giants on whose shoulders I've been lucky enough to stand: Drs David Willis, Maggie Bennington-Davis, and Teri Pettersen, whose patient teaching and mentorship helped set me on this path; the members of the Academy on Violence and Abuse, whose early feedback encouraged me and shaped my work—particularly Drs David Corwin and Tasneem Ismailji; and the pediatricians I've worked with through the American Academy of Pediatrics, who are a constant source of wisdom and inspiration—particularly Drs Nadine Burke Harris, Andy Garner, Marian Earls, Denise Dowd, and Heather Forkey. And of course, my coauthor, Amy, deserves a special callout for her partnership, wisdom, creativity, and friendship.

Most importantly, I want to recognize all the relationships in my personal life that give shape and form to my ability to be resilient: Paul, for enduring hundreds of tempests in teapots on the home front and always gently holding my heart in his hands; my "work spouse," Rebecca, for reminding me to be proud and for always having my back; Jackie and Paul, for their care and constant cheerleading; and my amazing circle of friends, who listened to the frequent babbling, regular ranting, and occasional boasting that this book-writing process brought out. My relationships with all of you make me a better human and, ultimately, a better clinician…and, for that, you have my heartfelt gratitude.

Amy King: I want to thank the countless professionals who have given me inspiration and vision for this work, the MOST important medicine. Especially, I want to thank Dr Dean Moshofsky and colleagues at the Children's Health Alliance. Thank you for inviting me into your spaces of healing and support and believing that, together, we could create a world where children and families are seen, heard, and supported in pediatrics. Also, thank you to Dr David Willis and Dr Nadine Burke Harris, who have been ombudsmen of my work and trailblazers for children and families.

I would be remiss if I did not acknowledge Drs Myrtle Scott, Ellen Brantlinger, and Marsha McCarty—3 brilliant mentors who shaped my intellectual history and passion for young children, children and families with extreme adversities, and family systems work, respectively. Your words and wisdom live inside of me and every individual whose life I have touched.

To my friends. R.J.—your brilliance, wit, partnership, and dedication to this work have been incredible to witness as I walk beside you on this journey. Thank you. And to my girlfriends, who raise me up, cheer me on, hold me close, and laugh with me. You are my family.

It is my relationships with the innermost circles in my life for which I owe the most heartfelt gratitude. My mom, who taught me the delightful feeling of unconditional love. You and me against the world, Mom. My dad, who taught me perseverance, competitiveness, and the blessing of being loved despite messing up. Thanks for choosing me. Sophia and Jack, my beautiful kids, who teach me, who forgive me, and who hold my entire heart. I am blessed to be your mother. Finally, my husband, Ryan—there is no other soul in the world who has healed my heart more than you.

About This Book

R.J. Gillespie, MD, MHPE, FAAP

There are no shortcuts to any place worth going.
Beverly Sills

Recently, in what has become a routine conversation in my practice, I learned that the mother of a 4-month-old had experienced 9 adverse childhood experiences (ACEs), plus 2 additional traumas, all of which added up to a pretty challenging childhood that resulted in years of therapy. As part of the conversation, I talked with her about positive childhood experiences (PCEs), including how they can be even more important in determining lifelong outcomes than the adverse experiences. I talked with her about setting intentions around her goals for her son, to think about which PCEs are most important for him to experience, and about how she was doing with making those experiences happen.

When I asked how her past experiences affected her parenting now, she had one question: "How do I make sure my relationship with my son is as strong as it can be?"

I love this question. It cuts straight to the chase, doesn't it?

When it comes to becoming a trauma-responsive practice, this is really the heart of the matter: How do we strengthen relationships and build resilience in our everyday interactions with patients, rather than simply take a trauma history and let the disclosure just hang out there in the open? If you've asked yourself this question in your practice before, you've probably had several different choices of how to respond:

- **Path A:** We're on a tight schedule here; we need to get back on course. Let's talk about using car seats and introducing solid foods. (In other words, *Yikes, I don't know what to do!*)

- **Path B:** That's not in my wheelhouse; let's refer to mental health or behavioral health. After all, relationships are complicated—some therapists spend years with people trying to mend their relationships. (In other words, *That's an important question, but I don't have the capacity to manage it in the course of a well-child visit.*)

- **Path C:** That *is* a complicated question, but we can break it down. Let's dig into what we know about the early relational health (ERH) and social-emotional (SE) development of a 4-month-old; give the parents a brief overview of attachment and how to recognize bids for attention, including what they can do with their child to support that developmental task; and follow up at the next visit to see how it went and give them a new intervention that matches the SE development of a 6-month-old. (In other words, *honor the importance of the question, tap into your existing skill set, and support the caregiver and family in their desire to be more resilient.* If this seems like a lot, don't worry: the actual script I use to talk about attachment and bids for attention is in an upcoming chapter.)

Our training, or at least my training, left me in a position to take either path A or path B. When I think back on my residency training, my rotation in developmental and behavioral pediatrics made up about 2 weeks out of the 3-year program, which I think is a common experience for clinicians of my generation.

Path C is where we want you to be by the end of this book. It's a more challenging approach, but it has the potential to make a huge difference in the lives of our patients and families. Furthermore, I think you'll find that doing this essential work (one of Amy's trainees called it "*the most* important medicine") will transform your relationship with your families and invigorate your practice by giving you a new perspective on your role in promoting the health and wellness of the families we serve.

The purpose of this book is to help you learn how to ask about trauma as part of your routine care for families and then know how to respond compassionately and effectively to disclosures of trauma. We're making the assumption that you are interested in becoming more trauma responsive in the care you're giving your families, which means getting more comfortable with assessing trauma histories in some way. More importantly, we want you to know what to do when the patient or caregiver says, "Yes, there's been a trauma," in whatever form they tell you. We want to reinforce that managing disclosures of trauma is in your wheelhouse. You don't have to engage in long-term therapy with the patient or caregiver, but you can start by supporting the family and by doing brief, developmentally based, efficacious interventions during well-child visits that support resilience and enhance relational health between kids and their caregivers.

To be clear, we believe that building resilience through these interventions is important for primary prevention (by building relational skills before a trauma happens to mitigate its effects) but can also be used as a secondary prevention (to build those skills in the context of a traumatic event). In either case, it's important to remember that when a family discloses trauma, you won't resolve it within a single visit; rather, you'll use that information to engage with the family as their parenting journey unfolds and support them over the years of well-child visits that follow the disclosure. We think about building resilience as hundreds of little doses of relational health support—starting early and continuing through the child's life.

Our goals, for ourselves and for you, are the following:

- Introduce the concept of the relational health history (RHH), including how the RHH comes together to form a comprehensive picture of a child and family's wellness.
- Create a culture change to support practical responses to trauma. Move practice from being trauma aware (*I understand the importance of trauma to my patients and families*) to trauma responsive (*I'm ready to do something about it*).
- Build your confidence in your abilities to assess and address caregiver trauma and other barriers to safe, stable, nurturing relationships (SSNRs).
- Feel confident in responding to disclosures of child/patient trauma.
- Make the work of responding to trauma meaningful for patients and families.
- Learn tools and interventions that build relational health between caregivers and their kids, that are actionable and can easily fit into well-child visits, and that help families prepare for, prevent, or recover from adversity.

We've conceptualized this work as being relationally focused, rather than adversity focused. Unavoidably, bad things sometimes happen to our patients and families, but we're in a position to build the relationships between caregivers and their children to prevent the effects of toxic stress. If you think about the taxonomy of stress (**Table 1**), the main difference between a tolerable stress and a toxic one is the presence of an SSNR that helps buffer the effects of that trauma. That's why we focus on building those relational skills with our families—to prevent the effects of toxic stress by building SSNRs between our patients and their caregivers.

Table 1. Taxonomy of Stress

Type of Stress	Description
Positive stress	Everyday pressure that pushes people to perform. Is usually temporary, promotes learning and adaptation, and has an activating effect.
Tolerable stress	Negative events (usually temporary or onetime) that activate our stress responses but are well buffered by coping strategies and the support of those around us, allowing us to return to our previous state of functioning.
Toxic stress	Chronic, repeated stresses—which are not sufficiently buffered by safe, stable, nurturing relationships—that overwhelm the capacity for coping. This level of stress is associated with physiological changes in the body.

Before you can start asking anyone about their trauma history, you'll need to have a strong foundation of knowledge and skills on which to build your response. This means spending some time preparing yourself and your practice before actually embarking on any assessment protocols within your office. We'll walk you through every step of the way.

Framing Concepts

What's in a Name?

In developing this book, we've gone back and forth about a simple piece of nomenclature that actually represents a lot of the controversy behind ACEs and trauma in primary care. Do we call it *screening* or *assessment* or *history taking*? *Screening* implies mutual discovery, meaning that both the clinician and the patient or caregiver are learning something new. But that's not accurate for trauma histories: only the clinician is learning something new. *Screening* also implies the use of a standardized, validated tool that helps in our diagnostic efforts with patients. For the purposes of our book, we use the term *screening* in the context of using such validated tools (specifically SE health, caregiver mental health, and social drivers of health [SDOH]), and *assessments* is used for areas of clinical inquiry that don't have a validated tool or may rely on history taking rather than using a tool at all.

Another terminology debate: Do we refer to it as *trauma, adversity,* or something else? When people hear *trauma,* they still sometimes think about emergency department visits—something that's broken or injured. Most importantly, how do we include the aspect of PCEs and give the process a strength-based approach? It's not just semantics; rather, it represents the complexity of this relatively new part of pediatric health care. For clarity, *adversity* generally refers to the negative events an individual might experience; *trauma* refers to the physical and emotional consequences of that adversity.

We also vetted a lot of different names to describe what we're talking about in this book and settled on the phrase *relational health history.*

As clinicians, we take a family history, a social history, a past medical history, and so on, so the best way to describe what we're talking about is to borrow that same framework. Think about the phrase for a minute: *relational health history* implies that we're talking about not just trauma or the negative events of the past but also the positive. It doesn't imply that you're using a specific written assessment tool—you might—but you might choose to use a series of history-taking questions to get you to the same point, or you might use a combination of the two, depending on the context. This term also accounts for the fact that the history is longitudinal and changes with time and with the circumstances of the patient or family, so it's an ongoing, flexible, and dynamic process that takes place over the life span of our relationship with the family. I think of the RHH as being made up of several related parts: what's happened to the family (past history of caregiver trauma and PCEs), what's happening now (caregiver mental health, SDOH), and how we support relational health for the future (resilience-based interventions to build 2-generational skills).

Note From Amy

I recently spoke with a mother who's a speaker and advocate for parents who've endured trauma. As she reflected on her childhood and becoming a parent, she pointed out that the relationship with her child's pediatrician was fraught with worry. She was a successful mom but terrified of parenting. And even more so, she was terrified that if her child's pediatrician knew how anxious she was, he would take away her girls. After all, she had experienced being removed from her mother at a young age; the fear was tangible. When we talked about this book and what it might mean to mothers like her, she wept. She said, "I felt so alone. I wanted someone to ask me what I was going through. But no one was asking. It would have changed so much for me." She was referring to the ongoing worry, guilt, and shame she was experiencing as a mom because of her early adversities.

Asking doesn't mean solving or therapizing. It means providing a space for less aloneness so you can focus on creating more positive experiences for families and increasing the quality of relational health. You already do this on so many fronts, and this space can be transformational for your patients. You can do this.

What Do We Mean by "Interventions"?

Throughout the book, you'll hear us talking about 100 little conversations to build relational health between caregivers and their kids. We refer to these as *interventions,* and we believe these interventions collectively build stronger families. We intend for these interventions to be started early, and done often over the course of a child's life, little by little.

In defining an "intervention," we're talking about taking a specific action to interfere with a potential outcome or course, and creating a condition or process to at least prevent harm caused by trauma, or, better yet, to improve functioning within families. In breaking this down, we think that the interventions we present throughout the book mitigate the harm of stressful events by building preexisting strengths into the SSNRs that our caregivers and kids experience by giving them actionable tools to promote ERH.

This work sounds like a lot, and it is; but as we've said, we think it's the most important medicine (you'll see that phrase repeated throughout this book). We have a hard time coming up with any part of medicine that is more important than building strong, resilient families. That said, the interventions are actionable and easy to implement. After all, we're primary care clinicians—we have a lot to cover in a visit—so none of the interventions will take you more than a few of your precious minutes during a visit. They're intentionally designed to be trauma informed and evidence based and to support and promote ERH—or heal it when it's been compromised. Implementing them is a direct response to what we're asked to do in the American Academy of Pediatrics (AAP) policy statement on preventing childhood toxic stress[1] and clinical report on trauma-informed care.[2]

Four Key Questions

When it comes to implementing any sort of screening or assessment tool or surveillance/history questions in practice, there are a few key questions I use to ensure that implementation is completely thought through from a quality improvement (QI) perspective:

- Why am I looking?
- What am I looking for?
- How will I find it?
- What will I do when I find it?

These questions will pop up throughout the book as we guide you through implementation of the different components of the RHH. In all fairness, I usually start with the end in mind—the "What will I do when I find it?" part—because if I don't have an adequate answer to this question, I'm probably doing harm by asking the questions in the first place. There is also a double meaning in the question when it comes to trauma. There's the practical part of the question of what I do for the patient and family in terms of resources and referrals, safety planning, and counseling and guidance; and there's the personal aspect of how I keep myself and my practice regulated, safe, and supportive for the patient and family. We'll explore each of these meanings throughout the book.

Tying Relational Health Histories to Medical Home Principles

Your success in implementing RHHs in practice is predicated on the idea that you are providing a medical home for the patient or family that you are assessing. If we're committed to the principles of the medical home for our patients and families, the idea of taking an RHH almost becomes a necessary component of the comprehensive, patient- and family-centered, whole-person care that the model is based on. In our opinion, it's hard to imagine being a true medical home without incorporating trauma responsiveness into our practice culture, including the use of RHHs to help us identify patients who need additional care and support.

The principles of the medical home were developed in the 1960s as a way of providing more comprehensive and organized care for children with special health care needs.[3] With time, medical home principles have evolved and changed, but these principles are still considered the gold standard for how we care for kids, particularly those who experience additional health care needs. In fact, medical home principles have become some of the core values of primary care clinicians. Children who have been exposed to toxic stress should be considered children who need the comprehensive, coordinated care provided by a medical home, because they may be at risk for poor health outcomes; they may need additional services, community-based supports, and referrals both within and outside the health care system; and they (and their caregivers) need and deserve more anticipatory guidance around developmental promotion, positive parenting skill building, and resilience skills. When thinking about medical home principles, how we care for kids who have additional service needs, and how that applies to kids or families that have experienced toxic stress, we break down the process into 5 steps:

1. Identify the population through screening or surveillance, and track them.
2. Assess the family and patient strengths, assets, and needs for services.
3. Make referrals.
4. Provide self-management tools.
5. Follow up on referrals and close communication loops.

You'll be able to expand on each of these steps using the chapters that follow, but for now, suffice it to say that you can't do this kind of work unless you're providing continuity for the family and building a supportive relationship with the family and caregivers first. In our state, we have a specific model of care called the Patient-Centered Primary Care Home[4] that comes with a detailed set of standards that practices must attest to; the National Committee for Quality Assurance has a similar set of standards that help define practical steps that should be taken to declare your practice a medical home.[5] If you haven't explored these kinds of processes, it's worth taking a look as part of your QI goals. Imagine asking a family or patient about their most personal histories if you're not the one who's providing continuous, family-centered care for the family or if you haven't developed workflows and processes that help track families needing additional help and support.

It Doesn't Start—or End—With ACEs

You'll hear a lot from us about ACEs; and of course, you've already heard a lot about them, which is probably why you grabbed this book to begin with. That said, we're going to dive into a lot more than just the traditional ACEs. There's a great conceptual diagram called the "pair of ACEs" that depicts a tree where ACEs are the branches, but adverse *community* environments—the other "ACEs"—are the roots of the tree.[6] The graphic implies that the traditional 10 ACEs described by Felitti and colleagues[7] are only part of the picture, but there are other traumas that can have the same kind of impacts. Of course, the 10 original ACEs described by Felitti and colleagues are particularly harmful because they happen within the context of the family that is supposed to buffer us from stress (now referred to as *intrafamilial adversities*), but stresses outside the family, including SDOH and other community and social contexts that impact children and families, are important considerations in exploring RHHs. Later we'll talk about expanded definitions of trauma, mostly from The National Child Traumatic Stress Network, that encourage you to think beyond these classic 10 ACEs.

Recent research indicates that PCEs are even more impactful on long-term outcomes than ACEs.[8] PCEs generally represent ways in which relational health between caregivers and children manifests during childhood, as well as within peer groups, communities, and schools. From a practical perspective, this means we can't, or shouldn't, assess traumas without giving equal, balanced consideration for assessing what's going well in the child's or family's life. We should spend as much time promoting PCEs as we do trying to prevent ACEs.

These 2 concepts mean that our attention to family wellness has to go beyond trauma assessments and include considerations of caregiver health and wellness (including peripartum mood disorders) and SDOH, as well as SE health promotion and screening for children. This may sound like a lot of screening and assessment tools, and it is. The more screening tools we introduce into practice, the stronger the tendency to treat them like a checklist: screen, pass/fail, refer, and move on to the next patient. Instead, think of how these tools integrate with each other and paint a picture of the child and family's overall wellness.

We see the whole set of screening tools against a backdrop of developmental health (**Figure 1**), with all these screening tools relating to each other and dictating different clinical workflows. For example, a visit with a child who has experienced trauma and has developmental challenges would lead to a different workflow than a visit with a child who has developmental challenges in the context of negative SDOH, and both of these would require different clinical responses than a visit with a child who experiences developmental challenges without these other contextual factors. Not only is the workflow different (as in what resources you refer to), but the way you engage the caregiver may be subtly different as well. All these different combinations of barriers to SSNRs should additionally trigger further evaluation of SE health.

Resilience Isn't Innate, But You Can Help Teach It

There's a myth about resilience: that people are born with it, and that's the main factor in how they manage difficult situations. There are even people who are starting to turn away from the word *resilience* because so many people equate resilience with "grit" or the idea of just "powering through." We think about resilience in a much different way; it's a skill that is developed longitudinally throughout life *within relationships*. The truth is, resilience isn't

FIGURE 1.

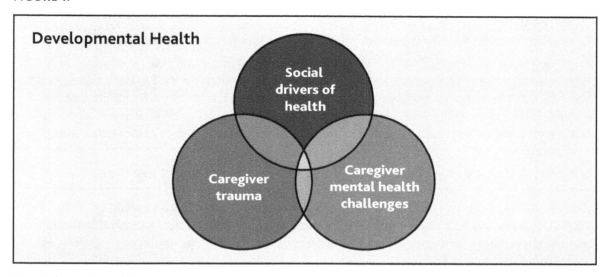

Integrated screening model.

innate—no one is born with it—but rather learned, developed, and fostered in the context of relationships. It continues to develop throughout a lifetime, as we learn to adapt and evolve from our day-to-day experiences, as well as the bigger life-changing events. In other words, no one is born resilient, but resilience—like SE learning, self-regulation, and self-efficacy—is achieved over time. And, over time, we see not that people are *always* resilient in every moment or in every situation but that they struggle, especially without buffering relationships, and that relational health is required to lean into resilience and foster it.

It's also important to consider that when you're teaching a resilience intervention, resilience is also created from and learned by the teacher, so empowering caregivers to teach resilience skills to their kids will also build the resilience of the caregivers themselves. A lot of the development of resilience begins in the early relationship between children and their caregivers, when they're spending the most time in our offices, so that's where we step in as clinicians who care for children. We recognize that you haven't been trained in your residencies to do this (neither was I), but we'll get you there.

The fundamental message to remember as you read through this book is simple: *You can do this.* Building relational health between children and their caregivers is well within your wheelhouse, even if you've not seen it that way before. Throughout the book, you'll be introduced to dozens of resilience-building interventions that are anchored in a developmental, trauma-informed context, so you'll be able to implement them in the course of your well-child visits with families. We're also going to help you reframe some of the anticipatory guidance skills you've already developed, to turn them into trauma-informed interventions. From my (R.J.'s) personal perspective as a mid-career physician, this will invigorate you and give your work some meaning that you may not have experienced before.

Structure of This Book

To support the SSNRs of our patients and families, we have a few core challenges to untangle as clinicians: reducing sources of stress in the lives of our kids and families, strengthening skills within families, and supporting responsive relationships for kids and their caregivers.[9] To help you on your journey, the book is divided into 4 parts:

1. Background Concepts: Building a Foundation for Trauma Responsiveness in Primary Care

2. Assessing Risks: Navigating Barriers to Safe, Stable, Nurturing Relationships

3. Building Caregiver-Child Relationships: Finding 100 Little Conversations to Build Connection

4. Building Clinician Skills: Incorporating "The Most Important Medicine" Into Practice

Part 1 will walk you through the controversies around the concept of "ACE screening" and illuminate why the AAP does not recommend screening children for ACEs. We'll talk through how to address barriers to discussing trauma in practice and how to get your practice ready to embark on this journey. We'll expand on our conceptualization of resilience and begin to prepare your colleagues and your organizations to embark on the journey toward becoming trauma responsive.

In Part 2, we'll explore the things that get in the way of caregivers being able to provide SSNRs to their kids. This will start with deepening your knowledge of ERH in the first place and give you the tools for assessing SE health for the kids in your practice. Assessing SE health is a 2-part process: there should be universal screening for all kids (using a validated tool) and ongoing surveillance for problems, *and* SE screening tools should be employed in the context of potential disruptions to SSNRs. We'll then move to the main barriers to caregivers being able to provide SSNRs to their kids—including caregiver depression and anxiety, SDOH, and caregiver trauma—and how to screen or assess for them in practice.

Part 3 will explore ways to enhance the caregiver-child relationship to "build the buffering" that helps mitigate the effects of toxic stress through 100 conversations that you'll have with your families over their lifetimes. This will include tweaking your anticipatory guidance to make it more relationally focused and learning how to design and use resilience-based interventions in practice. We'll discuss how to use these skills in the context of supporting kids who have experienced trauma and how to do safety planning and care coordination for these families as well. In the last chapter of this section, you'll see how we pull it all together into a roadmap for how to implement RHHs in the first 6 years after birth.

Finally, in Part 4, we'll discuss the clinical skills that you'll need to make this all work. You're already an awesome listener (We have faith in you!), but we'll talk about the importance of honing your listening skills, as well as discuss how to take care of yourself and your colleagues as you engage in this challenging work. And we're encouraging you to bring your whole self into this work, because we know it will make you feel more competent and decrease burnout. This section will also include an emphasis on QI skills that you'll need to motivate change within your practice and address how to sustain what you've implemented in your trauma-responsive work.

This book is based on our real-world experiences with addressing and responding to trauma in our practices; our perspectives are complementary as a primary care clinician and a psychologist. We see this book as an interdisciplinary collaboration, and we've written it with a conversational approach that represents how we tend to interact with patients and clients (and each other). With that in mind, when one of us writes a chapter, you'll see the other give perspectives on the material and vice versa in either a "Note From Amy" or a "Note From R.J." We're also presenting a lot of interventions you can implement in practice that will help build relational health with your families: you'll see the symbol in the margin to the left of this paragraph whenever we describe an intervention, just to help highlight them. Chances are, you already are doing some interventions with your families, so ours are meant to expand your toolbox and complement what you're doing rather than replace what's working well in your individual practice.

Our hope is that you will find this book practical. We can't give you all the answers about how taking an RHH will work in your practice, since every practice setting is different. At each step of the way, we include questions to help stimulate thinking about how you can adapt the information to your unique environment. We've included tools and scripts in the appendixes to help you tailor to your own specific needs. Remember that becoming trauma informed, taking RHHs, implementing trauma assessment tools, and utilizing resilience-building interventions in practice is a journey, not a destination. We're providing you with a roadmap to set you on your way, but the journey is all yours.

References

1. Garner A, Yogman M; American Academy of Pediatrics Committee on Psychosocial Aspects of Child and Family Health, Section on Developmental and Behavioral Pediatrics, and Council on Early Childhood. Preventing childhood toxic stress: partnering with families and communities to promote relational health. *Pediatrics*. 2021;148(2):e2021052582 PMID: 34312296 doi: 10.1542/peds.2021-052582

2. Forkey H, Szilagyi M, Kelly ET, Duffee J; American Academy of Pediatrics Council on Foster Care, Adoption, and Kinship Care; Council on Community Pediatrics; Council on Child Abuse and Neglect; and Committee on Psychosocial Aspects of Child and Family Health. Trauma-informed care. *Pediatrics*. 2021;148(2):e2021052580 PMID: 34312292 doi: 10.1542/peds.2021-052580

3. What is medical home? American Academy of Pediatrics. Updated May 23, 2022. Accessed March 18, 2024. https://www.aap.org/en/practice-management/medical-home/medical-home-overview/what-is-medical-home

4. Patient-Centered Primary Care Home Program. Oregon Health Authority. Accessed March 18, 2024. https://www.oregon.gov/oha/hpa/dsi-pcpch/Pages/index.aspx

5. Patient-Centered Medical Home (PCMH). National Committee for Quality Assurance. Accessed March 18, 2024. https://www.ncqa.org/programs/health-care-providers-practices/patient-centered-medical-home-pcmh

6. Ellis WR, Dietz WH. A new framework for addressing adverse childhood and community experiences: the Building Community Resilience model. *Acad Pediatr*. 2017;17(7)(suppl):S86–S93 PMID: 28865665 doi: 10.1016/j.acap.2016.12.011

7. Felitti VJ, Anda RF, Nordenberg D, et al. Relationship of childhood abuse and household dysfunction to many of the leading causes of death in adults: the Adverse Childhood Experiences (ACE) study. *Am J Prev Med*. 1998;14(4):245–258 PMID: 9635069 doi: 10.1016/S0749-3797(98)00017-8

8. Bethell CD, Gombojav N, Whitaker RC. Family resilience and connection promote flourishing among US children, even amid adversity. *Health Aff (Millwood)*. 2019;38(5):729–737 PMID: 31059374 doi: 10.1377/hlthaff.2018.05425

9. Cohen SD. *3 Principles to Improve Outcomes for Children and Families.* Center on the Developing Child at Harvard; 2021. Accessed March 18, 2024. https://developingchild.harvard.edu/resources/three-early-childhood-development-principles-improve-child-family-outcomes

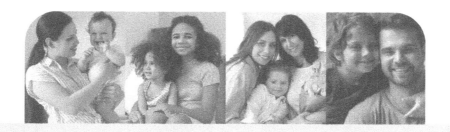

PART 1

Background Concepts: Building a Foundation for Trauma Responsiveness in Primary Care

We're going to begin our journey into supporting early relational health (ERH) with some background concepts that will help frame the interventions you'll be learning about throughout this book. These are key areas to explore in depth as a practice. First and foremost, we believe that understanding and inquiring about parent and caregiver trauma is an important component of relational health histories (RHHs); this is likely new work for you and your practice. We'll start by helping you understand potential pitfalls about assessing trauma in practice, starting with a discussion of the controversy around ACE screening specifically, since components of that debate apply more broadly to assessing trauma in practice.

Since you're likely embarking on this journey with the rest of your practice, we'll then talk about how to address commonly perceived barriers to discussing trauma and other sensitive subjects in clinical practice. While the conversation focuses primarily on barriers to discussing trauma in practice, remember that negative social drivers of health are also a form of trauma and that parent and caregiver mental health is another sensitive subject, so the perceived barriers apply to these aspects of RHHs as well.

We'll then address how to prepare your practice to be more trauma responsive and, ultimately, more compassionate toward patients and families. You may need to consider doing some training for your practice partners on trauma-informed care, depending on where you are on this journey; we'll provide a little guidance for how to approach training your colleagues and staff.

Finally, we'll turn our attention to resilience and explain why helping families build resilience is well within the pediatrician's wheelhouse. When taken all together, this book's interventions for building ERH between caregivers and children create a curriculum for how to enhance well-child care in the first 6 years after birth with a resilience-building focus. Amy will present her 6 guiding principles (3 for clinicians and 3 for parents and caregivers) for addressing resilience in practice. In our clinical work, we focus on teaching parents and caregivers how to build resilience in their children specifically because this process builds resilience in the teacher (ie, the caregiver) at the same time. This approach is key for building ERH, which we'll cover in depth in Part 2.

Chapter 1

The ACE Debate and Ethical Considerations

R.J. Gillespie, MD, MHPE, FAAP

Practice two things in your dealings with disease: either help or do not harm the patient.
Hippocrates

I have a heckler.

At this point in my career, I've done dozens of conference presentations about my work in assessing caregiver ACEs, but in the early days, I kept running into the same person at a lot of my lectures. They always asked highly critical questions about what I was doing—both in front of the audience and afterward in the post-lecture question and answer sessions. Their tone felt aggressive, sometimes mocking, and always put me on the defensive. *Why are you using* that *tool? How can you think* that *intervention is helpful?* Then the comments started showing up on blogs about my work: *That resilience questionnaire they're using is a disaster!* along with comments about how our approach should be changed in a dozen different ways. It felt like a continuous assault on what I saw as meaningful, important work. Honestly, it felt brutal.

When we started our work, there weren't a lot of practice-based models for how to approach trauma, let alone how to do a relational health history (RHH) in primary care, so I knew we were out on a limb. I sometimes left those conferences questioning our entire approach. Looking back, we started asking parents and caregivers about ACEs before a lot of this debate came to light, so we had put ourselves in a rather precarious situation by taking this path. Eventually, I had to take my own advice that I give to parents when they see a behavior in their kids that they don't like: you can get furious, or you can get curious. In the end, what my heckler did for me was to encourage me to dig deeper and deeper into why I'm doing the work I'm doing, how I can continually improve, and how I can best support my families. Ultimately, my heckler wasn't alone; the process of translating ACEs science into practical workflows in primary care is hotly debated.

We're going to start here by addressing this debate and why there are concerns about how or even if we approach trauma in primary care practice, particularly with the idea of "ACE screening." To be clear, the American Academy of Pediatrics does not recommend screening children for ACEs; the American College of Preventive Medicine agrees that we should not routinely collect ACE surveys on patients.[1] Not everyone agrees with this position,[2] but it's important to understand the background of this debate before you start asking questions about trauma in practice because some of the same debate points about screening for ACEs apply to asking about trauma generally. That said, given the impacts of trauma on relational health, inquiring about trauma is potentially a key component of an RHH; my personal practice has been to try to understand how trauma in parents and caregivers may impact their current parenting decisions and skills (more on this later). Inquiring about caregiver trauma histories has been recognized as a "promising practice"[3] and is a potential avenue for moving upstream in supporting early relational health in families. Assessing when trauma has happened to a child can potentially help us understand the roots of some behavioral and mental health concerns, somatic symptoms, or school difficulties; this is best addressed by asking caregivers and children about any scary or upsetting events rather than pulling out the ACE survey itself.

To answer the first question in implementation that we talked about in the Introduction—"Why am I looking?"—it's important to understand the specifics about this controversy.[4] Before you embark on any changes within your practice, think deeply about why you're interested in taking an RHH in the first place. If your reason is to capture payment for a screening tool, to satisfy an intellectual curiosity, or to "join the movement" that's going on in health care, we're going to encourage you to dig deeper. This is partly to ensure that your reasons for doing the assessments align with the ethical principles of health care, but it's also to prepare you for the hesitancy or resistance you might encounter in your practice or your patients.

In this chapter, we'll talk about the roots of the debate around trauma assessments in practice and then discuss how the basic tenets of health care ethics inform how asking about trauma in the context of an RHH can be meaningfully conducted in practice. From there, we'll talk a little bit about the public health approach to ethics related to trauma and trauma-informed care (TIC) and then tie all of this back to the implications for the pediatric medical home.

The Debate About ACE Screening

So, why is there a debate? One of the principal reasons for debate about ACE screening in particular is that the ACE questionnaire wasn't developed as a clinical tool but rather as an epidemiological tool (ie, as part of population health research) to explore correlations between childhood trauma and later lifelong health at the population level. At an individual level, an ACE score doesn't directly predict outcomes, partly because it doesn't assess the balancing factors of resilience and PCEs. It has been described by Robert F. Anda, one of its original authors, as a "relatively crude measure of cumulative childhood stress exposure that can vary widely from person to person."[5] The ACE score also doesn't recognize the type, intensity, or frequency of the traumas: an ACE score of 1 may represent a parental divorce, or it may represent years of recurring sexual abuse—and these 2 traumas may have very different effects on an individual's well-being.

Reducing an individual to an ACE score, with a specific cutoff for what represents a significant score, may in some cases miss serious and important histories and in other cases overestimate the effects of multiple traumas. In fact, researchers have found that ACE scores have poor accuracy in predicting which children will have later health problems and which ones won't.[6,7] Even something as seemingly common as parental divorce may result in very different experiences for patients. In the context of an amicable divorce, with 2 supportive parents in different households, that ACE may not have the same impact as when a single caregiver is facing constant financial instability and isolation or when a divorce is characterized by constant yelling and fighting. An ACE score also doesn't assess the timing of the traumas relative to a child's neurodevelopmental stage, with earlier traumas potentially having more profound impacts on a child's physiology and long-term wellness.[8,9] This is thought to be due to the rapid brain growth in early years, how dependent this brain growth is on a child's environment, and the context of the presence or absence of nurturing relationships that are intended to provide buffering experiences in the early years.

Because the ACE survey doesn't take resilience and relational health into account, it is considered a deficit-based model, which is another major criticism of the survey itself; research suggests that the presence or absence of PCEs is more powerful for driving outcomes than ACEs themselves.[10] At a clinical level, it's still unclear how adding an assessment of resilience or PCEs will improve the accuracy of deciding which patients or families need an intervention and which don't. However, one of the main reasons that ACE scores are minimally predictive of future outcomes is that ACEs can be buffered or balanced by safe, stable, nurturing relationships (SSNRs) or by early development of resilience skills that happen in the context of SSNRs. In other words, knowing that a trauma occurred in a person's life doesn't actually imply anything about their level of functioning; practitioners must take the next step beyond simply asking a history and into an assessment of the symptoms and consequences of that trauma, whether by follow-up questions in the case of caregiver RHHs or by specific symptom screeners if children have experienced trauma.[11] More important than assessing consequences of trauma, putting a focus on promoting PCEs and building relational health is primary prevention of toxic stress; by doing so, we're following Dr Heather Forkey's catchphrase, "Instead of summing the suffering, we should be building the buffering." Ultimately, this goal of "building the buffering" by intentionally supporting SSNRs in practices is the whole purpose of this book.

The ACE survey itself is also criticized for missing some important traumas,[12] and as such, it can be somewhat limiting in how trauma is defined. I once had a patient whose family had moved from a gang-controlled town in Mexico. The 8-year-old in the family was having some pretty drastic anxiety because his grandma was still living in that area, and he was (with good reason) worried about her safety. Technically, community violence and forced emigration aren't included in the ACE questions, but it's clear that those are significant traumas that were impacting my patient's wellness. It was also a reminder to me that the original ACE survey may introduce a degree of cultural bias into our conversations about trauma. For example, the traumas that affect our immigrant and refugee families are completely excluded from the list of potential adversities; in these populations, a different set of questions would need to be added in order to completely assess their needs.[13] Traumas that happen outside the family unit may not only have impacts on the child who witnesses the traumas but also end up distracting caregivers from their caregiving; the results may be similar to ACEs because the ability of caregivers to buffer relationships may be impaired.

Bullying, racism and prejudice, poverty, and medical trauma are other examples of potentially harmful experiences that may be missed if histories are not explored in other ways, as was the case for a father in our practice with a single ACE of parental separation. His comment to the ACE questions was "This survey seriously underestimates how difficult things really were." The National Child Traumatic Stress Network identifies over 2 dozen different traumatic events that may affect children,[6] but as you can imagine, it's difficult to get one screening tool to capture all potential sources of trauma that a patient or family might experience unless an open-ended question is included, like "Did anything else scary or upsetting happen?" to help capture other traumas we might have missed.

There are also concerns about whether or not primary care clinicians can provide evidence-based interventions (or referrals for interventions outside of primary care) in the event of a disclosure of trauma. Some of this concern revolves around what therapies will actually improve outcomes, but more importantly, these therapies may not exist in all communities or practice settings. Therapeutic modalities such as trauma-focused cognitive behavioral therapy, attachment and biobehavioral catch-up, and other dyad interventions have been shown to be effective in addressing the effects of early childhood trauma, but access to these therapies may not be available in all areas. However, within this debate is the assumption that the primary intervention for trauma is a mental health or therapy-based intervention. Parenting classes, support groups, mentoring programs, home visitation, programs that alleviate poverty, and other community-based services may also provide solutions for patients and families, depending on the clinical context.

Note From Amy

So often, when talking with pediatricians about intervening with families, I tell them, "You're already doing this!" Throughout the book, we'll point out how subtly and more directly you're providing trauma-responsive interventions that strengthen and support families. Sometimes, it's how you talk; other times, you're providing a specific tool. We'll point these out along the way so you can gain confidence that there's so much you're already doing. And just know, there are straightforward ways to provide support, in your office, every day.

Principles of Health Care Ethics

While understanding the debate is important, with careful and thoughtful planning, and with appropriate preparation of your clinicians and staff, trauma surveys or surveillance questions can be an integral part of an overall trauma-informed transformation of your practice. Right now, we're going to talk about the ethics of assessment tool implementation. In the next chapter, we'll discuss common real-time barriers to using assessment tools in practice and how to address them, so you're prepared to talk about them with your practice partners. We'll start with the 4 basic tenets of health care ethics[14]—non-maleficence, benevolence, autonomy, and justice—and how these principles influence your process for assessing and addressing trauma (**Table 1-1**). Be aware that while creating a space to address trauma is often healing, in individuals who have experienced a lot of traumas, we may inadvertently re-traumatize a person (thereby doing harm). Asking permission to delve into this history and being clear about the patient's choice in answering the questions (autonomy) are probably the 2 most important principles to adhere to in order to prevent re-traumatization.

Table 1-1. Connecting Ethical Principles to Trauma Assessments

Health Care Ethics Principle	How It Applies to Trauma Assessments
Non-maleficence ("First do no harm")	• Commit to supportive conversations about the assessment tool. • Before implementation, develop a plan for response. • Avoid labeling. • Protect confidentiality as much as possible.
Benevolence	• Connect patients and families to services that will help. • Create a culture of safety within your office.
Autonomy	• Give patients a choice about completing assessments. • Get patient and family feedback about how the assessment tool is being used.
Justice	• Use trauma-informed care to help achieve health care equity. • Be mindful of what power and privilege are brought to the clinical visit.

Non-Maleficence

As you remember, the first principle of health care ethics—non-maleficence, or "First do no harm"—is one of the cornerstones of how we practice. It is possible to do harm to a patient or family by asking about trauma histories, particularly if you don't have the right mindset about asking or if you don't have a clear plan about what you intend to do with the information obtained by taking the history. In a powerful editorial,[15] one author described the experience of being asked about past traumas in a medical intake form. After disclosing a history of abuse, she was surprised that the health care professional never acknowledged or addressed that history, even though she endorsed it multiple times over several visits. To be fair, a lot of clinicians may get stuck at the point of not knowing what to say; this reinforces the point of not implementing an assessment if you don't know what you'll do with the results. To help you craft a meaningful response, we'll talk about scripting for your response to disclosures, and how to address disclosures clinically, in Chapter 10, Supporting Families That Have Experienced Trauma, and Chapter 12, The Art of Listening.

There is an inherent message in a practitioner's silence in the context of a disclosure of trauma. If a patient discloses a trauma history and we don't respond to that disclosure, we're telling the patient that we don't think the history is important, that we don't believe the patient, that we can't handle the disclosure because it's too distressing or uncomfortable, or that the patient is simply not safe disclosing that history to us. It reinforces the social stigma that many people with trauma histories, particularly survivors of sexual abuse, already experience in relation to their trauma. Silence is often seen as a violation of trust,[16] particularly in the context of a disclosure of trauma. If we violate trust, we are unlikely to ever have a patient or caregiver make important disclosures in the future. It's hard enough for a survivor to undergo the process of building a personal narrative around a history of abuse, so when a story isn't responded to by the listener, it may be seen as safer to simply lock that story away again.

There is a broader ethical conversation related to screening, which asserts that a screening or assessment tool is useless (and potentially harmful) if you don't have a clear answer about what you're going to do with the information.[17] For example, you can develop an amazing test for a rare genetic disease, but if you don't have a viable treatment for those patients who test positive, you may do harm by performing the test because of the distress a patient could feel from being given a diagnosis they can't do anything about. When it comes to assessing trauma in primary care, you can avoid doing harm by having a clear plan in place for what you're going to do with the disclosures you experience. There will be a lot more on developing your clinical response in the chapters to come.

One of the potential risks to patients and families is the idea of being labeled based on their trauma. People are so much more than their ACE score; care must be taken to avoid reducing human beings to such reductionist labels. Instead of labeling patients or families as mere "trauma survivors," think about the idea of "radical acceptance." This is a Buddhist principle that states that we recognize our own experiences and how they influence the way we see others, and we then embrace what we see with kindness and compassion. In other words, as clinicians we suspend our judgments of others and accept them for who they are—the foundation of empathy. We've all met people whom we make snap subliminal judgments about—that they're dangerous, unstable, crazy, uneducated, or whatever. This comes from our own implicit biases and highlights the need for us to approach questions about trauma and adversity with humbleness about the things we're carrying into the conversation. Radical acceptance would encourage us to recognize how our own biases paint a picture in our mind about that individual and to recognize that the picture we've painted is *our own baggage* and has nothing to do with them. In fact, exercising compassion with our patients and families is a powerful yet under-recognized tool that improves quality of life, self-efficacy, adherence to treatment plans and recommendations, and control of symptoms.[18]

Note From Amy

Here's an empathy-building exercise that gets to R.J.'s point about radical acceptance. Imagine that every day, we all pick up 2 suitcases: In one hand, we hold our short-term stressors. Perhaps that's an unpaid bill, a medical concern, a recent fight we've had with a loved one, or concerns about our job. In the other hand, we pick up our long-term adversities—difficulties or traumas that may have affected us for weeks or even years. Some traumas we may have discussed; some are unknown to others. Every day, we pick up all these adversities and carry them around. *We carry our baggage.* When we interact with others, we're walking toward another human, dragging along our baggage, about to engage in a conversation. If we're not aware of the heaviness we carry, or if we personalize what someone else may be carrying, we will be harsh and judgmental toward that person, wondering, *What's wrong with them?* If instead we wonder, with curiosity, what they might be carrying, or have compassion for ourselves that we're carrying a heavy load, we'll be more empathic.

The idea of avoiding labeling patients includes how we protect confidentiality (when able) when we're documenting disclosures of trauma. If we write an ACE score, details about a trauma history, social drivers of health (SDOH), or other sensitive information in our clinical record and then send that record to a specialist or another practice, we've "outed" a caregiver or family without their consent. Care must also be taken to avoid labeling in our problem lists, billing documentation that is sent to insurance companies, and after-visit summaries. My personal practice is to document trauma disclosures in a confidential section of my electronic health record, so I can see it when I'm in a visit but it doesn't print into notes or follow the patient if their records are sent to another clinician outside my practice. That leaves any decisions about disclosures up to the patient or family, but I have that information to help guide my clinical decision-making when I need it.

Avoiding harm doesn't apply just to our patients; staff and clinicians may also experience harm. The idea of secondary trauma, or "the emotional duress that results when an individual hears about the firsthand trauma experiences of another,"[19] is an important consideration before embarking on any assessment process. Given the prevalence of trauma in the general population, you should assume that staff and clinicians may also have their own trauma histories and may be triggered by doing this kind of work. Staff and clinicians should be prepared for this potential outcome, offered choice and power in how they participate in the trauma assessment process, and given strategies for how to address their own wellness. That said, self-care can't be presented as yet another thing on their to-do lists in an already busy clinic environment; wellness and well-being need to be addressed at an organizational level and become embedded within the culture of the clinic and organization. We'll talk more about this need in Chapter 13, Self-Care and Sharing Our Humanity, and Chapter 14, Addressing Physician Overwhelm.

Benevolence

As you know, the second ethical principle, benevolence, refers to the idea of "doing good." Beyond just avoiding harm to our patients, our actions should in some way improve their lives or be of benefit to the family. That means a clinical assessment of, and response to, trauma needs to offer some benefit to patients or families, build a skill or asset within the family, or address a specific concern they have in their health or wellness.

Some of this benevolence comes from the process of educating families about trauma and resilience, giving a space to be heard, validating the importance of the experience, and removing stigma associated with the events. Traub and Boynton-Jarrett[20] described 5 modifiable resilience factors in primary care, or things we can do within clinical practice that will help build up families in the face of trauma. One of those key factors is trauma education, or helping patients and parents understand the effects of trauma and what we can do about them. When discussing trauma with parents and caregivers, I've frequently found that they are relieved by just being asked the questions. They know their past was difficult and want more than anything to be able to do better for their own children. When trauma is left as a stigmatized, not-for-polite-conversation topic, these kinds of childhood hurts can be left to fester. Caregivers are usually relieved that someone is bringing up the conversation and that someone is willing to help them work through forging a different path for their children.

Benevolence may also come from connecting families to needed or desired resources or from coaching families on resilience interventions. Positive parenting skills are another of those modifiable resilience factors that we can impact in practice. One of my colleagues in the Defending Childhood Initiative once told me that "kids who have experienced trauma need developmental promotion times 10." In other words, all the things we do to promote development, child-caregiver attachment, and resilience need to be amplified in kids who have experienced trauma. Similarly, parents and guardians who have experienced trauma may need 10 times the usual dose of skill building, which is something we can offer with confidence. This developmental and positive parenting promotion, though, is best in frequent, small doses—depending on the caregiver's readiness, interest, and need.

Doing good also comes from creating a culture of safety within your practice, which enables healing and recovery. This is the inverse of the harmful message of silence: openly talking about trauma in small, manageable doses helps destigmatize the topic and gives patients and families the space to heal. Without creating a safe space, conversations about adversity won't really happen, and this reinforces the harms done to patients rather than helps with healing. We'll talk a lot about listening throughout the book, but for now, suffice it to say that when clinicians spend time listening to their patients, we can become powerful forces in healing.

The importance of having some sort of a plan for what to do with trauma disclosures can't be overstated. It's our best chance to help turn a difficult past into a promising future.

Autonomy

By now, you've surely heard plenty about being patient centered, and hopefully, that's one of your clinical values. When it comes to assessing trauma, it's vital to give patients and caregivers "choice and voice" in the assessment process. This means we have to pay attention to patient choice, informed consent, privacy and confidentiality, and transparency.

If you are using an assessment tool in your clinical practice—for a sensitive subject such as trauma or SDOH—remember that the person completing the tool always has a choice about whether to answer the questions or not. Be explicit about this. In my mind, the goal of using assessment tools is never about forcing a disclosure; rather, it's about letting patients and caregivers know that the door is open if they ever need to have tough conversations in my office. They may choose to disclose today, at some future visit, or maybe never; but they know that they can if they should ever choose to. In a study of parental perspectives about disclosures of ACEs and unmet social needs, this was aptly described as "disclosure is a longitudinal process, not a discrete event."[21] After implementing parent and caregiver trauma assessments in my practice, I've had dozens of conversations at subsequent visits—unprompted by me—about domestic violence, food insecurity, personal losses, financial problems, and other family stressors. To be clear, I don't always know the resources off the top of my head, or have a handy solution to all the problems, but I can always lend an empathetic ear, reflecting how these problems may impact health and wellness, or provide context for parenting or challenging childhood behaviors. Then I can get help from one of my care coordinators in tracking down necessary resources and schedule a specific follow-up with my families to connect them with these resources.

Remember, too, that parents and caregivers need some autonomy in how and when the results of any assessment tools are discussed. It's extremely difficult for a caregiver to talk about their trauma history if a grandparent is present, for example, or to talk about social drivers if an older child is in the room listening. In my practice's assessment tools for caregiver trauma and SDOH, we added some boxes to let caregivers communicate how they want to discuss the results: now, later by phone, or not at all. If needed, we can have older kids go back to the waiting room, or sit with one of the medical assistants, to allow for a private conversation with the caregiver if needed. That way, we're respecting autonomy as much as we can.

As part of a quality improvement (QI) process within your office, it's wise to engage patients and families to give feedback about the process of conducting trauma assessments as part of an RHH, both before implementation and as the process is underway. There's a saying originally from disability advocacy that has been adopted as well in patient-centered care, "Nothing about me without me," which is meant to highlight the importance of integrating the patient perspective into any QI effort. It is worth the time to ask parents—both informally and in a structured way—how they perceive the screening efforts, their opinions on the tool itself, their comfort with completing the tool, and whether the tool leads them to a better understanding of either their own health and wellness or how to better engage with their kids. If you have a family advisory panel in your practice, have them review any assessment tool and your proposed workflow before you start to use them. In fact, that's where my practice got the idea to let caregivers decide how and when assessment tools are reviewed: parents were the first ones to point out how difficult it is to talk about some of these sensitive subjects in front of older children. We'll talk more about family feedback in Chapter 16, Sustaining Trauma-Responsive Practices.

Justice

Full disclosure: I'm a white guy (maybe you picked this up already).

From a practical perspective, that means that every time I walk into an exam room, I'm wielding power and privilege *whether I intend to or not*. I'm also carrying my own implicit biases (subconscious attitudes, beliefs, and preferences for certain groups that I identify with that are based on how, when, and by whom I was raised and educated) that impact how I interact with the world. We all have them. As much as I try, I will never fully understand the lived experiences of some of my patients, and I will never have historical trauma as part of what influences the way I interact with the world around me. Some patients and families have really good reasons to distrust the health care system; structural racism is embedded in the way our health care system was developed and in how it continues to be maintained and utilized, which means the health care system has the potential to be traumatizing in itself.

That doesn't keep me from trying to do better. It means I will always be learning how to weave cultural awareness into my daily practice and learning how families bring their own culture and experiences through my office door, which influences how they perceive and process traumatic experiences or what it means to live in relationship with each other and within a community. It also means I have to be careful with how I interact with the families in my practice, or at least mindful about how I may come across to them, and that I have to accept that the power dynamic between a white male physician and my patients will always be a potential barrier unless it's front and center in my mind with all my patients.

Am I forcing my patients into talking about something they aren't comfortable discussing? Am I creating a situation that will result in a patient being labeled (or feeling like they're being labeled)? Am I inadvertently wielding power in this interaction? Are my families fearful about me reporting them to a government agency based on my discovery of their past traumas?

ACEs drive health disparities; TIC has been recognized as a powerful tool for potentially reducing these disparities. Differences in health outcomes are driven by community and interpersonal violence, SDOH, and structural racism, making them all social justice issues. Because of its impact on social justice, trauma care must be intertwined with equity—one of the 6 dimensions of quality identified by the Institute of Medicine.[22] In that way, the ethical principle of justice would suggest that adopting a TIC approach in practice is an essential first step to achieving equity. A National Academy of Sciences roundtable[23] appropriately identified that "most illnesses and behaviors that contribute to health disparities are correlated strongly with individual-, family-, and community-level trauma; trauma continues to be an obstacle to successful treatment of many common illnesses; and clinics and environments of care often mirror the trauma experienced by patients and can themselves be traumatizing."

That said, given that assessing trauma and inadvertently labeling patients are also intertwined, justice can be violated as easily as it can be supported by taking an RHH. Trauma-informed care must be adopted with the intention of connecting patients to evidence-based resources that promote healing and resilience and providing a calm and nurturing environment in which patients seek care. Patient choice, and patient confidentiality, must be protected to the best of our abilities. When talking about trauma, we must be clear about which disclosures would result in a report to child protective services and which wouldn't (more on this in Chapter 11, Pulling It All Together). Furthermore, if TIC is viewed as a deficit model (finding out "what's wrong" with a patient) rather than as a strength-based approach (finding out "what's strong" with a patient), then the health care system is likely perpetuating trauma rather than addressing it effectively. At the end of the day, we need to understand how trauma may be affecting a family in addition to building family strengths, but even in the absence of a trauma disclosure, we can help reinforce what is strong with a family. In other words, simply assessing for trauma without also assessing for strengths or resilience is purposely looking at only one side of the coin.

Social drivers screening tools, including trauma assessments, are included in the primary care clinician's toolbox because of the social justice aspect of effectively using these tools. If you think about Maslow's hierarchy, it's hard for a patient or family to achieve higher levels of motivation if their basic physiological and safety needs are not being met. If you're not familiar with this model, Maslow described a pyramid of needs, starting with physiological and safety needs at the base of the pyramid, which need to be satisfied before moving on to psychological needs (like self-esteem, connection, and relationships), which in turn must be met before growth needs like creative outlets and achievement of personal goals.[24] Using a screening tool for food insecurity, for example, has the core purpose of helping families obtain healthy and nutritious foods (physiological needs) so they can move up on the hierarchy and achieve better things for their children and family. Taking an RHH can partially address the next level in the hierarchy, safety, to again help families get closer to achieving their growth needs.

If you haven't participated in any trainings in diversity, equity, and inclusion (DEI), then do so. And then do another one. If you don't know where to start, review the chapter The Intersection of Culture and Trauma in Forkey, Griffin, and Szilagyi's book *Childhood Trauma and Resilience: A Practical Guide.*[25] A few toolkits that might be useful are *Raising the Bar,* sponsored by the Robert Wood Johnson Foundation,[26] and *A Toolkit to Advance Racial Health Equity in Primary Care Improvement,* from the California Improvement Network.[27] I've personally been journaling through Layla Saad's *Me and White Supremacy*[28] workbook in an attempt to address some of my implicit biases…it's challenging, sometimes overwhelming, but worth the effort. Strive to approach your patients from a place of humility—that you don't necessarily understand all the things that they are facing in their current lives or all the things that they carry from the past.

I do believe that TIC really is social justice work, if it's done in a way that supports fairness and elevates families that have been marginalized—by helping them break down structural barriers to their care and helping them meet their needs. All of this requires that we give patients choice and voice about whether they disclose any aspects of their relational health to us; otherwise, we may be perpetuating the historical harm that the health care system has inflicted on many of the people in our care.

Public Health Ethics

In an overview written by Shanta Dube,[29] the principles of public health ethics are outlined in the context of whether or not ACE screening should happen in primary care practices. In that article, Dr Dube gives the opinion that we are "ready to proceed with caution." The first and most important reason is that information is power. We know the potential effects of early childhood trauma, we know that supporting SSNRs helps buffer adversity, and we know that population-level prevention of trauma would mitigate a lot of the health risks that patients live with. Sharing that information with families may help set them on a road to healing and recovery, or it may inspire them to provide more positive experiences for their children. In fact, one of the identified evidence-based, modifiable factors in resilience in pediatrics is trauma education for patients and families, which is all about teaching patients about the effects of trauma and the potential healing of building resilience. Conversely, withholding information from patients may be unethical, so if we know about trauma and its effects and don't share that information with patients, we may be doing harm. We'll talk about some scripts for universal trauma education—which all families deserve as a preventive practice—in Chapter 8, Revamping Anticipatory Guidance.

If information is power, then the implication is that taking an RHH has to also incorporate education about trauma. Part of the opportunity that is implicit in structured screening tools is the educational message that comes along with the screening tool itself. By implementing a tool, sharing it with your families, and discussing the result, you have an opportunity to open a conversation about the importance of trauma and SSNRs to health and wellness. That means you can't implement a tool without committing to discussing not only the results (whether the tool results in a disclosure or not) but also the context in which you are asking the questions. My typical process is to give an elevator pitch before I even look at the results of the tool; in the best of circumstances, that happens before the tool is completed so I can reinforce the caregiver's choice to opt in or opt out of the tool. We have a cover letter that explains the purpose of the tool (see Appendix F for our full assessment survey), but when you're a caregiver wrestling a kid into a doctor's office, the cover letter often doesn't get read before you just start answering the questions. In this elevator pitch process, the caregiver is given a better understanding of why I'm asking the questions. Several times I've had a caregiver take the assessment tool back and change some of their answers, resulting in more disclosures.

Garner and Saul[30] organize our responses to toxic stress into 3 public health levels—primary, secondary, and tertiary prevention—and screening tools can play a role in all 3 levels. In their framework, primary prevention is about supporting SSNRs, secondary prevention is about identifying barriers to SSNRs, and tertiary prevention is about repairing relationships when they have become strained or compromised.

Part of primary prevention when it comes to toxic stress is maintaining a focus on universal resilience building in our anticipatory guidance (more on this in Chapter 8, Revamping Anticipatory Guidance), but primary prevention also includes the universal psychoeducation we give our patients and families about the effects of trauma and resilience by explaining the context for the assessment tool. Secondary prevention comes down to identifying patients with increased risk due to exposure to toxic stress or to disruptions in SSNRs. Obviously, assessment tools are used for this specific purpose—to help identify risk. Once risk is identified, tertiary prevention is about intervening on behalf of those patients or families that have experienced toxic stress and have physiological or psychological consequences of that exposure by referring them for evidence-based treatments. For this reason, disclosures of trauma should be followed up by additional assessment for current safety and an assessment of potential sequelae of the trauma exposure.

Conclusions

Universal screening for ACEs in primary care is still controversial. The ACE questionnaire itself isn't evidence based for use in clinical settings, as it has poor predictive value for outcomes at an individual level. This is an important consideration when deciding how to assess trauma histories in caregivers and families as part of RHHs. When deciding on a clinical process for assessing trauma as a part of taking RHHs in primary care, careful consideration must be given to how the clinician will avoid doing unnecessary harm to patients and families, using an ethics framework. That said, with appropriate planning, assessments for caregiver and family trauma can become an integral part of being a trauma-informed and trauma-responsive practice.

Questions to Consider

1. What is your primary reason for engaging in this work of addressing trauma in your practice? Does your reason align with ethics principles?

2. What is the primary outcome you're hoping to improve by starting to take RHHs?

3. What are your initial thoughts on how you will respond to disclosures of trauma? Can you commit to staying engaged with families that have disclosed trauma?

4. Which trauma disclosures will result in mandated reporting? How will you communicate this to caregivers and families?

5. What practice and personal changes do you need to make to prepare yourself for meaningful conversations about trauma before beginning?

6. What mechanisms do you have for getting feedback from patients and families about conducting trauma assessments? Do you have a parent advisor, family advisory panel, or other mechanisms for getting formal review of your assessment protocols?

7. How do trauma assessments fit into the work you've already done in your medical home journey? How are these assessments similar to screening tools you've done in the past? How are they different?

8. How have you, or your practice, addressed DEI? How will you ensure that your practice has a foundational understanding of providing equitable care for the populations you serve?

References

1. Sherin KM, Stillerman A, Chandrasekar L, Went NS, Niebuhr DW. Recommendations for population-based applications of the Adverse Childhood Experiences study: position statement by the American College of Preventive Medicine. *AJPM Focus*. 2022;1(2):100039 doi: 10.1016/j.focus.2022.100039

2. Gordon JB, Felitti V. The importance of screening for adverse childhood experiences in all medical encounters. *AJPM Focus*. 2023;2(4):100131 doi: 10.1016/j.focus.2023.100131

3. Forkey H, Szilagyi M, Kelly ET, Duffee J; American Academy of Pediatrics Council on Foster Care, Adoption, and Kinship Care; Council on Community Pediatrics; Council on Child Abuse and Neglect; and Committee on Psychosocial Aspects of Child and Family Health. Trauma-informed care. *Pediatrics*. 2021;148(2):e2021052580 PMID: 34312292

4. Finkelhor D. Screening for adverse childhood experiences (ACEs): cautions and suggestions. *Child Abuse Negl*. 2018;85:174–179 PMID: 28784309 doi: 10.1016/j.chiabu.2017.07.016

5. Anda RF, Porter LE, Brown DW. Inside the Adverse Childhood Experience score: strengths, limitations, and misapplications. *Am J Prev Med*. 2020;59(2):293–295 PMID: 32222260 doi: 10.1016/j.amepre.2020.01.009

6. Baldwin JR, Caspi A, Meehan AJ, et al. Population vs individual prediction of poor health from results of adverse childhood experiences screening. *JAMA Pediatr*. 2021;175(4):385–393 PMID: 33492366 doi: 10.1001/jamapediatrics.2020.5602

7. ACEs and toxic stress: frequently asked questions. Center on the Developing Child at Harvard. Accessed March 18, 2024. https://developingchild.harvard.edu/resources/aces-and-toxic-stress-frequently-asked-questions

8. Lupien SJ, McEwen BS, Gunnar MR, Heim C. Effects of stress throughout the lifespan on the brain, behaviour and cognition. *Nat Rev Neurosci*. 2009;10(6):434–445 PMID: 19401723 doi: 10.1038/nrn2639

9. Smith KE, Pollak SD. Early life stress and development: potential mechanisms for adverse outcomes. *J Neurodev Disord*. 2020;12(1):34 PMID: 33327939 doi: 10.1186/s11689-020-09337-y

10. Bethell C, Jones J, Gombojav N, Linkenbach J, Sege R. Positive childhood experiences and adult mental and relational health in a statewide sample: associations across adverse childhood experiences levels. *JAMA Pediatr*. 2019;173(11):e193007 PMID: 31498386 doi: 10.1001/jamapediatrics.2019.3007

11. Keeshin B, Byrne K, Thorn B, Shepard L. Screening for trauma in pediatric primary care. *Curr Psychiatry Rep*. 2020;22(11):60 PMID: 32889642 doi: 10.1007/s11920-020-01183-y

12. Amaya-Jackson L, Absher LE, Gerrity ET, Layne CM, Halladay Goldman J. *Beyond the ACE Score: Perspectives From The NCTSN on Child Trauma and Adversity Screening and Impact*. National Center for Child Traumatic Stress; 2021

13. World Health Organization. Adverse Childhood Experiences International Questionnaire (ACE-IQ). January 28, 2020. Accessed March 18, 2024. https://www.who.int/publications/m/item/adverse-childhood-experiences-international-questionnaire-(ace-iq)

14. Gillon R. Medical ethics: four principles plus attention to scope. *BMJ*. 1994;309(6948):184–188 PMID: 8044100 doi: 10.1136/bmj.309.6948.184

15. Austin AE. Screening for traumatic experiences in health care settings: a personal perspective from a trauma survivor. *JAMA Intern Med*. 2021;181(7):902–903 PMID: 33938929 doi: 10.1001/jamainternmed.2021.1452

16. Agarwal S, Prakash N. Psychological costs and benefits of using silent treatment. *J Res Humanit Soc Sci*. 2022;10(4):49–54

17. Shickle D, Chadwick R. The ethics of screening: is 'screeningitis' an incurable disease? *J Med Ethics*. 1994;20(1):12–18 PMID: 8035433 doi: 10.1136/jme.20.1.12

18. Trzeciak S, Mazzarelli A. *Compassionomics: The Revolutionary Scientific Evidence That Caring Makes a Difference*. Studer Group; 2019

19. National Child Traumatic Stress Network. Secondary traumatic stress. Accessed March 18, 2024. https://www.nctsn.org/trauma-informed-care/secondary-traumatic-stress

20. Traub F, Boynton-Jarrett R. Modifiable resilience factors to childhood adversity for clinical pediatric practice. *Pediatrics*. 2017;139(5):e20162569 PMID: 28557726 doi: 10.1542/peds.2016-2569

21. Selvaraj K, Korpics J, Osta AD, Hirshfield LE, Crowley-Matoka M, Bayldon BW. Parent perspectives on adverse childhood experiences & unmet social needs screening in the medical home: a qualitative study. *Acad Pediatr*. 2022;22(8):1309–1317 PMID: 36007805 doi: 10.1016/j.acap.2022.08.002

22. Agency for Healthcare Research and Quality. Six domains of healthcare quality. US Department of Health and Human Services. Reviewed December 2022. Accessed March 18, 2024. https://www.ahrq.gov/talkingquality/measures/six-domains.html

23. National Academies of Sciences, Engineering, and Medicine. *Improving Access to and Equity of Care for People With Serious Illness: Proceedings of a Workshop*. National Academies Press; 2019 doi: 10.17226/25530

24. McLeod S. Maslow's hierarchy of needs. Simply Psychology. Updated January 24, 2024. Accessed March 18, 2024. https://www.simplypsychology.org/maslow.html

25. Ocampo Rosales A. The intersection of trauma and culture. In: Forkey HC, Griffin JL, Szilagyi M, eds. *Childhood Trauma and Resilience: A Practical Guide*. American Academy of Pediatrics; 2021:141–152 doi: 10.1542/9781610025072-ch12

26. *Raising the Bar: Healthcare's Transforming Role*. Accessed March 18, 2024. https://rtbhealthcare.org

27. Manchanda R, Do R, Miles N. *A Toolkit to Advance Racial Health Equity in Primary Care Improvement*. California Improvement Network, California Health Care Foundation, Healthforce Center at UCSF; 2022

28. Saad LF. *Me and White Supremacy Workbook*. 2018. https://blm.btown-in.org/uploads/1/1/8/6/118615243/me_and_white_supremacy_workbook__final_book_.pdf

29. Dube SR. Continuing conversations about adverse childhood experiences (ACEs) screening: a public health perspective. *Child Abuse Negl*. 2018;85:180–184 PMID: 29555095 doi: 10.1016/j.chiabu.2018.03.007

30. Garner AS, Saul RA. *Thinking Developmentally: Nurturing Wellness in Childhood to Promote Lifelong Health*. American Academy of Pediatrics; 2018 doi: 10.1542/9781610021531

Chapter 2

Addressing Barriers

R.J. Gillespie, MD, MHPE, FAAP

If there is no struggle, there is no progress.
Frederick Douglass

When my practice decided to start talking about caregiver trauma as a part of taking relational health histories (RHHs), there was one physician in the office who declined to participate. At first, I was really hung up on the idea of trying to convince him that this was the right thing to do; I tried to think of different ways to persuade him that we really were helping families by doing this work. But his heart just wasn't in it, so he chose to stay on the sidelines.

In the end, that's OK. I'd rather have clinicians be all in than have someone make a half-hearted attempt at these conversations, because that's where you have the potential to do harm. You may have someone in your practice for whom the barriers to asking about or assessing for trauma may seem insurmountable, but listening to their perspective and responding to their needs will ultimately strengthen the process you set up.

Barriers to taking an RHH can be thought of from 2 interrelated perspectives: that of the clinician and team implementing the assessment tool or surveillance questions and that of the caregiver or patient who is being asked to complete the tool and thereby disclose trauma to the pediatrician. Both parties must be comfortable with the idea and process of assessing relational health for it to be effective, so it's wise to consider these valid perspectives before implementation and proactively decide how to respond to the concerns and objections you're likely to hear.

I had a colleague in quality improvement (QI) once tell me that he loved the "naysayers"—the people within a practice who responded to proposed changes with negativity or just flatly refused to engage in a QI project. That sounds frustrating when it's your job to implement changes in a practice, but the truth is, there's a lot you can learn from the people who always dig in their heels. Anticipating their reasons for refusal will help you address those barriers at the outset and allows you to work through obstacles before your naysayers have a chance to even bring them up. When people say no to a change, Grenny and colleagues identify 2 fundamental reasons why: a lack of motivation and will or a lack of knowledge and skill.[1] The approaches will differ depending on this context. There's a phrase from Collaborative & Proactive Solutions that "children do well when they can."[2] To put a twist on it, *people* do well when they can, which includes your practice colleagues. Try to approach naysayers in your practice with curiosity and compassion. Think about which of those perspectives the resistance comes from.

When asked, clinicians typically identify a handful of common reasons why they can't complete yet another assessment or screening tool in their practice, particularly related to those tools that address trauma and other sensitive issues: not enough time, lack of confidence, fear of caregiver rejection of the tool, worries about "kicking a hornet's nest" or having a visit go completely sideways, and not having resources or not knowing what to do with a positive response.

Parents and guardians will also have concerns about completing an assessment tool—validating a common clinician concern—so stepping into the caregiver's shoes during your planning process will inform how the implementation takes place. Caregivers may have their own reasons for declining a conversation about trauma in a clinical visit; they are often concerned about what will be done with the information, whether they are safe disclosing trauma to their clinician, and whether the information is fundamentally important or relevant to the clinical visit.

In the rest of this chapter, we'll explore each of these barriers, where they may be coming from, and tips for how to address them. Some of the tips are reminders about clinical tools that you may already have at your disposal, just reframed with a trauma lens in mind.

Note From Amy

These barriers are similar to ones that come up when we talk about building resilience through interventions during office visits. We'll dive into these later, but for now, know that you're already doing so much of this! You don't have to be a therapist to talk about trauma; in fact, just beginning to ask and then listen is supportive and an intervention on its own. When I talk with doctors about their experiences, they often reflect that the conversation went a lot more smoothly than they had initially feared and that patients felt heard and cared for.

Time

A common concern with any new process introduced into an office is lack of time. This objection may come from either a place of motivation/will ("Asking about trauma isn't relevant to my practice, so I don't want to spend precious time on it") or a place of knowledge/skill ("How do I effectively manage the visit given that I have limited time to get through all my patients?"). Looking at the literature, we know that the average conversation after a disclosure of trauma is a lot shorter than people think. In pediatric primary care practices that ask parents about their ACE history, the conversation was estimated to take about 3 to 5 minutes at the most.[3] That may seem like a lot given the short time we have for visits, but it may be the most crucial time you spend in the visit that day; the advice or plan that you create will probably be different from what you anticipated but may be of immense value to the family. A common finding across pediatrics, family medicine, and OB-GYN practices is that the vast majority of the time[4,5] (75% of the time in Glowa and coworkers' study[4] in family medicine), the immediate plan wasn't changed by a disclosure of trauma, which is part of why it doesn't generally take as long as you would think. Remember that the disclosure is usually only news to the clinician asking the questions; the patient already knows what happened to them. Of course, these disclosures are sensitive and shouldn't be approached in a rushed or hurried manner—if there's a disclosure, you have to spend the needed time with the family. From Trzeciak and Mazzarelli's book *Compassionomics,* we learn that the average amount of time it takes to convey all the benefits of compassion—including better patient outcomes, patient satisfaction, adherence to treatment plans, utilization patterns, and less burnout of health care professionals—is a mere 40 seconds.[6] I think that's good news: despite how busy we are, we can spare 40 seconds listening with compassion to our patients.

One of the most important tips for managing time is the idea of triage. We often come into patient encounters with a set agenda of all the things we need to accomplish in that limited amount of time. If there is a disclosure, stop and think about what actually needs to be addressed today and what can be rescheduled for another visit or communicated in another way—but keep the family's agenda at the top of your triage list. We do our assessment tools during a well-child visit, so if there's a disclosure, I'm not necessarily going to spend time talking about our usual anticipatory guidance subjects like using car seats or avoiding walkers. My immediate concern (other than addressing the family's agenda items) is to address the trauma itself and to assess the family's immediate safety and needs. We'll talk more about this when you get to Chapter 10, Supporting Families That Have Experienced Trauma, but for now, just note that a simple safety plan includes 4 primary steps:

1. Assess child and family safety: Are there immediate threats to the child or family, such as ongoing domestic violence, abuse, or community violence? Are there immediate social drivers that need to be addressed? Will any of the disclosures necessitate a call to child protective services? How is the emotional wellness of the patient or family?

2. Account for assets, resources, and resiliencies in the family: Does the family have a support network that can be called on? What coping strategies are they currently using, and what skills can we teach to bolster resilience?

3. Use follow-up tools (or history questions) for assessing social-emotional (SE)/mental health and development or potential trauma-related somatic symptoms in patients as needed.

4. Connect with appropriate resources: parent coaching/positive parenting skill building, peer support groups, mental health clinicians, dyadic therapies, social service clinicians/resources, home visitation, mentorship programs, and others.

Once safety and immediate needs are addressed, schedule a follow-up visit or phone call to address other outstanding issues that need more time. Patients immediately forget 40% to 80% of medical advice given during a visit,[7] so it's important to be selective about what you address in these critical visits anyway; overloading them with too much information won't really benefit anyone.

We all have busy schedules. Some days it seems impossible to keep up; adding "one more thing" to do can feel overwhelming. That said, there are visits that naturally feel easier to add to than others. When my practice was deciding when we would implement caregiver ACE assessments, one of the considerations was to assess which visits naturally felt like they had more time by looking at a screening grid, which is a list of which forms and screening tools were being used at each visit. When we started implementation in 2013, the grid looked something like what you see in **Figure 2-1**.

FIGURE 2-1.

2 weeks	2 months	4 months	6 months
None	Caregiver depression Food and diaper insecurity	None	Caregiver depression
9 months	**12 months**	**15 months**	**18 months**
Developmental screening	Lead screening TB screening Caries risk assessment	None	Developmental screening Autism screening Caries risk assessment
24 months	**30 months**	**36 months**	**48 months**
Autism screening Caries risk assessment	Developmental screening	Caries risk assessment	Lead screening TB screening Caries risk assessment

Sample screening grid. This grid illustrates the screening tools implemented at different well-child visits during the first 4 years after birth. TB indicates tuberculosis.

To be clear, the *Bright Futures* recommended screening grid has changed and expanded a lot since then. We are advised to use a validated tool for SE health and function at every visit. As we added more tools, such as food insecurity screening, SE screening, and expanded caregiver depression screening to all visits up to the 6-month well-child visit, the grid started to look pretty full. Given that the developmental and autism screening tools were pretty lengthy and necessitated a specific conversation about the results, adding another tool at one of these visits would have been a recipe for disaster in terms of time management. We also thought about what conversations naturally took more time during a visit, such as the first immunizations at 2 months and the conversations around feeding and solid foods at 6 months. Talking about trauma and other sensitive topics at the 2-week visit felt inappropriate given that we were still developing our relationship with the family at that early appointment (although it's a great time to start asking about how a caregiver is planning to raise their child). The natural fit for adding an additional tool looked like either 4 or 15 months; since there weren't other tools to discuss at those visits, there was some natural space to add a big conversation if needed. We wanted to have the conversation early enough to influence parenting in a positive way, so we chose the 4-month visit as the time when we implement our new tool. Creating a similar grid for how questionnaires are used in your office will help you make logical decisions that will aid in time management.

Another important concept in managing time is to provide teaching scripts and conversation prompts to direct the conversation after a disclosure. Having some simple phrases to validate the importance of the conversation, along with questions to use as a follow-up to a disclosure, helps keep the subsequent discussion more focused. Felitti and Anda described major positive changes in utilization patterns among trauma survivors by asking one simple question—"How did this affect you later in life?"[8]—which resulted in decreased emergency department visits, hospitalizations, and unnecessary primary care visits. Presumably this question helps patients begin to integrate their experiences, allowing the logical brain to start sorting out the emotional reactions to the experience. For example, in screening parents and caregivers for their trauma histories, I always start by thanking the respondent for their disclosure to validate the importance of the conversation. This can't be emphasized enough—it's a tough decision to make a disclosure, so honor the risk the parent or caregiver has taken. I then use 3 follow-up questions:

1. Do any of these experiences still bother you now?
2. Of those experiences that no longer bother you, how did you get to the point that they don't bother you anymore?
3. How do you think these experiences affect your parenting now?

The first question gets at safety and helps assess whether there are any immediate mental health needs for that caregiver. The second is really a question about resilience: What are the personal traits, experiences, or safe, stable, nurturing relationships (SSNRs) that helped facilitate recovery, and are those resilience factors still something the caregiver feels they possess? The third is a question about integrating experiences and helping caregivers who survived trauma to perhaps begin to be more aware of their parenting goals and approach parenting with more intention and mindfulness. If you're responding to trauma disclosures in older kids and adolescents, you can modify the question to something like "How do you think these experiences affect you now?" By having these 3 questions in mind before the visit, I am able to direct the conversation toward a positive, constructive end in most cases. The questions you use as conversation prompts may vary depending on context, so modify these examples as needed.

Clinician Confidence

Lack of confidence comes almost exclusively from a knowledge/skill perspective, although there is an element of motivation/will behind it as well. As far as the latter piece goes, many clinicians will try to convince you that trauma belongs in the domain of mental health rather than primary care; thus, they aren't motivated to implement trauma assessments in their day-to-day work. My response to this is that I'm not a cardiologist, but I still use my stethoscope; and these days, we use a lot of mental health screening tools to explore depression, anxiety, or attention-deficit/hyperactivity disorder in our patients and provide resources and referrals, so trauma isn't really that different from other everyday tasks that we take care of in practice.

It comes down to acknowledging your role in assessing trauma, social drivers, and mental health concerns. With your cardiac exam, if you find an abnormality, it isn't your job to patch a ventricular septal defect or perform a cardiac catheterization to close a patent ductus arteriosus. It's your job to recognize the problem, explain the interim plan to the family, and get the patient sent to the appropriate specialist or resource.

To be fair, the conversations around trauma seem like difficult ones—but remember that we have difficult conversations with families all the time. We've learned how to sit with families in their grief, fear, or confusion around medical problems. I've had 3 kids in the past 20 years who I identified as having a brain tumor; you can imagine how scary those conversations were for everyone. Again, it wasn't my job to remove the tumor, calculate chemotherapy doses, or give rehabilitation therapies in any of those cases. My job was to identify the problem, emotionally support the family, explain the interim plan, and connect the patient to appropriate resources. The process is the same in trauma conversations.

Ultimately, clinical confidence—as with any form of confidence—comes from knowing what to do. When it comes to trauma conversations, the most important thing you can do is to listen, which means that the most important skill you need in your toolbox is, in fact, already there. The Survivor Voices study, a survey of trauma survivors conducted by The Trauma Healing Project in Eugene, OR, provides some important findings about the power of listening[9]:

- When survivors said they had been listened to with compassion, they were 2.9 times more likely to report being mostly or completely healed.

- When survivors believed that people understood the impact of trauma on their lives, they were 2.2 times more likely to report being mostly or completely healed.

- When survivors believed that people knew how to help them heal, they were 2.3 times more likely to report being mostly or completely healed.

In other words, healing for trauma survivors came from someone being willing to listen, so you already know what to do. Many of the classic ACEs represent disruptions in the relationship with caregivers—in other words, authority figures in the child's life—so when an authority figure (including a medical professional) can listen with compassion, we can turn the tables on the trauma narrative and become vital factors in families' healing and resilience.

As with anything in medicine, confidence comes with time and experience. In family medicine studies,[4] confidence levels were measured before and after the implementation of the ACE survey, and as expected, confidence gradually improved with time. One way to facilitate confidence is to brush up on motivational interviewing (MI) skills.[10] One of the primary principles of MI is to "abandon the righting reflex," which is the tendency to want to fix whatever problem is set in front of us. It's what we're trained to do, so it's ingrained in our mind to jump straight to solutions. Motivational interviewing would suggest that the solutions to many patients' problems can be found in open-ended questions and reflections back to the patient. Most of the time, patients have some ideas about what they need to do, or what resources they're interested in pursuing, if they're actually asked and given the opportunity to think about it. If we're leaning on our tendency to want to fix things, that means we probably are already thinking through solutions in our heads during the conversation and not actually listening.

Motivational interviewing uses the mnemonic RULE as one way to frame how we navigate conversations around trauma: **R**esist the righting reflex, **U**nderstand and explore the patient's motivations (or the context of their day-to-day lives), **L**isten with empathy (there's that listening part again), and **E**mpower the patient, encouraging hope and optimism. This framework reminds us to spend time understanding what patients want and need out of their health care, starting with an assessment of a parent's or patient's understanding of trauma and its effects. Sometimes the patient's needs include not talking about their trauma (that may be our motivation, but their wishes should trump ours if there's that kind of discordance), so know when to let the conversation go if someone isn't ready to talk about their past. Be sure the family knows you're open to conversations in the future if they should choose to talk about it further, and think about the work you do with that family as delivering a lot of small doses rather than trying to resolve everything in a single visit.

Hope is also part of the communication techniques outlined in the American Academy of Pediatrics (AAP) toolkit *Addressing Mental Health Concerns in Pediatrics,*[11] which was developed as a way to respond to mental health concerns that are raised in practice. It can also be applied in thinking about our approach to trauma disclosures; the HELLPPP mnemonic[12] can be used as a framework to build confidence around navigating these difficult conversations:

- **Hope:** Increase the family's hopefulness by describing your realistic expectations for improvement and reinforcing the strengths and assets you see in the child and family.
- **Empathy:** Communicate empathy by listening attentively.
- **Language:** Use the child's or family's own language to reflect your understanding of the problem.
- **Loyalty:** Communicate loyalty to the family by expressing your support and your commitment to help.
- **Permission:** Ask the family's permission for you to move into more in-depth questions or make suggestions for further evaluation or management.
- **Partnership:** Partner with the child and family to find agreement on achievable steps that are aligned with the family's motivation.
- **Plan:** Establish a plan (or incremental first step).

The message of hope is a particularly important one when it comes to conversations around ACEs and other traumas: conveying to families that ACEs are not destiny helps in the healing process and is supported by our efforts to build resilience in families and kids.

Reflective practice is the idea of spending time, either alone or with other clinicians in our office, reflecting on what went well or not so well in our interactions with patients.[13,14] It's meant not as a process to judge you for things that went less than ideally but rather as a QI process of thinking about the words you used, the conversation questions you tried, or other aspects of the patient interaction that can be improved on in future visits. Our mental health and social work colleagues have reflective practice and reflective supervision as mandatory and routine parts of their job—just the natural ways they do things in practice. What a powerful idea! The clinicians in my office had a couple of lunch and learn sessions where we sat and talked about some of the more challenging trauma conversations that we'd experienced to get advice, learn each other's teaching scripts, and generally compare notes about difficult interactions. We'll talk about this more in Chapter 16, Sustaining Trauma-Responsive Practices, but for now, recognize that this process of reflective practice is immensely helpful for building confidence.

Note From Amy

Having these conversations with colleagues is critical. The more you uncover and talk about trauma with patients and their families, the more likely you are to experience secondhand trauma. Supporting each other, seeking outside consultation, and practicing scripts help process the stories you're hearing. Processing stories helps our bodies work through the trauma we've heard and been exposed to. When we do so, we're much less likely to internalize the trauma ourselves, which can ultimately lead to overwhelm and burnout for physicians. So, seeking consultation and support early and often is key to treating vicarious trauma.

Kicking the Hornet's Nest

It will happen: There will be a visit where the conversation after a trauma exposure gets big. Someone will get emotional, and it may feel like you'll never get out of the conversation. Thankfully, it's really not that frequent in real-world practice, and at the end of the conversation, you will have a much deeper understanding of the patient and family. In all likelihood, if you're mindful in your approach, you'll have helped more than you can imagine. This fear of a challenging conversation is a corollary of the lack-of-confidence barrier, so be ready to address what to do. Being prepared for difficult conversations involves knowing why they happen and avoiding making assumptions about why the interaction went awry.

Visits may go sideways if the clinician doesn't quickly assess the nature of the interaction after a disclosure. In their book *Crucial Conversations,*[15] Joseph Grenny and colleagues explain that a crucial conversation is one in which opposing opinions, strong emotions, or high stakes are at play; certainly, trauma conversations are crucial in this respect. A clinician may feel that a person's trauma history is their business, whereas the patient or caregiver may not (opposing opinions); strong emotions are usually involved when it comes to trauma; and patients or families may perceive the conversation as high stakes if they perceive a threat, such as believing that a disclosure might result in repercussions. When a person feels threatened in a conversation, they retreat into "silence or violence"—not actual physical violence but sarcasm, anger, deflection, or other ways of avoiding the conversation or expressing distress. It's important to be attuned to the person's body language and social cues that might indicate they've retreated into silence or violence by assessing whether the conversation is regulated or not.

After a disclosure of trauma, identify whether a person is regulated, as in engaged in the conversation and asking and answering questions, or the person is dysregulated, as in distressed, upset, crying, angry, or shut down. If a caregiver (or patient) is regulated, they don't feel threatened by the conversation, so you can proceed with education, advice, and an offer of resources. Conversely, if you start unloading advice and education on a caregiver who is dysregulated, they just aren't going to hear you. In those cases, it's best to stay calm, listen with empathy, provide support, and pledge your partnership as you navigate the implications of that trauma together. A person who is dysregulated may still need some degree of mental health support, but ask permission from the person before offering mental health resources. You can often start with a simple script, like "That sounds like it was a difficult experience. What do you think would be helpful now?" If the caregiver or patient volunteers that mental health help would be useful, you're already there. If not, a gentle follow-up question of "Do you think a counselor would be helpful right now?" might open the door to the idea.

The caregiver isn't the only one who might get dysregulated: there will be days when you're the one who is triggered or upset. My personal "canary in the coal mine" that tells me I'm not doing well is either complete silence or sarcasm (Why choose between silence or violence when you can do both, right?); when I recognize those patterns in myself, it tells me I need to be paying attention to my own self-care. In the long run, if you're the one who is dysregulated or if you're having a day when you just can't address another challenging conversation about trauma, call it out. It's far better to acknowledge the importance of the conversation and to make a plan to address it with the family at a separate time. It can be as simple as saying, "This is a really important conversation, and I want to think about how to best help you. Would it be OK for us to talk about this at a later time?" If you make that kind of a plan with the family, be sure to follow through.

It's important to also try to recognize why the caregiver is dysregulated. I had one mom who, completing our parent ACE assessment tool, was quietly in tears as she wrote in her answers. To start with, she was one of those patients who had answered no to most of the ACE questions until I reiterated the purpose of the tool—in a nutshell, that it was to help me understand her past to be able to coach her better in her parenting. She said, "Well, in that case…"; took the tool back; and answered yes to 4 of the ACEs…and then the tears came with full force. Talking through her story, she revealed that she had grown up in a household with such severe domestic violence that on multiple occasions, she'd thought her mother was going to die in front of her, her father was verbally and physically abusive to her and to her sister, and her father also experienced alcoholism. Mom then told me that her sister was now married to the same kind of abusive man, and her own oldest daughter (whom I had never met) was 16, pregnant, and living back in Mexico with extended family.

Through the tears, this mom's final comment was "I just want better for my child than what I had."

The mom's tears were completely understandable. They really were a combination of a deep-seated wish to be a better parent and relief that someone had asked so she didn't have to privately worry about repeating the mistakes her parents had made. I find that most caregivers who experienced childhood traumas have a fear in the back of their minds that they're going to make the same mistakes their parents did; after all, what was modeled to us as children formulates our own parenting tendencies. They're usually relieved to have someone bring that out in the open in a nonjudgmental way. In this case, I had an opportunity to offer hope and pledge partnership (Remember the common factors approach?) in helping the mom understand positive parenting as she raised her infant. It was the beginning of a longitudinal conversation over all the subsequent visits, and it was an opportunity to build some amazing parenting skills with her child. It was also the beginning of a much deeper and stronger patient-clinician relationship between us.

Another mom was visibly tense when I walked into the room. She had been reading the assessment tool while sitting in the exam room, and it obviously upset her. I said, "Ah, I think we need to talk about that tool." Her terse response was "Yes. We do." Once I had explained the tool to her, that I intended to use it to help her navigate through her parenting challenges and that it would be treated with the strictest confidence, she visibly relaxed. She had thought we were going to "call an agency" on her—that a disclosure meant I was going to report her to social services or I would deem her a "bad parent" because of her past. Once we cleared the air, we were able to have a meaningful conversation about her childhood traumas and started laying the groundwork for how we'd address positive parenting for different ages as her child developed. If I had gone in with my own agenda, instead of "reading the room" and addressing the source of the distress right away, it would have resulted in a much more difficult conversation: any advice or counseling I offered would have been disregarded, she likely would have been angrier because I contributed to her feelings of isolation and being misunderstood, and she probably would have left my practice altogether.

The point is that neither of these initially dysregulated parents needed mental health support per se, and not every instance of someone who is hurt or angry about a trauma assessment can be reduced to "You need to go to counseling" as a response. It's really going to depend on where that individual is in their process of healing and integration of their experiences; in fact, I offered mental health support in the second case and the parent declined. If you see a dysregulated parent, try to understand the context of what you're seeing so you don't make an inappropriate assumption about what they need. When you recognize the emotion in the room, that's what you should try to respond to—not the behavior that accompanies the emotion. In all, I've referred a parent or caregiver for a mental health service only a handful of times as a result of our screening process and only when we mutually agreed that it would help or if a caregiver asked for that service specifically. When in doubt about whether someone thinks a mental health referral will be helpful, ask.

The process in these difficult conversations is similar to Dr Bruce Perry's Three R's[16] that we use for kids who are having a tough time, like in the middle of a tantrum—regulate, relate, reason—only we're using those same skills to help support an upset parent. Regulation comes from the clinician keeping calm and in control, rather than reflecting back the caregiver's or patient's distress. Listening attentively and keeping the environment calm and supportive are the necessary first step. Then you try to relate to the patient or caregiver, expressing an understanding of and validation for their emotions. Only then can you take the third step of reasoning with the person giving the disclosure, which includes helping them understand the reasons for being asked the trauma questions, reassuring them of their safety, and reminding them that their privacy will be protected to the best of your ability. *Crucial Conversations* refers to this as "step out, make it safe, then step back in."[15] Taking that first step back to allow for the tough emotions to be expressed and processed always helps defuse the situation.

Lack of Resources

Clinicians are frequently (and validly) concerned that they won't have appropriate referral resources to use in cases of trauma disclosures, especially when embarking on any sort of trauma or social drivers of health (SDOH) assessments in practice. Depending on your community, this may be an all-too-real situation, but it also depends on how you think about what resources you might need and how often those resources come into play after a disclosure of trauma.

Remembering that in most cases, the immediate plan is not changed by a disclosure[4]—again, it's news to the clinician but not to the patient or family—and also remembering that not all disclosures need a mental health referral depending on the nature of the situation, it's important to think about what resources you might need depending on the type of tool you use. In my practice, we asked caregivers who were screened for trauma histories what resources they were most interested in receiving.[3] The most common responses were parenting classes, parent support groups, and more information about trauma and its effects. This finding mirrors both the policy of the AAP,[17,18] which states that we should be supporting positive parenting, and the core modifiable resilience factors in primary care: supporting and building positive parenting skills and improving trauma knowledge. Since trauma knowledge and counseling on positive parenting are already in your skill set (or will be enhanced by the time you're done reading this book), in some cases you might be the only resource the family needs—and yes, you can do this.

This information about what parents and caregivers request for resources influences what you'll need on your list of referral sources. In addition to knowing what evidence-based mental health and dyad therapies are available in your area, you should know what parenting classes, support groups, and other skill-building resources are available in your area. I also keep a list of websites and apps that support parenting and parent skill building, because the way that caregivers choose to access this kind of information may vary according to their schedules and ability to attend in-person parenting classes. Home visitation programs can also help support caregivers who need to develop parenting skills; when my practice asked if caregivers wanted to engage in home visitation programs, they generally said no, but I think this is primarily due to a misunderstanding of the role of this type of program. In families that have experienced trauma, as well as within some cultural groups, there is a distrust of "governmental agencies," so home visitation may be seen as invasive or even risky. Clear communication about what these programs can offer may be needed.

We'll talk more about finding resources in upcoming chapters, but for now, know that many communities have developed clearinghouses for parenting resources, such as Help Me Grow (www.helpmegrow.org), Unite Us (https://uniteus.com), Aunt Bertha (https://helpfinder. auntbertha.com), 211Info, or United Way. If these programs exist in your area, they can often provide a single point of referral for all these resources. After all, it's a lot easier to have someone else manage your list of resources than to have to track them yourself. You may also be able to find resource lists for specific types of traumas, such as the Futures Without Violence programs (www.futureswithoutviolence.org), which keep lists of intimate partner violence resources by county, or the Postpartum Support International (www.postpartum.net) lists of resources (managed by state) for peripartum mood disorders. Consider that for some families, mentorship programs may also be useful, such as Big Brothers/Big Sisters programs or Boys & Girls Clubs; these programs are designed to help children and teens develop SSNRs outside the home. There are also toolkits that have been developed for some of the specific SDOH screeners that have algorithms for what types of resources you might need, such as food insecurity or the Safe Environment for Every Kid tools (https://seekwellbeing.org). These algorithms will walk you through how to find specific resources in your community. We'll go further in depth into finding resources in Chapter 10, Supporting Families That Have Experienced Trauma, and Chapter 15, Implementation Nuts and Bolts.

To manage resources in your practice, the first step is to ask parents what resources they think would be most helpful and ask permission before doing any specific referrals. Once a referral is made, it's a good medical home practice to follow up with the family at a later date to see whether the resource offered was accessible and useful to the family. This means that some manner of referral tracking is required; it may be as simple as a paper log of what referrals you have made, a computer-based spreadsheet, or a note in the patient's medical record. If you have a care coordinator in your practice, these resources will probably be managed by them. You likely won't be able to anticipate every resource request or need identified by a family. Remember that it's OK to say, "I don't know"; establish a plan for finding out the information or tracking down the requested resource; and then get back to the family at a later date. We'll talk about all these points about referrals and referral tracking in more detail in Chapter 10, Supporting Families That Have Experienced Trauma.

Caregiver Acceptance of Trauma and SDOH Questionnaires

Since discussing trauma in practice can be such a sensitive topic, there is a fear that caregivers will not be willing to complete an assessment tool, either about themselves or about their child. The last thing we want as clinicians is to anger or offend someone; and there's a lot of worry about whether or not asking about trauma can, in fact, be re-traumatizing or triggering to the person completing a survey. It's important to consider what's at stake for a family when they disclose trauma to their child's pediatric clinician; keeping this perspective in mind will influence the workflow that you adopt. How caregivers accept an assessment tool depends greatly on how you set up the workflow in practice.

Focus groups that asked parents how they felt about trauma questions revealed some positive results.[19] First, and most importantly, parents are generally comfortable with questions about trauma; it turns out that they clearly understand the importance of the issue and are interested in breaking the cycle of adversity from one generation to the next. In studies of home visitation clients,[20] most parents were not at all or, at most, slightly uncomfortable with being asked the ACE questions, a response partly dependent on how high their ACE score was and whether or not they were experiencing depression. In that study, only 3% reported feeling extreme discomfort with being asked the ACE questions. In a family medicine study, no patient refused the ACE screening tool during their clinical encounter.[4] Generally, parents see their child's pediatrician as a "trusted change agent" who can help support them in their parenting skills and strongly support screening for ACEs as a means for getting connected to needed services.[19] Finally, parents don't even mind the results being recorded in the medical record.[19]

That said, trust and transparency are vital. In another series of focus groups, parents in low-income households were asked how they felt about sensitive questions, specifically around SDOH.[21] In these focus groups, parents emphasized the need for a trusting relationship first, before being asked questions that seem personal or intrusive. When it comes to social drivers, and perhaps services related to trauma, many caregivers don't think of their child's pediatric clinician as the person to go to get help. Asking such questions requires a culture shift on the part of both the caregiver and the practice itself. Most importantly, caregivers state that a clinician shouldn't "ask just for the sake of asking"; that is, if you're asking only because you're curious or because you're being reimbursed for a specific screening tool but are not prepared to help, then don't embark on any assessment process. The conclusions drawn from this study are the following:

- Clinicians should be transparent about why they're asking the questions and what they're going to do with the information.
- A plan needs to be in place to address positive results.
- A culture change in practice is needed to help caregivers feel comfortable with being asked these questions.

There are several tips for helping with acceptance of screening and assessment tools, starting with the scripting around the tool. When front desk staff (or whoever) hands the tool to the caregiver, have scripting available that explains not only what the tool is for but also that it is universally given to all families in your practice. It's important to avoid the impression that you are targeting a specific family because of socioeconomic status, race and ethnicity, or other demographic information; rather, communicate that you ask the questions of all families in your care. Include a cover letter that addresses the nature of the tool, what you intend to do with the information, and how you will protect patient privacy and confidentiality.

Be clear that caregivers have a choice about whether or not they complete the tool in the first place. Remember that the purpose of a screening tool is not to force a disclosure but to provide an open door for having conversations about trauma in your practice. Declining an assessment tool, or choosing not to answer history questions, is always an option.

Discussing every assessment tool, whether the tool includes a disclosure or not, facilitates caregiver acceptance of the tool in the first place. My first QI project was working on the state-wide implementation of developmental screening tools; when talking to practices in follow-up, I learned that some physicians from the trainings had a stack of completed tools on their desk that they would review at the end of the day when they were completing their charting. They were frustrated by then having to call families back to discuss the results of the screening tools— meaning they had not talked about the tool at all during the actual visit. It created a much more challenging workflow to track down the families and provide them with resources after the visit, but more importantly, it meant that the tool itself was met with silence at the time of the visit. It not only reflected a missed opportunity for teaching and engagement but minimized the importance of the tool itself. Needless to say, you can't do that with trauma assessments. That said, remember that the common factors approach includes permission, so be sure to ask permission to discuss the tool further with the family.

When addressing the assessment tool with the family, as we've mentioned, it's important to start by thanking the parent or caregiver for completing it, regardless of what the results say. This helps validate the importance of the conversation and acknowledges the difficulty they may have experienced in answering the questions. If you're having one of those days when you're too dysregulated or running too far behind to address the trauma, still thank the caregiver, make a plan for addressing the tool in the future, and follow through.

Conclusions

Although there are real barriers to addressing caregiver trauma in practice, most of them can be addressed by anticipating the challenges you will face and planning how to overcome them. Preparing for resistance to screening and for the naysayers in your office before embarking on implementation will help facilitate the process of incorporating tools in practice by helping develop either knowledge and skill or motivation and will in trauma-informed care. Similarly, maintaining a focus on the parent and caregiver perspective of how trauma screening is perceived will alleviate some of the resistance from families. The most common barriers of time, confidence, lack of resources, fear of upsetting a caregiver, or caregiver acceptance of screening tools can be alleviated through some practical techniques and steps, including reframing some of your current clinical skills for the context of conversations about trauma.

Questions to Consider

1. How do you think your colleagues will respond to the idea of implementing trauma assessments? Will your colleagues say yes or no? What reasons will they give for saying no to a screening tool? What about the rest of your clinical team?

2. Do your clinical visits allow enough time to adequately address new assessment tools while you're with a patient? Are there visits that naturally have more time or space to implement tools or surveillance questions? What do you normally do when you're falling behind in your workday (because we all know it's happened), and how will you plan to accommodate for conversations about trauma that "get big"?

3. What training opportunities would most benefit your practice before implementation to improve clinician and staff confidence? Do you need more training in MI? Trauma-informed care?

4. What opportunities can you create in your office (or with other colleagues) for reflective practice? Will you be able to regularly meet to talk about challenging cases and how you managed them?

5. What support or training would be helpful for managing difficult conversations?

6. What resources (or, better yet, resource clearinghouses) exist in your community? What relationships do you have with those resources? Are they prepared to take new referrals based on your specific assessment protocol?

7. What scripts, cover letters, or other communications need to be developed to help explain screening or assessment tools to families? What mechanisms do you have in place to get feedback from families, both formal and informal?

8. How will you ensure privacy while people are completing assessment tools?

References

1. Grenny J, Patterson K, Maxfield D, McMillan R, Switzler A. *Influencer: The New Science of Leading Change*. 2nd ed. McGraw Hill; 2013

2. Kessler E. Ross Greene on challenging behavior. Smart Kids With Learning Disabilities. Accessed March 18, 2024. https://www.smartkidswithld.org/getting-help/emotions-behaviors/ross-greene-on-challenging-behavior

3. Gillespie RJ, Folger AT. Feasibility of assessing parental ACEs in pediatric primary care: implications for practice-based implementation. *J Child Adolesc Trauma*. 2017;10(3):249–256 doi: 10.1007/s40653-017-0138-z

4. Glowa PT, Olson AL, Johnson DJ. Screening for adverse childhood experiences in a family medicine setting: a feasibility study. *J Am Board Fam Med*. 2016;29(3):303–307 PMID: 27170787 doi: 10.3122/jabfm.2016.03.150310

5. Flanagan T, Alabaster A, McCaw B, Stoller N, Watson C, Young-Wolff KC. Feasibility and acceptability of screening for adverse childhood experiences in prenatal care. *J Womens Health (Larchmt)*. 2018;27(7):903–911 PMID: 29350573 doi: 10.1089/jwh.2017.6649

6. Trzeciak S, Mazzarelli A. *Compassionomics: The Revolutionary Scientific Evidence That Caring Makes a Difference*. Studer Group; 2019

7. Kessels RP. Patients' memory for medical information. *J R Soc Med*. 2003;96(5):219–222 PMID: 12724430 doi: 10.1177/014107680309600504

8. Felitti VJ, Anda RF. The relationship of adverse childhood experiences to adult medical disease, psychiatric disorders and sexual behavior: implications for healthcare. In: Lanius RA, Vermetten E, Pain C, eds. *The Impact of Early Life Trauma on Health and Disease: The Hidden Epidemic*. Cambridge University Press; 2010:77–87

9. Cortez P, Dumas T, Joyce J, et al. Survivor Voices: co-learning, re-connection, and healing through community action research and engagement (CARE). *Prog Community Health Partnersh*. 2011;5(2):133–142 PMID: 21623015 doi: 10.1353/cpr.2011.0020

10. Rollnick S, Miller WR, Butler CC. *Motivational Interviewing in Health Care: Helping Patients Change Behavior*. Guilford Press; 2008

11. Earls MF, Foy JM, Green CM. *Addressing Mental Health Concerns in Pediatrics: A Practical Toolkit for Clinicians*. 2nd ed. American Academy of Pediatrics; 2021. Accessed March 18, 2024. https://publications.aap.org/toolkits/pages/Mental-Health-Toolkit

12. American Academy of Pediatrics. Mnemonic for common factors communication methods: HELP. 2010. Updated May 2017. Accessed March 18, 2024. https://downloads.aap.org/AAP/PDF/Mneumonic_for_Common_Factors_Communication_Methods_Help.pdf

13. Koshy K, Limb C, Gundogan B, Whitehurst K, Jafree DJ. Reflective practice in health care and how to reflect effectively. *Int J Surg Oncol (NY)*. 2017;2(6):e20 PMID: 29177215 doi: 10.1097/IJ9.0000000000000020

14. Zachary LJ. *The Mentor's Guide: Facilitating Effective Learning Relationships*. 2nd ed. Jossey-Bass; 2011

15. Grenny J, Patterson K, McMillan R, Switzler A, Gregory E. *Crucial Conversations: Tools for Talking When Stakes Are High*. 3rd ed. McGraw Hill; 2022

16. Perry B. The Three R's: reaching the learning brain. Restorative Practices Whanganui. Accessed March 18, 2024. https://restorativepracticeswhanganui.co.nz/wp-content/uploads/2018/06/3-Rs-reaching-the-learning-brain-Dr-Bruce-Perry.jpg

17. Garner AS, Shonkoff JP, Siegel BS, et al; American Academy of Pediatrics Committee on Psychosocial Aspects of Child and Family Health; Committee on Early Childhood, Adoption, and Dependent Care; and Section on Developmental and Behavioral Pediatrics. Early childhood adversity, toxic stress, and the role of the pediatrician: translating developmental science into lifelong health. *Pediatrics*. 2012;129(1):e224–e231 PMID: 22201148 doi: 10.1542/peds.2011-2662

18. Garner A, Yogman M; American Academy of Pediatrics Committee on Psychosocial Aspects of Child and Family Health, Section on Developmental and Behavioral Pediatrics, and Council on Early Childhood. Preventing childhood toxic stress: partnering with families and communities to promote relational health. *Pediatrics*. 2021;148(2):e2021052582 PMID: 34312296 doi: 10.1542/peds.2021-052582

19. Conn AM, Szilagyi MA, Jee SH, Manly JT, Briggs R, Szilagyi PG. Parental perspectives of screening for adverse childhood experiences in pediatric primary care. *Fam Syst Health*. 2018;36(1):62–72 PMID: 29215906 doi: 10.1037/fsh0000311

20. Mersky JP, Lee CP, Gilbert RM. Client and provider discomfort with an adverse childhood experiences survey. *Am J Prev Med*. 2019;57(2):e51–e58 PMID: 31253559 doi: 10.1016/j.amepre.2019.02.026

21. Schleifer D, Diep A, Grisham K. *It's About Trust: Low-Income Parents' Perspectives on How Pediatricians Can Screen for Social Determinants of Health*. Public Agenda, United Hospital Fund; 2019. Accessed March 18, 2024. https://www.publicagenda.org/reports/its-about-trust-low-income-parents-perspectives-on-how-pediatricians-can-screen-for-social-determinants-of-health

Chapter 3

Getting Your Organization Ready: Creating Compassionate Pediatric Practices

Amy King, PhD

> *Do the best you can until you know better. Then when you know better, do better.*
>
> **Maya Angelou**

"What if we're not ready?"

"What if our MAs, front office staff, or administration don't understand what we're looking for or why we're doing this?"

"Have we given everyone at our organization tools to be aware of what trauma looks like and how it presents?"

My experience from training health care professionals is that knowing *about* trauma is different in practice from knowing *what to do about* trauma. Beginning to implement trauma-informed care (TIC) can be daunting, especially for the thoughtful clinician who values the information *and* wants to know how to respond thoughtfully. That was certainly the experience of the physicians I worked with at the Children's Health Alliance (CHA), in Portland, OR. These thoughtful considerations guided the rollout for this group as we began to create a roadmap to becoming trauma responsive, asking about relational health histories (RHHs) and previous adversities, and creating resilience for patients.

The research of late gives us an unprecedented opportunity to learn and implement changes in pediatric practices based on science and knowledge about early relational health and childhood adversity. We are beginning to understand how early childhood development is affected by these factors and creates a cascading sequelae of long-term outcomes. This understanding provides a bedrock of guidance for how practices can intervene and support families in primary care. With the urging of Dr Nadine Burke Harris and other pioneers in the field of trauma research, clinicians have begun to address adversity in medical homes.

In 2021, the Center on the Developing Child at Harvard put out a policy statement[1] pointing out that blending the science of what we know regarding child development and the core capabilities that resilient adults have, practitioners can use the information to improve outcomes for children and families. The authors outline 3 core principles of development that can be used to "redesign policy and practice" (**Figure 3-1**):

1. Support responsive relationships for children and adults.
2. Strengthen core skills for planning, adapting, and achieving goals.
3. Reduce sources of stress in the lives of children and families.

FIGURE 3-1.

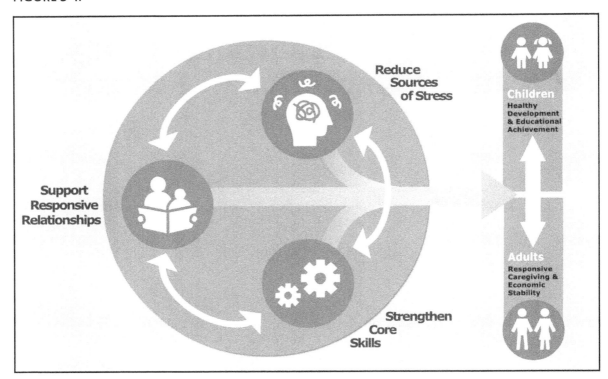

Three principles to improve outcomes for children and families. These principles, grounded in science, can guide policymakers and program developers as they design and adapt policies and programs to improve outcomes for children and families.

From Cohen SD. *3 Principles to Improve Outcomes for Children and Families.* Center on the Developing Child at Harvard; 2021. Accessed March 18, 2024. https://developingchild.harvard.edu/resources/three-early-childhood-development-principles-improve-child-family-outcomes.

Over the course of this book, we will review practical ways to improve outcomes for children and families, as encouraged by this research. When we look at ways to support relationships between children and adults and strengthen core skills, as the policy authors point out, we're building resilience in relationships for children. We'll explore this in Chapter 6, Understanding Early Relational Health, as we discuss the importance of early relational health histories, and in the next few chapters, we discuss practical ways to increase capabilities to address trauma. In Chapter 15, Implementation Nuts and Bolts, we talk about how to use applied implementation to strengthen these core skills so families are better served and policies/programs are in alignment with practices that help families thrive. In this chapter, we're focusing on 2 things: how we create trauma-informed environments in pediatric care to reduce stress for children and families and how to create an environment of supportive professionals who are trauma responsive. This chapter gets at 2 of the 3 principles to improve outcomes for children and families, so let's take a look.

What does it mean to be trauma informed? If a trauma-responsive practice is our destination, how do we get there from here? This chapter provides 2 different, but cooperative, maps: one for your organization as a whole and one for the individual clinicians and staff who make up your organization. To date, there are not universally accepted definitions of TIC; rather, there are models of what it takes to become a more aware, responsive, compassionate, and sensitive practice or organization. We will offer some models that may feel helpful as you venture on this path to becoming more aware of trauma and adversities that affect your organization and patients.

Creating Maps of Safety

Our patients and families get the most benefit from their care when their environment and the people in it are safe. Caregivers and children with histories of trauma are hypervigilant to their environment. Seeking out and assessing safety is a survival mechanism for them, a primal instinct.

When organizations and individuals act in trauma-responsive ways, when they convey an understanding of how trauma presents and behave in ways that create safety, interactions with patients look different and more intentional. I explain this to individuals: "Our brains are constantly making maps. Maps of what feels safe and maps of what feels threatening. If we're to restore a sense of safety, we must become a 'map of safety' for our patients by interacting with them in ways that recognize and reduce symptoms of trauma." When we empower staff and create a mutual understanding that *how* they interact with patients will determine the outcome, interactions shift. Consider the following statement in terms of how our patients perceive safety with us:

> If we are safe, our system is open and available for connection. If we are not safe (and this is subjective) our brain switches into a defense stance. It could be alert-orienting or full-blown aggression or dissociation. Defensive strategies prioritize protection NOT connection. —Robyn Gobbel, LCSW[2]

What I emphasize to health care professionals is that *our patients and their caregivers determine whether or not we are safe as professionals; we do not.* Through our interactions, we *earn* the perception of safety. Often, as professionals, we represent inherent threats to our patients: previous interactions with clinicians, complex medical procedures, dismissive staff, systemic traumas of people of color, and skepticism of health care all create barriers for our patients to feel safe in an office visit. It's *our* job as professionals to become a map of safety for our patients and their families through our behaviors and words.

It's worth mentioning that the goal of implementing RHHs is not the disclosure itself. Rather, it's creating a cultural shift in the organization—one that shows empathy, support, and sensitivity to what patients have endured. It is truly up to individuals and families whether or not to disclose and if their map of safety indicates that they feel safe enough to do so. Our hope is to educate families about the connections between early adversity, later health, attachment, and intergenerational trauma. The choice about when, how, and if they talk with their clinicians is up to them.

Becoming a map of safety is possible. It's empowering. And we know how to do it:

1. *Show empathy.* When talking with caregivers, this means acknowledging that life has overwhelming moments, parenting is hard, and being a provider for your family can be burdensome. For patients, it's important to let them know that you believe they're doing the best they can. After all, as Pollastri, Ablon, and Hone point out, kids and caregivers do well when they can.[3]

   Recognize that some people come from a background that hasn't prepared them for positive coping techniques. Some examples include the following:

   ● Intergenerational trauma and lack of a positive parent role model

   ● Their own history of trauma or abuse

   ● Relationship or environmental issues that the practice may not be aware of

   ● Not knowing what positive parenting interactions look like

   ● Not understanding important themes of development that increase resilience, such as play, attachment, and attunement

2. *Show respect.* If you create an environment of acceptance and nonjudgment, your patients will know that you have an open mind regarding their story, knowing you may not be aware of the trauma they have experienced. One way to do this is by demonstrating respect for a family's expertise of their own lived experience. When you partner with patients instead of assuming knowledge or understanding of their experience, you're demonstrating respect. When you acknowledge biases you may have as an individual (eg, race, socioeconomic status, ability, sexual orientation) and how they affect your work as a clinician, you create an environment for diverse children and families.

3. *Support the patient and their family.* Encourage them by letting them know that they are not to blame for the trauma they've experienced and that, sometimes, situations happen that are out of their control. Give patients and caregivers choices. When families have experienced trauma, they experience a great deal of loss of control. Put patient needs over organizational needs. Know local resources for trauma-informed counselors, community health workers, and community referrals. Finally, communicate with empathy and in a family's choice of language whenever possible.

4. *Provide safety.* Providing both physical and emotional safety for families is the foundation of creating maps of safety. Physical safety begins with your waiting room and is reflected throughout your clinic. Signs and posters should welcome all patients and clearly communicate that your clinic accepts them. It also means that staff reflect the community in appearance and language that is spoken. Physical safety includes providing choices, using separate spaces for privacy when needed, acting predictable with movement, getting down on your patient's physical level, and allowing other safe adults to be present. Being emotionally safe means being predictable and trustworthy: if you offer to reach out or provide a resource or support, be sure you follow through. It also means that all staff are embodying principles of TIC.

Essential Steps for Organizations

In their book *Childhood Trauma and Resilience: A Practical Guide*, Forkey, Griffin, and Szilagyi provide a wonderful summary for trauma-informed systems of care within the pediatric setting.[4] They lay out principles of trauma-informed work and offer a series of concrete "steps to implementation" that practices can begin to utilize. That work is also supported and reflected in the American Academy of Pediatrics (AAP) clinical report on TIC.[5] Importantly, these authors point out that becoming a trauma-informed environment takes time and dedication. We won't belabor their work here, but we will point you to it as a resource. Here, we'll focus on complementary models that offer implementation and organizational assessment tools, moving practices along the continuum from trauma aware to trauma informed. For the purposes of this book, we're using the working definition of TIC from The National Child Traumatic Stress Network (NCTSN)[6]:

> A trauma-informed child and family service system is one in which all parties involved recognize and respond to the impact of traumatic stress on those who have contact with the system including children, caregivers, and service providers. Programs and agencies within such a system infuse and sustain trauma awareness, knowledge, and skills into their organizational cultures, practices, and policies. They act in collaboration with all those who are involved with the child, using the best available science, to maximize physical and psychological safety, facilitate the recovery of the child and family, and support their ability to thrive.

The Missouri Model of TIC breaks down 4 straightforward phases to consider during implementation: *aware, sensitive, responsive,* and *informed.*[7]

Aware

We would advocate that all organizations *increase their awareness of trauma* within every role at their clinic. We accept that trauma is ubiquitous and that all families we work with have experienced adversities.

In my work with CHA, we increased awareness for organizations through what we called *compassion-informed care training,* or CICT. At the time, many of the clinics we worked with felt hesitant to use the term *trauma-informed training* because they did not want to imply that after a 90-minute staff workshop, the clinic would be trauma informed. Rather, we were raising awareness and increasing compassionate practices. Compassion-informed care training focused on raising awareness of the nature of trauma and how it presents and increasing compassion for patients and their caregivers regarding trauma histories. The training also increased awareness of how staff might be activated (ie, triggered) as well. We worked through case scenarios so each person throughout the organization might better recognize how trauma manifests and think about how to respond with more compassion. The end result was greater empathy and insight for patient care.

The following key elements helped ensure the success of this program:

- We ensured that the meetings took place during work hours and that employees were paid for their time.
- The meetings were mandatory, but the level of participation was by choice.
- We identified clinic champions early on—people who were committed to the work and could be available for resources and support.

We were intentional in setting up trainings in this way. The high value of the trainings meant that we wanted them to take place during the workday and ensure that folks were paid. Yet, at the same time, we wanted to model trauma-informed practices ourselves and recognize that not all staff would be comfortable participating in ways that might be activating for them, so the level of participation was by choice. Finally, identifying champions in-house allowed for ongoing support and touch points. This meant we solicited buy-in from key leaders and stakeholders to support our efforts.

Sensitive

According to the Missouri Model, the next step after awareness is for organizations to *increase their sensitivity* to trauma-informed principles and possible ways to overcome trauma. This happens through meetings, modeling, and education. In my work with CHA, we provided a great deal of information regarding how trauma presents in children and adults, both caregivers and colleagues. We challenged employees to rethink how they interpreted difficult patient behavior and encouraged clinicians to differentiate between trauma and other presenting medical issues. The shift from "What's wrong with that person?" to "I wonder what happened to that person…" was a vital part of becoming more sensitive.

Here's how I often introduce this concept. Imagine I'm interacting with someone at work today, perhaps someone in the front office. Usually, "Claire" acts friendly and engaging. But today, she's short-tempered and snappy when I ask for help or support. My natural inclination is to think, "Geez, what's the matter with Claire? Why is she so grumpy? I never did anything to her." But responding in a more sensitive, compassionate way means I reframe my question toward "I wonder what's going on with Claire (maybe her child is sick, she didn't sleep well, or she's carrying a worry I don't know about) and I wonder how I could help brighten Claire's day or take something off her plate." Or, more simply, I do not take Claire's behavior personally. **Box 3-1** offers a script that I use as an analogy for being trauma sensitive.

Box 3-1.
The Suitcase Analogy for Being Trauma Sensitive

Imagine that every day we wake up and pick up 2 suitcases. We do this whether or not we're aware of doing so. Think of these suitcases as our personal "baggage." The suitcase in our right hand holds our short-term or acute stressors. Perhaps the stressors are a late bill, a worry for a loved one, a recent argument, or concern for our job. Short-term may be earlier that day, or it may be a few months ago. In the suitcase in our left hand, we hold our trauma or adversities. Having experienced any of the trauma we've referred to so far feels heavy in that suitcase. Those traumas may have occurred recently or many years ago.

Now imagine that multiple times per day, we're going to have interactions with other people, be that our staff, patients, friends, or caregivers. On our best days, we're aware of the weight of our suitcases; therefore, we give ourselves and others compassion and grace. On other days, we feel judgmental, easily frustrated, or triggered because, often, the way we behave or interact when we feel "weighted down" is less than charming.

To be sensitive to trauma means that we're aware that we all carry suitcases, and that includes every person we interact with daily. When we say to ourselves, "I wonder what feels heavy to this person?" or "I am/they are carrying a lot today," it allows us to recognize that trauma and stress are ubiquitous and to respond with compassion.

During this phase, our aim was to educate clinic staff regarding their own trauma responses. We engaged in a brief reflection exercise by asking all of them to be aware of factors that might crop up for them because of the families and environments in which they had grown up. We had them privately take the ACEs Too High (https://acestoohigh.org) questionnaire so they knew their own ACE score. The goal here was for staff to see the types of questions we were asking of patients and caregivers and have an opportunity to reflect on some of their own experiences that naturally become activated in doing this work. It opened up incredibly vulnerable and honest conversations about themselves and the patients they were interacting with. R.J.'s trainings with the Oregon Pediatric Society took this part of the training one step further. They had participants complete the questionnaire and asked them to "get ready" to disclose the score to their neighbor. Rather than actually doing so, they used it as an opportunity for reflection about how disclosing such information felt and how it might help them gain empathy and sensitivity for a patient's perspective in disclosing such personal information.

You can see that as we progress along the continuum from trauma aware to trauma sensitive, we're increasing empathy through reflective practices.

Responsive

Once staff are more aware and sensitive to the prevalence of trauma and how it presents, they can begin to shift their response to patients, families, and each other. A parent comes in, harried and breathless, for her child's appointment. She's 15 minutes late. Before the training, a front desk employee might have thought, "Geez, how hard is it to be on time? You've known about this appointment for a month." But having developed greater sensitivity, she responds differently, thinking, "I wonder if her bus was late or if she couldn't get out of work." And instead of being exasperated with the parent, she offers her a glass of water and reassures her that she and her child can still be seen. As the authors of the Missouri Model point out, responding to trauma differently means *everyone* at the clinic does so, embodying a model of "This is how we treat patients." Forkey, Griffin, and Szilagyi offer 14 practices that can be implemented to create such a culture (**Box 3-2**).

Box 3-2.
14 Steps to Implement Trauma-Informed Care in Pediatric Settings

1. Educate all clinicians, staff, and leadership about trauma, patient engagement, nurturing caregiving, and resilience promotion.

2. Practice every step of a health visit and assess for physical, psychological, and emotional safety.

3. Review office resources on parenting and trauma.

4. Review family engagement.

5. Notice and note experiences of kids and families.

6. Offer simple choices.

7. Explain what will happen during the visit.

8. Practice positive engagement and strength-based history-taking skills.

9. Partner with caregivers and youth.

10. Screen with intention.

11. Utilize trauma as a differential diagnosis.

12. Provide psychoeducation.

13. Give messages about how to heal from trauma.

14. Follow up.

Derived from Forkey HC, Griffin JL, Szilagyi M. Trauma-informed systems of care. In: *Childhood Trauma and Resilience: A Practical Guide.* American Academy of Pediatrics; 2021:187–198.

It goes beyond patient care as well. How clinicians and staff relate to each other, how clinicians respond to parents and talk with them about trauma, and how staff treat each other are all seen as aftereffects of a responsive approach. Going back to the Harvard Center on the Developing Child, these practices decrease stress for families and support responsive relationships. We encourage an organization that aims to be trauma responsive to begin to put quality improvement measures in place in order to track what's working well and what effects the new practices are having on organizational wellness and patient care.

Informed

In the final phase of the Missouri Model, organizations fully implement trauma-informed practices, review their policies to ensure compliance with trauma-informed principles, put behaviors into practice, and monitor the impacts of changes that are made. As mentioned earlier, the AAP clinical report reflects this endeavor,[5] suggesting that trauma-informed practices are found across an organization—including, but not limited to, policies affecting leadership, policy overall, financing, collaboration with outside resources, and evaluative practices—and include parent and caregiver voice.[4] It's important that organizations identify a clinic champion (or more than one!) so this important work does not go by the wayside. We would encourage several champions across roles so that practices have accountability, thought partners across roles, and buy-in from key stakeholders. When you create internal champions within clinics, you're setting your clinic up for success by being deliberate about having a group of people committed to this practice. Adding in patient voice or a parent advisory board to get feedback about their office practices also proves beneficial. Again, a system is never "done" and labeled as "trauma informed"; rather, it's a continuous feedback loop of reflection and practice. It is an iterative cycle. What we would be disappointed to see is if the "trauma-informed binder" gets put on the shelf and lost with other well-intended endeavors.

In later chapters, R.J. will offer some thoughts on measuring your efforts, including how to conduct a Plan-Do-Study-Act cycle. There's also the GNOME approach, which is a helpful tool for designing an educational curriculum.

Designing Educational Curriculum: The GNOME Planning Tool

Note From R.J.

With any luck, you'll be able to find people in your area who do TIC training for clinics and their staff, but if you find yourself on your own, the tool I use for designing curriculum is the GNOME planning tool. GNOME is an acronym for **G**oals, **N**eeds, **O**bjectives, **M**ethods, and **E**valuation; it can be used for anything from a quick 1-hour lecture to a full conference if need be.

Your curriculum will almost write itself if you spend time thinking about the first 2 steps in the planning tool. In the context of the GNOME planning tool, Goals refers to the overall purposes of your learning curriculum, in the form of broad statements that describe what you're trying to accomplish in your training. These goals will vary based on where you are in your journey to being a trauma-aware or trauma-responsive organization. In the beginning, you may need to simply educate staff and clinicians on trauma and its effects on health and wellness. Further down the road, you may be working on relational skills in the context of disclosures, enhancing positive parenting skills, or practicing difficult conversations. In this model, Needs refers to the needs of both the instructor and the learner: What does the instructor need to convey to the audience, and what does the audience need to know or be able to do by the end of the training?

Once you've considered these 2 pieces, the Objectives should almost write themselves. The objectives should be clear statements about what you intend for the learners to be able to do by the end of the presentation. In education circles, objectives are categorized by Bloom's Taxonomy[8] and range from simple recall (lower-order objectives) up to synthesis and creation based on what has been learned (higher-order objectives). If you start the objective with the phrase "By the end of this training, learners will be able to" and then insert an active verb based on the taxonomy, you've written a decent objective.

Methods refers to how the curriculum will be delivered. The goals, needs, and objectives that you've determined up to this point will often dictate the methods that you use: If you are trying to impart knowledge and information, you're probably going to stick with a didactic lecture. If you're trying to improve skills, you may need some small group discussions, role-play, or other interactive methodologies.

Evaluation is how we know that the curriculum worked in achieving the intended objectives. Back in our school days, that would have been a test or a term paper, but most of the time, it's an evaluation form that's done at the training (You've seen them a million times at this point, right?). Be sure to anchor the evaluation to the specific objectives; that can be as simple as "Were objectives A, B, and C met?" with a Likert scale response, but including some open-ended questions is a good idea for taking your clinic to the next phase in their TIC journey...including asking the participants what they want to learn about next.

There's a worksheet for this planning tool in Appendix B, in case you need it.

Assessing Organizational Readiness

A map to understand and assess readiness for organizations would be great, no? How do we know where to dive in? Are we ready? Can we pull back and look at what we need to know based on where we are regarding trauma-informed work? Two organizations have provided valuable tools to assess organizational readiness and assessment: Trauma Informed Oregon[9] and The NCTSN.[10] Trauma Informed Oregon created a TIC screening tool using the phase language from the Missouri Model (discussed earlier in this chapter).[9] In it, they lay out key indicators within each phase that an organization can reflect on to guide intervention and training opportunities and continue to raise awareness. (See **Figure 3-2**.)

The NCTSN also offers an organizational assessment tool that many practices may find helpful. They identified 9 domains to create a trauma-informed organization (**Figure 3-3**). The 9 domains of The NCTSN Trauma-Informed Organizational Assessment are the following:

1. Trauma Screening

2. Assessment, Care-Planning, and Treatment

3. Workforce Development

4. Strengthening Resilience and Protective Factors

5. Addressing Parent/Caregiver Trauma

6. Continuity of Care and Cross-System Collaboration

7. Addressing, Minimizing, and Treating Secondary Traumatic Stress

8. Partnering With Youth and Families

9. Addressing the Intersections of Culture, Race, and Trauma

To note, The NCTSN assessment tool is intended for any organization that serves children and families. Both the Trauma Informed Oregon and NCTSN tools are free for organizations to utilize. An important aspect of utilizing any tool to assess organizational readiness and offering the reflective practice of "Where are we and how can we improve?" is to clearly incorporate patient voice and intersections between individual, historical, and intergenerational trauma.[4,6] In their article, Moreland-Capuia and colleagues[11] have created a questionnaire to measure the degree of an individual's trauma-informed knowledge and positive attitudes toward trauma-informed systems change, as well as trauma-informed practices in the workplace. It's the first of its kind that looks specifically into culturally responsive, trauma-informed models. We encourage all organizations to use one or more of these free resources to continuously monitor and reflect on trauma-informed practices.

Essential Steps for Individuals

In addition to organizational readiness, we need to look into clinician and staff readiness. As stated earlier in this chapter, it begins with education around components of trauma-informed work and phases of trauma awareness. Once initial groundwork is laid, a paradigm shift begins. Often it starts with a clinic champion or a clinician who exudes commitment to this work. Here's an example of how one pediatrician, and soon his clinic, was affected by increased awareness of parental trauma, childhood trauma, and trauma-informed work. Please note that the physician's words indicate "following these ACE scores." We want to advocate that ACE surveys, or other ways for inquiring about caregiver trauma, are only part of the RHH, but we have added his comment because of how transformational this process was for his clinic, like so many.

> Once we started to recognize the degree to which adverse childhood experiences affect growth and development, performance in school, frequency of illness, ability to bounce back from illness, and overall well-being, we recognized the importance of identifying and following these ACE scores.... It has dramatically improved our practice in that every visit we have the opportunity to address those root causes that prevent children from thriving.
> —Evan Buxbaum, MD, Redwood Pediatrics[12]

In my work with nurse managers at dozens of busy pediatric clinics, one of them indicated several times how much more meaningful her work felt. She reflected that becoming aware of

FIGURE 3-2.

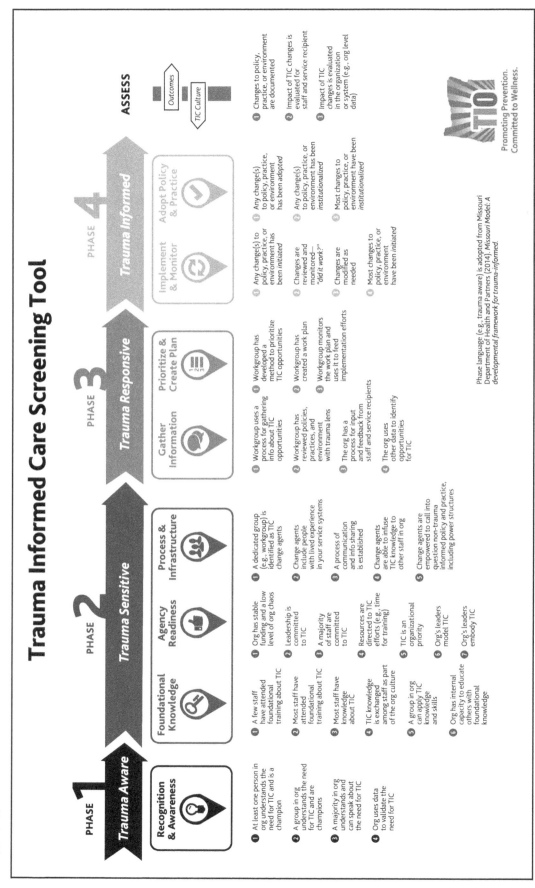

Trauma-informed care screening tool. info indicates information; org, organization; TIC, trauma-informed care.

From Trauma Informed Oregon. *Trauma Informed Care Screening Tool.* 2018. Accessed March 18, 2024. https://traumainformedoregon.org/implementation/implementation-and-accountability-overview/screening-tool.

FIGURE 3-3.

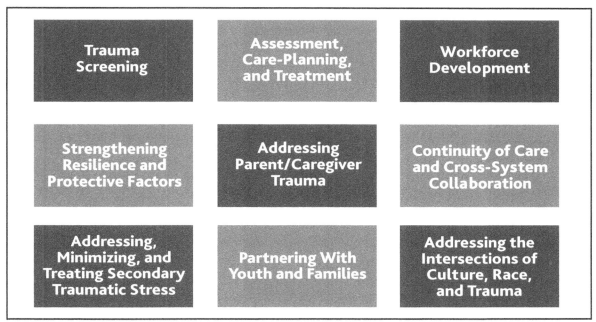

Nine domains to create a trauma-informed organization.

Used with permission from the National Center for Child Traumatic Stress, NCCTS Service Systems Program. (Published October 28, 2020.) *NCTSN Trauma-Informed Organizational Assessment. National Child Traumatic Stress Network.* https://www.nctsn.org/trauma-informed-care/nctsn-trauma-informed-organizational-assessment.

how trauma presents in children and in families helped her in direct communication and in her approach for education and offering resources. Several clinicians, once reluctant, have shared how significantly trauma-informed training has impacted them.

> I feel completely confident delivering this information even though I'm not a behavioral health clinician.
> —Kristan Collins, MD

The goal in sharing personal stories and testimonials from champions such as Evan and Kristan is to create and encourage a sense of readiness. And I would add that even clinicians who were hesitant or did not feel ready have a greater feeling of competency and willingness, knowing that their skepticism is normal and the outcome is positive.

Responding to Barriers and Creating Safe Work Environments

At times, using the voice of other clinicians is not sufficient. Late adopters of TIC need concrete data on how this type of investment will affect their practices. There is a plethora of research around workplace wellness and trauma-informed systems. Research indicates that staff want to bring their "whole self" to work and not compartmentalize themselves from their jobs. For some staff, personal issues and challenges they're facing outside the workplace can have a significant impact on their well-being. A workplace that encourages awareness of trauma, not just for its patients but also for its staff, will be better suited to meet the needs of its employees. Certainly, working in a health care organization can be inherently activating. And while we might hope that individuals within our organizations would reach out for help through programs such as employee assistance programs, only about 5% of them actually do.[13] So, if an organization is committed to trauma-responsive practices, its entire culture feels more supportive. This leads to greater productivity, less absenteeism, higher morale, and greater retention due to lesser burnout. We'll discuss this at length in Chapter 13, Self-Care and Sharing Our Humanity, and Chapter 14, Addressing Physician Overwhelm.

Moreover, if we look into cost savings of TIC training in pediatric settings and parallel the knowledge that early trauma can predict long-term impacts on a person's life, we can begin to see the imperative need to invest in trauma-informed training. As Forkey, Griffin, and Szilagyi point out,[4] if we even look at just 2 negative outcomes to childhood trauma, foster care and involvement with the legal system, billions of dollars are spent within those systems. The goal of trauma-informed systems, per the Substance Abuse and Mental Health Services Administration, is to *realize* the widespread impact of trauma, *recognize* the signs of it, *respond* by integrating trauma-informed practices, and *resist* re-traumatizing individuals.[14] Certainly, the data support the significant outcomes from childhood trauma and the need for pediatric clinics, as partners in care, to respond compassionately.

The work of Traub and Boynton-Jarrett lays out another complementary blueprint for creating trauma-informed pediatric medical homes.[15] Before any trauma assessments (or what we're calling *relational health histories*) are implemented and these delicate questions are asked of families, these authors point out that training for *all* pediatric staff is imperative. Their work shows that less than 20% of pediatricians report having adequate knowledge of either pediatric trauma or how to assess for or treat posttraumatic stress disorder. Earlier in this chapter, we discussed ways to prepare your organization, but certainly research supports that organizational readiness is necessary before collecting information about RHHs. Here and in **Table 3-1**, we'll highlight the components from Traub and Boynton-Jarrett's work that focus on clinicians and staff readiness. We're adding a few comments that reflect and support how this might look, best practice, in a pediatric office.

1. *Train all pediatric clinic staff in the principles of TIC.* This means everyone, or as I tell them, "Front office to back office, top of the organization chart to the bottom. Everyone matters."

2. *Customize pediatric health care to the needs of the family.* Often, so much time is focused on well-child checklists that the needs of the family or presenting concerns are missed. We'll touch on this more later, but suffice to say, when we respond to what's really happening in families, it enriches our relationship with families and builds trust.

3. *Assess pediatric patients for trauma, resilience, maternal psychopathology, family functioning, and family violence.* Here, we want to support questionnaires and discussions that ask about RHHs (not solely adversity or ACE surveys) including caregiver history of trauma, current stressors, and overall family health. We also want to encourage clinics to ask about PCEs anytime they're inquiring about relational health.

4. *Employ nonphysicians to conduct psychosocial screening and offer education to families about healthy development, recovery, and self-care skills.* This means partnering with mental health professionals, care managers, nurses, and medical assistants, as well as community health workers or social workers whom you may have access to in your organization.

5. *Create a medical home for children with ACEs, emphasizing strong relationships with families, regular care clinicians, and individualized care.* We would encourage a medical home clinician to ask about any history of childhood trauma. Safe, stable, nurturing relationships are the beginning of enabling healing and creating positive experiences for children and families.

6. *Integrate behavioral health into the pediatric office.* We recognize that not every practice has integrated behavioral health. When that's not possible, be sure to reach out to referral networks and community health workers and be sure that clinicians are familiar with resources in the community that offer efficacious treatment.

7. *Offer group-based parenting education and support that emphasizes trauma recovery and resilience.* Although not every practitioner is able to offer group appointments, there may be a behavioral health clinician within your practice, or one with whom you could partner

Table 3-1. Usual Care Versus Trauma-Informed Medical Home

Care Component	Usual Care	Trauma-Informed Medical Home
Medical health care	History and physical exam	History and physical exam Clinicians trained in trauma-informed care Daily huddles with other clinicians Care provided in patient's primary language
Behavioral health care	Separate Usually not trauma informed	Integrated within the primary medical team Daily huddles with physicians and other clinicians Trauma informed, team based, engagement focused
Relational health histories	Trauma/resilience assessments rare	Relational health histories that look for adverse *and* positive experiences Referral and integrated case management reflective of family need Strength based Culturally sensitive
Anticipatory guidance provided	Anticipatory guidance regarding age-appropriate risk reduction and parenting	Anticipatory guidance beyond risk reduction and parenting to include the following: trauma education; coping tools, mental health tools; resilience-building factors; and positive parenting
Case management	Usually none provided at the pediatric office	Integrated team-based case management with regular follow-up
Referrals for community-based services based on family/patient needs and preferences	Referrals made, but no ongoing communication with service clinicians or attempt to surmount obstacles to obtaining services	Relationships and communication with community-based service clinicians ongoing Staff with knowledge of community resources that helps families troubleshoot and overcome obstacles Referrals made to service providers who speak the language and support patient culture
Parenting support	Not usually offered except for brief conversations during well-child visits	Trauma informed Strength based Integrated into care Culturally sensitive
Peer support	Not usually offered	Trauma informed Integrated into care Patient voice and experience elevated Culturally sensitive
Educational advocacy	Not usually offered	Educational advocacy Caregiver education

Adapted from Traub F, Boynton-Jarrett R. Modifiable resilience factors to childhood adversity for clinical pediatric practice. *Pediatrics.* 2017;139(5):e20162569.

through an outside organization, who could offer parenting education and support with a trauma-responsive lens.

8. *Offer peer-based group education and anticipatory guidance to children and families with multiple ACEs about trauma and self-care to foster resilience and increase social support.* We want to emphasize that practices ask about any type of trauma, including intrafamilial trauma. And discussions about resilience and social support should occur at every encounter.

9. *Familiarize pediatric staff with resources in the community and make individualized referrals for children and families.*

10. *Be cognizant of barriers to engagement facing families of children with trauma histories—perception of mental health, family stress, cultural messages about trauma and mental health, and lack of social supports.*

Hopefully you can see that, beyond organizational readiness, a great deal depends on the readiness of individuals as well.

Note From R.J.

The ideas of creating a safe work environment and promoting staff wellness and self-care are intertwined in my mind. We'll talk more about the idea of self-care in upcoming chapters, but one of the problems I've always had with the idea of self-care is that it's often perceived as something that clinicians and staff have to do on their own time, rather than something that needs to be embedded within office practices. Unfortunately, a lot of self-care also focuses on escapism (getting away from the thing that's provoking your stress) rather than fixing the system that created the problem in the first place.

As part of your process of training your office in trauma-responsive care, pay attention to how you embed self-care into the process. In my office, we've encouraged the idea of "stress buddies" (some people call them "battle buddies"[16])—that is, someone in the office whom each staff member feels comfortable talking with when things are particularly challenging. If staff have someone they can decompress with after a challenging interaction, it makes the work environment healthier and safer. The stress buddy gives everyone a person to air grievances with who isn't a member of management, which often feels safer to staff.

Personally, I have a "work spouse." Normally on the days we're both in the office, she and I will be in the module between patients charting, talking with our respective nurse and medical assistant, and asking each other clinical questions. We're each buried in our laptops, working on our own tasks...but every once in a while, we really need to just get something off our chests about work, difficult patients, or something in our personal lives that we're having a hard time letting go.

I once walked out of a particularly tough interaction. About a year prior, a mom had disclosed domestic violence to me and shared her struggles with getting her husband help and managing her children's behaviors that were clearly a result of seeing violence in the household. Now, suddenly, Dad had just died. Both the mom and the teen son were struggling with a complex mix of grief and relief at the same time. Sitting with them, talking through that complicated emotional state, and figuring out resources and referrals felt, well, messy. I had recently experienced my own sudden loss of a family member, so my own emotions were flooding in.

I walked out of the room and found my work spouse at her laptop, charting away. I felt like it was under my breath when I said, "Wow, that was triggering." But it was like I said magic words: she stopped what she was doing, fully faced me, and said, "What happened?" She knows me and my personal life well enough to have known the connections I'd drawn in my own brain, so she saw me authentically, heard me compassionately, and really understood where I was coming from.

Imagine if instead I had just moved on to my next appointment while carrying that with me. What would the next patient have seen and experienced from me? Or imagine if I worked in an office where my partners were too concerned with their own schedules and flow to take a minute to help a colleague who was struggling. A lot of practices, particularly ones where compensation is based on production, become competitive and adopt an "everyone for themselves" kind of mindset, which is the opposite of being a trauma-informed or trauma-responsive practice.

In my mind, this is part of the goal of creating a compassionate, trauma-responsive office: that everyone feels safe, supported, and cared for—from patients to staff to clinicians.

What kind of office do you want to practice in?

Practical Pearls

Nothing swayed clinicians and staff more during our trainings than case studies. When we discussed how trauma presents in patients, in children, and in ourselves, our audience was reflective and empathic. When we discussed secondary trauma for health care professionals and discussed how trauma is ubiquitous within health care organizations, staff and clinicians felt seen and heard. When we encouraged them that every single person in an organization can be a present, supportive adult in a child and family's life, staff felt empowered to make a difference. As we mentioned earlier, knowing *about* trauma and knowing *what to do about* trauma are different in practice. Borrowing the phrases from the Missouri Model, becoming trauma *aware* and having skills to be *responsive* are 2 different levels.

> **Children are better able to thrive when we lighten the load on their parents so they can meet their families' essential needs, and when policies and programs are structured in ways that reduce stress rather than amplify it. —Harvard Center on the Developing Child[1]**

In addition to case studies, a few other factors had significant impact on clinicians' perception around trauma and staff empowerment for responding to trauma.

Understanding How Our Brain Protects Us

When staff and clinicians understand that it's a biological imperative for our brains to respond to trauma in protective ways, a massive dose of empathy can be provided. It reminds me of a parent I encountered who I thought was angry at me for running late between appointments. He came off as mean, terse, and guarded, and his mannerisms felt disrespectful to me. But once I found out (by simply asking) what else was going on, he said he felt worried his child would be slighted on time since I was running late. Our interaction went something like this:

Me: Hi there, sorry I'm running late, come on in [*as I escorted the family back to my office*].

Parent: Well, it's about time. You know, it doesn't make a good impression. I don't know what you're doing back there.

Me: [*sitting down on the same level as the parents/child with "warm eyes"*] I'm sorry. It's hard when clinicians run late. I was helping another teenager with a medical emergency. Tell me, what's going on for you right now? You seem upset.

Parent: [*voice elevated and shaky*] Well, it's already past 2:00 pm now, and we only have so much time with you!

Me: I see, you're worried we won't have enough time.

Parent: [*exasperated*] Exactly!

Me: How can I reassure you right now?

Parent: You can tell me my kid is just as important and my questions will be answered.

Me: OK. Let's do this: I'm going to put a note out front so people know I'm running late. I promise you, you'll still have your full time with me and won't be rushed. And if we get toward the end of our time, even if I'm running late for my next appointment, we'll make a follow-up within a couple of days. How's that sound?

Parent: Great. Thanks.

Me: I can tell you care about your child and want his needs met. That's what I want too. When crises come up with other patients, like the teen before yours, I will run late. And I'll do that for you and your child too. You're important to me.

I could literally see Dad's shoulders move down and worry wash away from his face. We then proceeded with the rest of our appointment, in partnership.

Van der Kolk points out that our brains' response to trauma is real, not disordered.[17] Brain changes are a genuine adaptation to an unhealthy or toxic environment. Noticing how the brain works and how it's cued for protection is another step in validating behavior that is rooted in trauma. In dangerous situations, a trauma response is protective, but often that response is generalized to situations that "feel dangerous" when they may not be. Only when we recognize that trauma responses are helpful and functional can we help a patient move from protective to more adaptive responses. Following are some examples of how trauma may present in patients and parents, from the work of Stephen Porges[18]:

- Interpreting neutral faces as angry
- Interpreting tone as hostile
- Feeling a sense of danger even in calm environments
- Staying in a state of alarm and hypervigilance
- Interpreting physical gestures of kindness as threats
- Carrying these patterns into many situations and relationships

Recognizing these manifestations of trauma shifts how we perceive patients, ourselves, and our interactions.

Note From R.J.

I think having an understanding of the neurobiology of trauma is a hallmark of a good, trauma-responsive office, and it helps staff and clinicians be able to understand why they're seeing what they're seeing.

However, it's important to help staff feel safe too. Some of these interactions are ugly and may feel hurtful, despite our best attempts to rationalize behaviors on behalf of someone who is behaving in a way that feels threatening or even abusive. In my experience, front desk staff and telephone advice nurses get the worst of it. There have been plenty of times the staff has told me about a challenging interaction that completely caught me off guard because the patient or family are always kind and reasonable once they're in the exam room. So how do we support the staff members who are treated this way?

It's an important first step for staff to be able to shift their thinking from "What is wrong with you?" to "What happened to you?" but there's a difference between understanding the behavior and simply accepting it. I think there's accountability to be had for people mistreating each other, and it can certainly be a fine line. I personally have zero tolerance for people cussing out my front desk staff, and I think it's important to create some boundaries when that sort of behavior takes place:

"I understand you're having a hard time right now, but I can't let anyone speak to my front desk staff that way. I will help you with addressing your needs, but let's take a minute to breathe first."

My office does have a policy that expresses our unwillingness to tolerate abuse from anyone; so if a patient, contractor, or other clinician is truly offensive to a staff member, our management team will call them out. We have a letter that gets sent to some people whose behavior violates this policy, reminding them to treat staff with respect and kindness. It's not only protecting the front desk staff and demonstrating that management has their back but also helping protect other patients in the waiting room who are hearing the aggression and may feel activated by it. It's possible to balance an expression of support for families with laying down firm boundaries; doing so is a key part of creating a safe environment for everyone.

Not Without Resilience

In future chapters, we will outline the importance of understanding resilience, incorporating resilience-based interventions into practices, and barriers to "treating trauma" through resilience interventions. As discussed in those chapters, no one is *born resilient;* resilience is built over time. For now, in regard to getting your organization ready and beginning to introduce trauma-informed practices, suffice it to say, while the term *resilience* may feel a bit overused at this point, we'll offer guidance on resilience and resilience-building interventions that have been shown to mitigate trauma and stress for children and families. In fact, being trained in the underpinnings of resilience, and how we might use knowledge about resilience to create buffering mechanisms for patients and families, has been shown to decrease physician burnout and increase feelings of competency.[19] As we circle back to the factors that authors from the Harvard Center on the Developing Child have led us to (discussed back at the beginning of this chapter), strengthening the foundation of resilience through supportive relationships and active skill building is exactly what we seek to do. Building resilience by promoting positive outcomes and buffering mechanisms for patients and families is, in fact, what the AAP has declared as a charge for clinicians.

> I was at the point in my practice, after 15 years, where I realized I would never get any better at taking care of asthma or treating an ear infection. And then, for the first time in a long time, I realized that I was going to be a better pediatrician because of this training and the resilience-building discussions I was having with patients and families. —Erika Meyer, MD

One thing we've both observed in our work is that each clinic has its own culture, and each clinic has varying degrees of readiness. So, it goes without saying that each individual has their own degree of readiness as well. We encourage you to see this work as iterative and revisit stages of readiness often, both for your organization and for yourself and the other individuals working within it.

Conclusions

As you can see, getting your organization ready to be trauma responsive is a multilayered process. It involves organizational components and individual components, as well as creating a plan to assess and measure readiness, process, and outcomes. If we start by creating safety within our organization for staff, colleagues, and patients and families alike and end with responding to barriers, we can shift from trauma aware to more trauma responsive. Then we will fold in factors of resilience to ensure that we're defining not just what trauma is but how to respond.

Questions to Consider

1. What stage of trauma-informed practice would you guess your organization is in: aware, sensitive, responsive, or informed?

2. What barriers to TIC does your practice face at this time?

3. We are all neurologically hardwired to protect ourselves. In what ways do you see this manifest in your patients? In their caregivers?

References

1. Cohen SD. *3 Principles to Improve Outcomes for Children and Families.* Center on the Developing Child at Harvard; 2021. Accessed March 18, 2024. https://harvardcenter.wpenginepowered.com/wp-content/uploads/2017/10/3Principles_Update2021v2.pdf

2. Gobbel R. *Raising Kids With Big, Baffling Behaviors: Brain-Body-Sensory Strategies That Really Work.* Jessica Kingsley Publishers; 2023

3. Pollastri AR, Ablon JS, Hone MJG, eds. *Collaborative Problem Solving: An Evidence-Based Approach to Implementation and Practice.* Springer; 2019 doi: 10.1007/978-3-030-12630-8

4. Forkey HC, Griffin JL, Szilagyi M. *Childhood Trauma and Resilience: A Practical Guide.* American Academy of Pediatrics; 2021 doi: 10.1542/9781610025072

5. Forkey H, Szilagyi M, Kelly ET, et al; American Academy of Pediatrics Council on Foster Care, Adoption, and Kinship Care; Council on Community Pediatrics; Council on Child Abuse and Neglect; and Committee on Psychosocial Aspects of Child and Family Health. Trauma-informed care. *Pediatrics.* 2021;148(2):e2021052580 PMID: 34312292

6. National Child Traumatic Stress Network. Creating trauma-informed systems. Accessed March 18, 2024. https://www.nctsn.org/trauma-informed-care/creating-trauma-informed-systems

7. *The Missouri Model: A Developmental Framework for Trauma-Informed Approaches.* Missouri Dept of Mental Health and Partners; 2014

8. Armstrong P. Bloom's Taxonomy. Vanderbilt University Center for Teaching. 2010. Accessed March 18, 2024. https://cft.vanderbilt.edu/guides-sub-pages/blooms-taxonomy

9. Trauma Informed Oregon. *Trauma Informed Care Screening Tool.* 2018. Accessed March 18, 2024. https://traumainformedoregon.org/implementation/implementation-and-accountability-overview/screening-tool

10. National Child Traumatic Stress Network. *Trauma-Informed Organizational Assessment (TIOA) Informational Packet.* Accessed March 18, 2024. https://www.nctsn.org/sites/default/files/resources/special-resource/trauma_informed_organizational_assessment_information_packet.pdf

11. Moreland-Capuia A, Dumornay NM, Mangus A, Ravichandran C, Greenfield SF, Ressler KJ. Establishing and validating a survey for trauma-informed, culturally responsive change across multiple systems. *J Public Health (Berl).* 2022 doi: 10.1007/s10389-022-01765-5

12. Casarez I. A paradigm shift: local physicians screening for ACEs have seen an adjustment in pediatric care. *North Coast Journal.* December 16, 2021. Accessed March 18, 2024. https://www.northcoastjournal.com/news/a-paradigm-shift-22270722

13. Agovino T. Companies seek to boost low usage of employee assistance programs. Society for Human Resource Management *HR Magazine.* 2019. Accessed March 18, 2024. https://www.shrm.org/hr-today/news/hr-magazine/winter2019/pages/companies-seek-to-boost-low-usage-of-employee-assistance-programs.aspx

14. Substance Abuse and Mental Health Services Administration. *SAMHSA's Concept of Trauma and Guidance for a Trauma-Informed Approach.* HHS publication (SMA) 14-4884. Substance Abuse and Mental Health Services Administration; 2014

15. Traub F, Boynton-Jarrett R. Modifiable resilience factors to childhood adversity for clinical pediatric practice. *Pediatrics.* 2017;139(5):e20162569 PMID: 28557726 doi: 10.1542/peds.2016-2569

16. Albott CS, Wozniak JR, McGlinch BP, Wall MH, Gold BS, Vinogradov S. Battle Buddies: rapid deployment of a psychological resilience intervention for health care workers during the COVID-19 pandemic. *Anesth Analg.* 2020;131(1):43–54 PMID: 32345861 doi: 10.1213/ANE.0000000000004912

17. Van der Kolk B. *The Body Keeps the Score: Brain, Mind, and Body in the Healing of Trauma.* Penguin Random House; 2015

18. Porges SW. Feeling safe is the treatment. In: Mitchell J, Tucci J, Tronick E, eds. *The Handbook of Therapeutic Care for Children: Evidence-Informed Approaches to Working With Traumatized Children and Adolescents in Foster, Kinship and Adoptive Care.* Jessica Kingsley Publishers; 2019

19. Moshofsky D, Stoeber A, Rumsey D. Targeting adverse childhood experiences by promoting resilience through anticipatory guidance: a quality project. Poster presented at: American Academy of Pediatrics National Conference and Exhibition; September 16–19, 2017; Chicago, IL

Chapter 4

Building the Case for Resilience

Amy King, PhD

If not me, who? If not now, when?
Rabbi Hillel

In 2015, a group of pediatricians asked if I would consult with them regarding how to respond to the ACEs study.[1] They had a couple of experiences that shaped this request. Many of them had seen Nadine Burke Harris' TED Talk, which had gone viral, and they'd been to a training from colleagues about the study and its effect on long-term health outcomes. One of R.J.'s colleagues had recently begun training pediatricians about childhood adversity across the state of Oregon and it was both eye opening and overwhelming. Additionally, Robert Block, past American Academy of Pediatrics (AAP) president, had recently stated that "ACEs are the single greatest unaddressed public health threat facing our nation today." The pediatricians I met with exuded compassion, as well as an intense desire to do something about childhood trauma and adversity.

As we talked, the request became clear: Could we find a way to work together to address childhood trauma? How would we do so? What would be the first step? And what step would be the most efficacious? Together, we decided we would intentionally craft a plan that afforded all of their offices to become more aware of the symptoms and signs of trauma, and more responsive to trauma, and then we would roll out a plan to educate pediatricians on tools that could boost resilience. In previous chapters, we discussed the importance of being intentional about implementation of screening for relational health histories (RHHs), social drivers of health (SDOH), postpartum depression, and the like, as well as creating trauma-informed clinics. This intentionality is required to begin building our patients' resilience, or what researchers are referring to as "buffering mechanisms" to mitigate adversity.

I'll never forget my conversation with this group of pediatricians. Dr Dean Moshofsky, a veteran pediatrician and trauma-informed superhero, said to me, "You know what I really want, Amy? I want a curriculum that would boost resilience at every well-child check, birth to adulthood."

My response: "OK."

"OK"?

My excitement for the cause overrode the limitations that a more rational response would have entailed. I naively accepted the challenge and set out to create just what was requested: a curriculum of trauma-informed, efficacious interventions for pediatricians to use at well-child visits. I blended my knowledge of integrated behavioral health care, trauma-informed practices, and short, population-health focused interventions along with my knowledge of efficacious practice for kids and families. (See Chapter 9, Designing and Using Efficacious Interventions to Support Early Relational Health and Heal Trauma, for full details on creating these interventions.)

And then, we dove in. This brave group of doctors and I met on a regular basis. It was like throwing spaghetti at the wall to see what stuck. Some ideas were met with excitement and piloted immediately. Others were pushed back with skepticism: "You want me to talk about *this*?" "How will that look?" "How much time will that take?" Often, the physicians asked for more: "I need a script," "I need notes," "I need a picture or graphic."

Nevertheless, these early adopters of trauma-informed care (TIC) in pediatrics soldiered on. They knew they would never feel comfortable with questionnaires about childhood adversities, SDOH, creating trauma-informed clinics, and asking more of themselves and their staff if they could not answer the question "Now what?" In practical terms, their internal dialogue went something like this:

- If I take this brave step of beginning to ask my patients about histories of trauma and adversity…
- If I trust that many of my patients and caregivers have experienced trauma and would benefit from validation and further discussion…
- If I voluntarily take on a greater role during my patient encounters…
- If I learn ways to recognize how stress and trauma present in my patients…
- If I trust that simply the act of asking and then listening can create acknowledgment for the families I care for…

…then I'd better have something in my back pocket to *do.* I'd better know how to *respond.* I want to be able to feel *helpful*—not just validating these experiences but knowing *what to do next.*

Can you identify with this line of thought? Let's talk about why resilience works and how it creates buffering mechanisms for patients and families. And let's talk about why the pediatric office visit is the ideal setting for education and guidance on tools to build resilience.

Defining Resilience

Although we wish that all children could grow in nurturing environments and never experience environmental, social, or physical stressors—not to mention the multitude of psychosocial stressors that are a part of normal growth and development—it's simply impossible. In fact, there's a great deal of research that indicates that a certain amount of predictable, tolerable stress in the presence of a supportive caregiver has a positive effect. Perry and colleagues point out that moderate, controllable, and predictable stress actually builds resilience.[2]

As we discussed in the Introduction, when the stressor is brief and short-lived, we refer to that as *positive stress*[3]; when the stressor is more serious but still temporary and buffered by supportive relationships, we refer to it as *tolerable stress.* For instance, when a toddler comes into your office for a well-child exam that includes vaccines (aka, "scary shots in my arm"), she may be quite stressed. In fact, as soon as the toddler becomes aware that there are shots, cortisol level increases. We see toddlers ask about shots even before the visit begins: "Ouch today?" During visits that include a poke in the arm, it can be stressful. However, a few important things are happening for this toddler. First, the environment is controlled. There are doctors and nurses buzzing about and, in the event that something goes awry with the vaccines, help is immediate. Second, the stress is considered a positive stressor because Mom has been informed of the pros and cons of vaccines for her toddler, she's been able to ask questions, and she knows the pain for her toddler is short-lived. Therefore, Mom can provide soothing comfort and remind the toddler that this will be short-lived. Plus, she has tools inherent to her to comfort and calm her child: feeding, rocking, cuddling—all invaluable to create experiences of resilience. Third, going through the visit is quite predictable. Because caregivers and toddlers see their pediatrician so frequently in the first 2 years, the regularity helps calm both the caregiver's and the child's nervous system. The 2 of them know, together, that visits to see their pediatrician are mostly great and supportive. Finally, the stress is moderate and short-lived. Again, this is referred to as *positive stress.* There is no significant medical procedure, no lifelong diagnosis, and nothing that would jeopardize the toddler.

Tolerable stress can also build resilience. Think of a child who's experienced a serious injury or witnessed a fatality, or the family experienced a home fire. The stress has a greater degree of activation in the child and more signs of danger. But if it is time limited and the child has supportive, reassuring adults to help them cope and soothe, the stressor is tolerable to the child. Positive and tolerable stressors build resilience because the child learns confidence and coping skills from experiencing the stressor, enduring it, and having a nurturing adult present for support and comfort. Both these stressors should be differentiated from toxic stress and complex trauma, which is what the ACEs study and The National Child Traumatic Stress Network refer to.

Given that we can't prevent all stressors from occurring, how do we shift to building personal and environmental strengths that buffer children from those adversities that they will, most certainly, face? Let's start by defining resilience. Zolkoski and Bullock define resilience as good mental and physical health despite the assails of early adversity—the ability to withstand, adapt to, and recover from adversities.[4] Resilience is not something a child is born with or predisposed to. Rather, woven into resilience is a multitude of factors including genetics, temperament, knowledge, past experiences, social supports, systemic supports, and cultural resources.[5-9] In other words, what creates resilience is multifaceted and intersects on many levels. Resilience intervention and research have progressed over the past 50 years. Previously, resilience research and implementation focused on preventing psychopathology and poor outcomes despite developmental risks. Recent studies, however, focus on how to promote resilience through prevention and intervention.[10] These studies include ways to promote positive outcomes and build or enhance buffering relationships with caregivers. The other important factor regarding resilience is that it is meant to be built within supportive relationships.

Resilience is multifaceted and determined by experience, culture, temperament, and social and systemic support. We are not meant to be resilient *all* the time in *every* situation. Some of us might find that we're resilient for periods when we have support and in situations where we feel safe. That's normal. Second, resilience is built *in relationships.* The best antidote for trauma and stress is a relationship with safe, stable, nurturing people with whom we can regulate our nervous system. Finally, resilience is built in communities and systems of support. When we look at research on resilience, it's those who feel seen and heard in supportive communities who feel resilient.

Describing Resilience

In a primary care visit, it's often helpful to have a script for how to talk about resilience. Many health care professionals I work with refer to resilience as the ability to "bounce back" from adversity. They use the metaphor of resilience as a basketball or boomerang. This is certainly helpful and describes an ability to recover from adversity. But it doesn't necessarily capture the ability to adapt, withstand, and change in the face of adversity. And it doesn't speak to the importance of resilience building within relationships. In speaking with clients who have endured extreme stress and trauma, I was once offered this analogy (the name has been changed to protect this client's confidentiality):

> After I was sexually abused, I tried to find a way to explain to my family how I was changed through the trauma I had experienced. I knew I was stronger and yet different. I knew I had found new purpose and yet would never be the same. Everyone wanted me to go back to being "like the old Sonja," but I knew I couldn't. I was forever transformed. But not in a bad way. I told them I feel a lot like a paper clip. Before, I knew my purpose and function. I knew who I was—I hold things together; I keep things organized. After I was abused, I changed. I was reshaped. I would never be "the old Sonja" because part of my innocence had been stripped away. And I had survived a horrific event. But I could be stronger and different and find new purpose. I was like a paper clip that had been reshaped. I could defend myself with a sharp point, I could pick a lock, or I could be a straight edge. In other words, I was still

a paper clip, but I had to find new meaning, new purpose—different but better and stronger. I had overcome a lot, and my new form had experienced change that helped me learn and survive.

Whatever analogy you choose, it's often helpful to have examples of what resilience might look like in your patients. Having this discussion can be quite empowering.

A plethora of research indicates that children with greater resilience have better developmental outcomes, despite early adversities.[9] In fact, new research shows that, despite early adversities, when there are safe, stable, nurturing relationships (SSNRs) available for children (ie, PCEs), the stressors and trauma can be mitigated through those connected relationships.[11] Multiple authors have outlined features of resilience for individuals. Today, we look at resilience as a mediating factor, a buffering mechanism, that reduces the impact of stress and trauma. The literature clearly outlines that resilience is the shielding mechanism to promote protective factors for children who've experienced trauma and can ultimately improve their health outcomes.[12-15] Ultimately, these individual and systemic variables can reduce negative chain reactions and even enable opportunities for recovery from traumatic experiences.[10] Wingo and colleagues[6] found that individuals who had experienced childhood sexual, emotional, and physical abuse experienced a less severe impact if they were found to be resilient. As well, many studies have shown that creating systems that promote resilience and coping can help children flourish.[4] This is all promising news. As we will discuss next, we provide education to clinicians about resilience and mitigating factors within the context of family and caregivers because that is the primary system where children live, especially in their first 3 years.

Resilience and Early Relational Health

When we discuss resilience within pediatrics, we're also talking about the importance of early relationships—namely, those with caregivers. In Chapter 6, Understanding Early Relational Health, R.J. outlines the importance of early relational health (ERH) and how it fits into universal interventions for all kids and families. A lot of trauma can happen to a family system before any professional is made aware of the family's hardships. The 2021 AAP policy statement "Preventing Childhood Toxic Stress: Partnering With Families and Communities to Promote Relational Health" stresses the importance of partnering with families and communities to promote relational health.[16] As research points to a deeper understanding of early attachment and development and the promotion of SSNRs, authors in this field recognize the importance that any model that looks to build resilience does so within the caregiver environment.

Much of the work around PCEs focuses on the relationship between children and caregivers across a child's life. The research indicates that promoting healthy relationships early on is the key to promoting connection that leads to resilience.[11,17] In fact, researchers point out that children who experience positive early relationships with caregivers thrive despite early adversity.[11] Also, researchers have learned that building those early relationships and supporting ERH promotes skills and tools that allow children to "flourish despite adversity."[16] In fact, work in the field of early education, child care, and home visiting programs has shifted significantly from focusing on child-only interventions and supports to bolstering care and education of parents and caregivers (see **Box 4-1** for an example illustrating how effective this can be). Researchers and practitioners in complementary fields of early intervention encourage supporting caregivers, involving them in intervention, and educating clinicians on how to support families.

Pediatricians can act as a catalyst early in a child's life, supporting their caregivers, building systemic supports, and providing education about features that build resilience. Those are taught first to the caregivers and then, as the child develops, to the child as well. They must be taught in a prescriptive manner to have the most efficacy—meaning, we must focus on what we know to be key developmental outcomes for children that boost resilience and must pair our support,

---

Box 4-1.
Case Vignette: Child-Caregiver Intervention

I still remember in the early months of my residency parents and caregivers dropping off children for therapy. The expectation to treat children alone, without a supportive adult, was pervasive. I had children as young as 5 years old, from the foster care system, dropped off via taxi for weekly therapy. As a young, outspoken clinician who hadn't yet been told to do otherwise, I started asking all caregivers, including foster parents, to stay for treatment. To observe. To ask questions. To coach and interact. At first, a mountain of barriers was presented: time, privacy, competing appointments. But I persevered and offered that the therapy might actually take less time to feel more successful if there was systemic involvement and caregiver participation. And *everything* changed. What I witnessed was that as children with trauma healed, caregivers healed too. And as caregivers healed, asked questions, and took small bites of information home, children flourished.

I'll never forget a sweet, freckle-faced 5-year-old whose only treatment goal was "to get messy." She'd been beaten and neglected so terribly that she was frightened of making messes or mistakes. But play is the job for 5-year-olds! So, I invited her foster mom in for our sessions. We made mud pies, smeared paint, and lathered our hands in bubbles. We made messes, cleaned up messes, and praised the girl for messes—all within the safety of her relationship with her caregiver. And, at home, they did the same; the skills translated and the safety became known. After a few months, with a gap-toothed smile, she told me she was ready to move on because she was OK to get messy.

---

education, and intervention with efficacious tools that support a healthy trajectory. We'll get deeper into this in Parts 2 and 3 of the book, but for now, let's talk about whether or not you can teach resilience.

Resilience Education

So, can resilience be taught? The short answer is yes. Resilience can be taught and modeled at every patient encounter. We would posit that tying resilience education to trauma education, RHHs, and well-child exams is exactly what helps pediatricians feel more competent when talking about stress and trauma, in general. Several authors cite the importance of education for children and families regarding trauma, stress, and responding to stress.[10] Furthermore, Streeck-Fischer and van der Kolk point out that it's important to do so because often children have very little insight into how their experiences shape how they act and react after experiencing significant trauma.[18] And before we create greater awareness in children, we must partner with parents and caregivers to bolster their knowledge about how trauma looks, how stress presents, and how behaviors that appear to be triggering or attention seeking might, in fact, be indicators of stress and overwhelm for a child. Caregivers and children need this point of acknowledgment before we rush in with tools to address their trauma.

> When one of my children was diagnosed with cancer, my younger child began taking care of her pretend babies, giving them medicine and taking them to the doctor. At first, I was saddened that the illness had become so pervasive in our home. I would try to redirect her or encourage her babies to "get better." When you pointed out that this was her way of coping and processing what we were all going through, it made so much sense! Now, I gently praise my daughter for being a great caretaker and we talk about how she feels about her brother being sick. It's helped see her behaviors as a way of adjusting and I can better support her. —Mom of a toddler

The authors of the AAP policy statement on preventing childhood toxic stress point out that several factors must be present to support this type of resilience education.[16] Pediatricians need enhanced training about SDOH, ERH, and resilience education (see Chapter 6, Understanding Early Relational Health). They also need sufficient time to talk with children and families, which means that payment reform and incentives are necessary.[19] This means doctors should advocate for themselves, both in terms of what they need individually and what kinds of structural reforms are needed to deliver the best care. Finally, they need a greater understanding about when and how to use opportunities to build on resilience.

There is no other group better suited for caregiver and patient education around well-being and resilience than pediatricians. Within the first 2 years after a child's birth, pediatricians meet with the child and family 10 times, at a minimum. They welcome families into their care within days of birth and continue to care for and create relationships with their patients for the child's lifetime. Over a child's life span, pediatricians develop a relationship with caregivers unlike that of any other professional. In fact, pediatricians interface with multiple children in one family and often multiple caregivers over the course of a child's life. They provide care, collaboration, and consultation about many aspects of childhood health—including, but not limited to, physical, emotional, social, and cognitive health. Crucially, pediatricians also have access to families and children to assess and address early adversity before any other professional in a child's life.

Pediatricians are well suited for teaching resilience and resilience-based interventions as part of anticipatory guidance in their practice. In fact, research supports anticipatory guidance around resilience-building tools, especially for children who have experienced trauma.[20] Using the pediatric visit to underscore the importance of trauma recovery and resilience building is crucial to child wellness.[10] In fact, the AAP encourages pediatricians to develop leadership roles in addressing toxic stress and early life adversity by tying education to patient encounters. However, as many others point out, pediatricians are often unsure of how to best move forward in teaching resilience to kids and families. In other words, just because they are in the best position to provide this type of education does not mean they feel equipped on the "how."

Anticipatory guidance is suited to foreseeing events that, without intervention and direction, might go awry. Additionally, you may identify areas where, without encouragement and guidance, caregivers or patients may miss opportunities to better respond to their child's experiences, stressors, or trauma that could benefit their long-term health. Resilience education related to stress, adversity, and trauma offers an opportunity to notice that the developmental trajectory of a child is off track and provide guidance to help the patient and family intervene. Traub & Boynton-Jarrett[10] identify 5 modifiable resilience factors that can mitigate the effects of stress and trauma: positive appraisal style and executive function skills, nurturing parenting, maternal mental health, good self-care skills and consistent routine, and understanding trauma. Again, there is no other professional who has the same access and opportunity to bestow information and provide support to parents and caregivers as a general pediatrician. In fact, even just the positive appraisal of caregiving by a clinician was associated with greater resilience in children.[21] Simply put, pediatric care is *the* place to deliver interventions that enhance resilience and mitigate childhood trauma and adversity.

> After teaching a mom about resilience during a visit, specifically about how emotions can flare up and how to respond, we discussed a tool you taught us about: "flipping your lid," from the work of Dan Siegel (see Chapter 8, Revamping Anticipatory Guidance). It changed everything for her. And I felt more competent too! I was able to help her with a new tool to de-escalate her child. The next day, I was perplexed when I saw the same family on my schedule. The mom proudly brought in her husband and said, "Teach him, we all need this." We went through the same technique again, and I could see Mom's learning deepening and Dad engaging, and I knew this family was changing.
> —Pediatrician's reflection

Models for Building Resilience in the Pediatric Office

One of the best-known models that lays out features of resilience for pediatric populations and pediatricians was created by Ken Ginsburg in his book *Building Resilience in Children and Teens,*[22] based on an amalgamation of research. Ginsburg outlines the 7 Cs—strengths for pediatricians and caregivers to pay attention to and build on to promote greater resilience in children: Competence, Confidence, Connection, Character, Contribution, Coping, and Control. (See **Box 4-2.**)

Box 4-2.
Ginsburg's 7 Cs

- **Connection:** Arguably the most important of the 7 Cs, Connection is the relationships that children and caregivers have to family, friends, and community supports.
- **Character:** How children are seen by others and how they know themselves.
- **Coping:** The ability to manage struggles and respond to environment or personal cues.
- **Competence:** A sense that a child has handled a situation effectively.
- **Confidence:** The belief the child has about their own abilities.
- **Control:** A child's sense that they can control an outcome or response.
- **Contribution:** Ways in which children give back to their world, their family, and their community.

Derived from Ginsburg KR, Jablow MM. Ingredients of resilience: 7 crucial Cs. In: *Building Resilience in Children and Teens: Giving Kids Roots and Wings.* 4th ed. American Academy of Pediatrics; 2020:39–48.

One amazing pediatrician I've worked with reflected on how she utilizes Ginsburg's 7 Cs in her pediatric office. Names are changed for confidentiality.

> I now ask all of my caregivers about character traits (one of the 7 Cs) they most wish for in their new babies as they grow and develop. We talk about why these traits are important and I encourage them to list a few. I also enter them into the child's electronic health record. Often caregivers say things like "I want my child to be happy," "I want my child to be smart," "I want my child to be a good self-advocate," "I want my child to be physically and emotionally strong." I validate all of these traits as wonderful character assets as I document them. Later, when the caregivers are struggling with behaviors during the child's toddler years, we reflect back on these early goals. I'm able to reframe defiant toddler behavior to "being a great self-advocate" or how toddlers only learn how to speak up for themselves and be "emotionally strong" if they practice refusal, defiance, and testing limits. It's a game-changer.

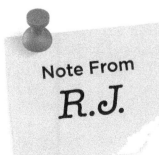

Note From R.J.

I have a poster on my wall with Ken Ginsburg's 7 Cs of resilience. It starts with a brief definition of what resilience means, followed by the list: Competence, Confidence, Connection, Character, Contribution, Coping, and Control. If you aren't familiar with them, it's a good idea to read up on them. It's a simple way to teach about resilience, and it's useful in clinical encounters for prompting a conversation about resilience:

"Do you see that list of the 7 Cs of resilience? What do you think that means, 'connected'? What can you do to help you feel more connected?" Bonus question for caregivers: "How about you—what can you do to feel more connected?"

"What kinds of coping strategies do you use?" or "What do you do as a coping technique to help you feel calm when you're stressed or upset?"

"What sorts of things are you doing to give back to your family, school, or community? That's what contribution is about." Bonus question for caregivers: "How are you making sure your kid's contributions are being recognized?"

If kids don't have a good handle on coping strategies, I usually build on the conversation by drawing 3 buckets of coping strategies on the exam table paper. I explain that there are good, neutral, and bad coping strategies. Bad coping strategies—like overeating, drugs, and alcohol—are things that might make us feel better for a little bit, but ultimately, they hurt our bodies. Neutral coping strategies—like too much screen time—put the stress off until later but usually don't get rid of it. Good coping strategies, on the other hand, usually help us feel better and also make us smarter, stronger, or wiser in some way—things like reading, exercise, meditation, breathing exercises, art, spending time with others, and so on.

If you put that kind of poster up, be sure you can accurately define each of the resilience factors, along with some backup recommendations you can make to help you navigate further conversations.

Another model that breaks down academic research into application and practice comes from the Center on the Developing Child at Harvard.[23] Their framework lays out 3 principles, based on research, that mitigate stress and trauma in children and families and move to build buffering resources and create resilient children:

1. Support nurturing relationships.
2. Reduce external stressors for families.
3. Strengthen core life skills.

Again, many reports and studies indicate that pediatricians are primed to use caregiver education and support to recommend ways that SSNRs can be enhanced. In fact, the emerging focus for pediatric care is to support and promote the relational health of families, recognizing pediatric care as the best venue to support and foster social-emotional (SE) health.[11] When clinicians understand the critical role of resilience education for caregivers and feel competent in bolstering these roles, they are acting to promote the necessary buffering resources that help children and families thrive.

Addressing Barriers to Resilience Education in Pediatric Settings

Models such as the ones we've just discussed are helpful in translating academic research into practical pearls for pediatricians. As we mentioned in Chapter 3, Getting Your Organization Ready: Creating Compassionate Pediatric Practices, pediatricians are already time strapped during well-child visits, so we don't want TIC to feel like an additional burden. The same is true when we begin to talk about implementing tools and teaching about resilience.

So, a few potential barriers have to be considered: first, skepticism about time and implementation; second, how and when to intervene; and finally, decreasing overwhelm by making it easy and accessible to navigate.

Skepticism

Many clinicians express skepticism about identifying trauma or adversity, pursuing education about trauma, and engaging in new practices that promote resilience and mitigate stress and trauma. Pediatricians note lack of time, lack of training, lack of reimbursement, and discomfort with the topic of trauma as significant barriers.[24-26] These are all valid concerns, certainly.

The AAP policy statement on preventing childhood toxic stress[16] indicates that a significant challenge of creating resilience in children is "a broad…spectrum of adversity [that] make[s] the formation of SSNRs more difficult." The job of pediatricians is to address these problems so resilience can be taught despite adversity.[11,16] This means that to nurture resilience, pediatricians must build and nurture their relationship with the support systems that children are in, mainly families and caregivers.

Garner points out that if we only look at measures of adversity, there are missed opportunities to support caregivers and early relationships—those that promote flourishing children.[16,27] In practice and training, I've found this to be true. If we only encourage pediatricians to become trauma informed and we don't bridge the gap between understanding and addressing, we create skepticism and overwhelm. But when we add training about buffering resources and resilience, we create more hope and energy for momentum.

> This is everything. Understanding and addressing trauma through resilience education is the most important aspect of medicine we are practicing. —Dr Ryan Hassan, Pediatrician

We would assert that if a clinic is aspiring to become trauma informed, they should also be ready to devote time and resources to resilience promotion.

How and When to Intervene

Often, when I'm in trainings, I remind pediatricians that they are already doing so much in terms of relationship building and strengthening families, and what we're talking about adding is simply making explicit to caregivers what the factors are that promote resilience. The authors of the AAP policy statement encourage pediatricians to build on foundational capacities that build resilience, stressing that these characteristics must be "modeled, taught, learned, practiced, reinforced, and celebrated."[16] In fact, the movement within pediatric training and focus is migrating toward skill building and coaching so that critical components of resilience are incorporated into office visits. The National Scientific Council on the Developing Child finds this to be the essential role of the pediatrician in encouraging positive health trajectories for children who experience the most disadvantage due to factors such as socioeconomic disparity, historical oppression, or intergenerational trauma, to name a few.[28]

My experience in training pediatricians is that if we encourage them to look at what they're already doing versus what they must add to an already full visit, then we can create momentum instead of overwhelm. When pediatricians understand that the most important work that's done within a well-child visit goes beyond health and safety and extends to a biopsychosocial model of health within early relationships, they're able to be more focused and curious.

One concept I encourage pediatricians to adopt is called "laying down your goals." It goes something like this: I ask them to think about a visit like planning for a trip. Their first instinct may be to treat it like a perfectly planned family vacation: every destination, attraction, and meal plotted out. But if they haven't also planned for a flat tire, a wrong turn, or running out of gas, then when a mishap occurs, they're going to feel lost and frustrated. If, instead, they see the pediatric visit more like a road trip that's spontaneous, they'll know the basics they need to cover (eg, the map, gas, clothes) but not feel wedded to the destination. If a caregiver says, "Hey, I know you wanted to go to Vegas, but I'm struggling over here in LA," then a doctor can compassionately say, "I'll meet you there." They temporarily lay down their goals, setting aside the vacation they planned (eg, helmet safety, developmental milestones) for the trip that's on the table (eg, recent divorce, school bullying, or dysphoria).

What this means is that training programs must underscore the importance of strong relationships between pediatricians and caregivers, nurturing and affirming positive interactions, and encouraging caregivers to have positive relational experiences with their children.[29] The AAP policy statement indicates the importance of layering interventions through a child's life and across systems. For instance, address SDOH when needed, respond with targeted treatments when necessary, and provide education regarding relational health and life skills at others. This obviously differs for each child or family.

Intervene soon and intervene often.

Note From R.J.

Yes—early and often! (Honestly, can we really say this too much?)

Remember that addressing SDOH and peripartum mood disorders and giving adequate resources for these things are also an intervention, which is why we spend so much time on these subjects in this book (see Chapter 7, Supporting Caregivers to Strengthen Safe, Stable, Nurturing Relationships). If caregivers are carrying these very heavy issues with them into a visit, there's little chance that any of the things we see as priorities are going to be meaningfully implemented by families.

And I love this analogy of meeting caregivers where they are, rather than taking over the agenda of the visit with our own list of things that need to be covered. Otherwise, you won't make much progress with the family with their journey to strengthen SSNRs, if they aren't engaged and if what you have to say doesn't meet their immediate needs. Besides, I've always liked LA better than Vegas anyway...

Making It Easy and Accessible

Overcoming the third barrier to resilience education means decreasing overwhelm by making anticipatory guidance around resilience accessible and straightforward. It also needs to be actionable and within the caregiver-child relationship—meaning, if the barrier is overwhelm (so much is going on in a visit), then the antidote is making guidance easy and accessible. After all, pediatricians are not the only people who want a prescribed tool they can implement. Caregivers need tangible tools as well. The authors of the AAP policy statement point out that focusing on the relationship between caregivers and children, as well as the relationship between physicians and caregivers, should be a central theme to all pediatric care. This focus on relational health is built on the assumption that SSNRs are the foundation that buffers adversity and builds resilience.[16] Therefore, pediatricians must partner with caregivers to impart and create actionable means to build resilience. Tools should focus on SE skills that lead to positive stress responses and create building blocks of resilience. The AAP policy statement stresses that relational health (requiring that caregivers are learning these skills too) is a universal imperative for children to fulfill their potential. The authors go on to outline 3 principles, which are defined as preventing childhood toxic stress responses, promoting resilience, and optimizing development, and indicate a need to develop "innovative strategies to promote SSNRs at the dyadic level, family level, and community level." All this work must be done within the context of nurturing caregivers and adults.

Conclusions

Although beginning to implement resilience-building strategies into your practice may seem daunting at first, we want to remind you that you're already doing so much of this. If we define resilience within relationships and pair that with the fact that pediatricians are primed to interact in the early caregiving relationships, then visits with you become a space for efficacious interventions. Discussing resilience as a balance to queries about childhood adversity creates greater competency and confidence in pediatricians. When we address the barriers and create more optimism and momentum for clinicians, they can readily engage in nurturing the most important relationships.

Questions to Consider

1. When you think about resilience or resilient patients, what qualities come to mind?

2. Can you identify ways you're already building resilience in your practice?

3. What types of scripts would be helpful to ease discussions with patients and their caregivers so you don't feel overwhelmed or like this is "one more thing" to attempt?

4. It's OK to be skeptical when it comes to TIC and building resilience. What worries might need to be addressed for you or your practice before you could enter into this work?

References

1. Felitti VJ, Anda RF, Nordenberg D, et al. Relationship of childhood abuse and household dysfunction to many of the leading causes of death in adults: the Adverse Childhood Experiences (ACE) study. *Am J Prev Med.* 1998;14(4):245–258 PMID: 9635069 doi: 10.1016/S0749-3797(98)00017-8

2. Perry BD, Pollard RA, Blakley TL, Baker WL, Vigilante D. Childhood trauma, the neurobiology of adaptation, and "use-dependent" development of the brain: how "states" become "traits." *Infant Ment Health J.* 1995;16(4):271–291 doi: 10.1002/1097-0355(199524)16:4 < 271::AID-IMHJ2280160404 > 3.0.CO;2-B

3. Center on the Developing Child at Harvard. Toxic stress. Accessed March 18, 2024. https://developingchild.harvard.edu/science/key-concepts/toxic-stress

4. Zolkoski SM, Bullock LM. Resilience in children and youth: a review. *Child Youth Serv Rev.* 2012;34(12):2295–2303 doi: 10.1016/j.childyouth.2012.08.009

5. Ungar M. Practitioner review: diagnosing childhood resilience—a systemic approach to the diagnosis of adaptation in adverse social and physical ecologies. *J Child Psychol Psychiatry.* 2015;56(1):4–17 PMID: 25130046 doi: 10.1111/jcpp.12306

6. Wingo AP, Wrenn G, Pelletier T, Gutman AR, Bradley B, Ressler KJ. Moderating effects of resilience on depression in individuals with a history of childhood abuse or trauma exposure. *J Affect Disord.* 2010;126(3):411–414 PMID: 20488545 doi: 10.1016/j.jad.2010.04.009

7. Wrenn GL, Wingo AP, Moore R, et al. The effect of resilience on posttraumatic stress disorder in trauma-exposed inner-city primary care patients. *J Natl Med Assoc.* 2011;103(7):560–566 PMID: 21999030 doi: 10.1016/S0027-9684(15)30381-3

8. Rutter M. Resilience as a dynamic concept. *Dev Psychopathol.* 2012;24(2):335–344 PMID: 22559117 doi: 10.1017/S0954579412000028

9. Rutter M. Psychosocial resilience and protective mechanisms. *Am J Orthopsychiatry.* 1987;57(3):316–331 PMID: 3303954 doi: 10.1111/j.1939-0025.1987.tb03541.x

10. Traub F, Boynton-Jarrett R. Modifiable resilience factors to childhood adversity for clinical pediatric practice. *Pediatrics.* 2017;139(5):e20162569 PMID: 28557726 doi: 10.1542/peds.2016-2569

11. Bethell C, Jones J, Gombojav N, Linkenbach J, Sege R. Positive childhood experiences and adult mental and relational health in a statewide sample: associations across adverse childhood experiences levels. *JAMA Pediatr.* 2019;173(11):e193007 PMID: 31498386 doi: 10.1001/jamapediatrics.2019.3007

12. Cicchetti D. Annual research review: resilient functioning in maltreated children—past, present, and future perspectives. *J Child Psychol Psychiatry.* 2013;54(4):402–422 PMID: 22928717 doi: 10.1111/j.1469-7610.2012.02608.x

13. Dozier M, Stovall-McClough KC, Albus KE. Attachment and psychopathology in adulthood. In: Cassidy J, Shaver PR, eds. *Handbook of Attachment: Theory, Research, and Clinical Applications.* Guilford Press; 2008:718–744

14. Cohen JA, Kelleher KJ, Mannarino AP. Identifying, treating, and referring traumatized children: the role of pediatric providers. *Arch Pediatr Adolesc Med.* 2008;162(5):447–452 PMID: 18458191 doi: 10.1001/archpedi.162.5.447

15. Bernard K, Meade EB, Dozier M. Parental synchrony and nurturance as targets in an attachment based intervention: building upon Mary Ainsworth's insights about mother-infant interaction. *Attach Hum Dev.* 2013;15(5-6):507–523 PMID: 24299132 doi: 10.1080/14616734.2013.820920

16. Garner A, Yogman M; American Academy of Pediatrics Committee on Psychosocial Aspects of Child and Family Health, Section on Developmental and Behavioral Pediatrics, and Council on Early Childhood. Preventing childhood toxic stress: partnering with families and communities to promote relational health. *Pediatrics.* 2021;148(2):e2021052582 PMID: 34312296 doi: 10.1542/peds.2021-052582

17. Bethell C, Gombojav N, Solloway M, Wissow L. Adverse childhood experiences, resilience and mindfulness-based approaches: common denominator issues for children with emotional, mental, or behavioral problems. *Child Adolesc Psychiatr Clin N Am.* 2016;25(2):139–156 PMID: 26980120 doi: 10.1016/j.chc.2015.12.001

18. Streeck-Fischer A, van der Kolk BA. Down will come baby, cradle and all: diagnostic and therapeutic implications of chronic trauma on child development. *Aust N Z J Psychiatry.* 2000;34(6):903–918 PMID: 11127621 doi: 10.1080/000486700265

19. Marsac ML, Kassam-Adams N, Hildenbrand AK, et al. Implementing a trauma-informed approach in pediatric health care networks. *JAMA Pediatr.* 2016;170(1):70–77 PMID: 26571032 doi: 10.1001/jamapediatrics.2015.2206

20. Fiese BH, Rhodes HG, Beardslee WR. Rapid changes in American family life: consequences for child health and pediatric practice. *Pediatrics.* 2013;132(3):552–559 PMID: 23918891 doi: 10.1542/peds.2013-0349

21. Savage-McGlynn E, Redshaw M, Heron J, et al. Mechanisms of resilience in children of mothers who self-report with depressive symptoms in the first postnatal year. *PLoS One.* 2015;10(11):e0142898 PMID: 26618860 doi: 10.1371/journal.pone.0142898

22. Ginsburg KR, Jablow MM. *Building Resilience in Children and Teens: Giving Kids Roots and Wings.* 4th ed. American Academy of Pediatrics; 2020

23. Cohen SD. *3 Principles to Improve Outcomes for Children and Families.* Center on the Developing Child at Harvard; 2021. Accessed March 18, 2024. https://developingchild.harvard.edu/resources/three-early-childhood-development-principles-improve-child-family-outcomes

24. Augustyn M, Groves BM. Training clinicians to identify the hidden victims: children and adolescents who witness violence. *Am J Prev Med.* 2005;29(5)(suppl 2):272–278 PMID: 16376730 doi: 10.1016/j.amepre.2005.08.023

25. Banh MK, Saxe G, Mangione T, Horton NJ. Physician-reported practice of managing childhood posttraumatic stress in pediatric primary care. *Gen Hosp Psychiatry.* 2008;30(6):536–545 PMID: 19061680 doi: 10.1016/j.genhosppsych.2008.07.008

26. Coker TR, Chacon S, Elliott MN, et al. A parent coach model for well-child care among low-income children: a randomized controlled trial. *Pediatrics.* 2016;137(3):e20153013 PMID: 26908675 doi: 10.1542/peds.2015-3013

27. Garner AS, Saul RA. *Thinking Developmentally: Nurturing Wellness in Childhood to Promote Lifelong Health.* American Academy of Pediatrics; 2018 doi: 10.1542/9781610021531

28. National Scientific Council on the Developing Child. Excessive stress disrupts the development of brain architecture. *J Child Serv.* 2014;9(2):143–153 doi: 10.1108/JCS-01-2014-0006

29. Katkin JP, Kressly SJ, Edwards AR, et al; American Academy of Pediatrics Task Force on Pediatric Practice Change. Guiding principles for team-based pediatric care. *Pediatrics.* 2017;140(2):e20171489 PMID: 28739656 doi: 10.1542/peds.2017-1489

Chapter 5

Guiding Principles of Resilience Education

Amy King, PhD

What we're learning here...is the most *important medicine.*
Dr Ryan Hassan

When we left off in Chapter 4, Building the Case for Resilience, I was rolling up my sleeves and getting down to work for physicians, creating efficacious interventions to build resilience in well-child exams at the request of the pilot group of pediatricians. Back and forth we went regarding what worked, what didn't, what felt seamless, what needed a script, what barriers we encountered, points of confusion, and ease of education. I created a formula to guide me and worked diligently to use tools that had steered me for years as a trauma-informed psychologist. Then, I blended that with my knowledge of behavioral health integrative work. Some interventions were created from my original ideas informed by therapeutic practices. Others were adapted from experts in the field. And yet, even after we had a solid handful of resilience interventions, I was not satisfied with the outcome. I was worried that we might haphazardly offer a new tool to a family without meeting a basic need or requirement—an agreed-on principle or practice through which these interventions were being delivered. Yes, I wanted the work to come from a trauma-informed space, but there was more to it. I wanted to have guiding principles in place *before* wielding advice to caregivers and youth with histories of trauma who were seeking support. It felt paramount to me that part of being trauma responsive meant identifying some core assumptions.

What are other factors we might consider?

When you think of offering tools and interventions to caregivers and children that reduce stress, mitigate the effects of trauma, and boost resilience, do any themes come to mind? Maybe this seems intangible to you so far, or maybe you're already doing it and you don't even realize it (That's my guess!). For me, the elements that rolled around in my mind included influences such as tools that are developmentally appropriate and have a solid evidence base as well as interventions that are practical and offset the likelihood for child abuse and maltreatment, build caregivers' competency, and bolster critical promoters of long-term health, like secure attachment and attuned caregiving. But I also considered individual factors such as professional demeanor, message, and delivery. What factors come to mind as you consider how you, personally, would deliver this information? I hope we can all provide a consistent message within our practices, a shared goal and belief that you already hold and can make explicit to caregivers: *We are in this together. I want what you want for your child. There's a foundation of trust we must have and a connection that's imperative between you and me and you and your child.*

So, let's focus on factors that would act as guiding principles.

We have learned the answers, all the answers:
It is the question that we do not know.
—Archibald MacLeish

Guiding Principles

A Formula to Guide Resilience Interventions

As previously mentioned, when I began to research and reflect on efficacious tools to use during well-child exams—tools and interventions that would address adversity, decrease symptoms of trauma, build relational health, and create more positive social-emotional (SE) development—I reviewed several domains. Then, I combined knowledge of child development, behavioral health integration, positive experiences for children and families, and trauma-informed practices, asking myself the following questions:

- *What is developmentally appropriate?* In other words, if we look at typical development at a given age, what might we expect to observe across all development, particularly SE development? When we know "what's going well and right," we can also begin to look for signs of distress or atypical development.

- *What are trauma-informed interventions?* In other words, what evidence-based interventions can we utilize that address adversity and build resilience within relationships? What do we already know to be efficacious, improve relationships, and promote mental health? And how can we offer brief interventions during a typical visit?

- *What themes build resilience in children and families?* For instance, we know from the literature that there are positive experiences that occur in a child's life that mitigate stress, individual coping tools that address mental health, and skills that build relational health and SE development. If we know these, how can we incorporate them into discussions and tools to offer children and their caregivers?

- *What does the world of trauma-informed therapy have to offer to behavioral health integration within primary care settings?* In other words, we need to think in terms of brief, efficacious, accessible tools that can easily fold into an already-busy well-child visit or encounter, in little bits, over time.

- *What do we know about the field of early intervention, parent education, and physician anticipatory guidance?*

- *What factors offset negative outcomes that would have occurred if we did not intervene?* Just as with guidance regarding putting infants on their backs to sleep yielded fewer infant deaths, we can provide education and resources regarding relational health and mental health that mitigate adversity and trauma.

- *How simple or complex must these tools be?* In my work with physicians, the simpler and easier it was for them to understand, the more easily they could communicate and feel helpful to their patients.

- *How do we message such tools?* We want to always communicate our message to parents in compassionate, nonjudgmental ways so we're seen as a partner in children's health. (We discussed this in Chapter 3, Getting Your Organization Ready: Creating Compassionate Pediatric Practices.)

These questions led me to a formula based on all these complex intersections to guide a selection of trauma-informed, resilience-building tools.

Here is the formula that has guided me. You'll see this again in Chapter 9, Designing and Using Efficacious Interventions to Support Early Relational Health and Heal Trauma, as we apply these principles and review several interventions that guide resilience building and well-being.

1. **Identify the significant tasks at each developmental or transitional stage.** In other words, if these tasks were not accomplished, how does that throw off healthy development or progression? For example, in the early childhood years, attachment, attunement,

co-regulation, play, and neurological development are key components to healthy, thriving children (**Table 5-1**). R.J. reviews the importance of this in Chapter 6, Understanding Early Relational Health. Once we've identified critical developmental milestones such as these, we can connect those milestones to resilience-building characteristics.

2. **Incorporate efficacious interventions that address chronic stress and trauma at each stage.** In other words, what research-based interventions can get those developmental trajectories on track should they go awry? Or, in best-case scenarios, how do we support and encourage healthy development when it's already present? For example, if a child and caregiver aren't experiencing secure attachment or the caregiver feels frustrated when their baby can't fall asleep, we must intervene with tools supported by research to support them and help get them back on track. And when we see a parent or caregiver successfully navigating tasks such as play-based development, we need to note the importance of this and point it out as a way to guide parents and educate them that they're building lifelong resilience for their child. Bolster and promote skills when they need help, and praise them when they're doing well.

3. **Combine developmental tasks with efficacious intervention.** The goal in marrying these two is to recognize the developmental/transitional task the child needs to accomplish and then intervene with appropriate support to mitigate trauma and/or boost resilience. It should feel like an observational exercise. Think of it as taking NOTES:
   - **N**otice what's happening in the room.
   - **O**bserve signs of caregiving that bolster resilience or interfere with relationship building.
   - **T**each one skill or **T**ell one story.
   - **E**nhance the visit depending on need.
   - **S**upport without shame; offering suggestions will decrease defensiveness.

4. **Provide interventions with a trauma-informed lens.** Another important dynamic to contemplate is that we might be in a position to do harm to groups or individuals. Part of being a trauma-aware health care professional and using research-supported tools is recognizing that some of the dyads with whom we work have experienced systemic trauma: Parents who've felt oppressed by our medical systems. Caregivers who have felt that clinicians have authority and judge their parenting practices. Groups of people who are desperate for solutions but unaware of intergenerational traumas.

Let's try an example to put this formula to work.

An 18-month-old comes in for a well-child visit. Dad is checked out, distracted, and impatient with the toddler. He uses a great deal of correction and appears frustrated. The toddler becomes tearful and begins acting out by pulling items out of drawers to gain Dad's attention. Dad uses

Table 5-1. Important Developmental Tasks That Boost Resilience and Well-Being

Age, y	Developmental Tasks
Birth–2	Co-regulation, brain development, attachment, attunement, play
2–5	Social-emotional development, positive discipline, family strengths, connection through secure attachment with adult caregivers, play
6–10	Regulation and coping, family strengths and connections, positive mental health, character development
11–14	Positive mental health, sense of self, peer relationships, problem-solving
15–18	Positive mental health, autonomy, peer and partner relationships, sense of future, self-worth

a harsh tone with the child, pulls the child away from the drawers, offers a toy, and goes back to scrolling on his phone. You note the strain on attachment and positive connection, 2 of the developmental tasks necessary for toddlers to thrive and gain resilience (Step 1). You offer a tool (ie, components of an evidenced-based tool such as Parent-Child Interaction Therapy [PCIT]; Circle of Security or Play-Based Therapy) that would promote a more secure attachment and a more attuned parent (Step 2). You give Dad some "homework" to play with his child every day, uninterrupted, for about 10 to 15 minutes and encourage Dad to reflect on how his relationship with his child feels. Of course, it's a great opportunity to model some of these skills and encourage positive, progressive steps toward attunement (Step 3). If you provide guidance regarding these types of interventions over the course of development with this dad and his child, at each visit or encounter, the relationship between Dad and his child is bolstered and the potential outcome of maltreatment or neglect is lessened (Step 4).

Note From R.J.

I love the principle that's embedded in this interaction of how we can help patients and families by creating SMART (**S**pecific, **M**easurable, **A**chievable, **R**ealistic, and **T**imely or time-specific) goals for them. We talk about this more in Chapter 8, Revamping Anticipatory Guidance, but this is a great example of how it actually works.

SMART goals have always been a part of quality improvement teachings, but they're a great clinical tool as well. There's such a big difference between "Play with your kid more" and "Spend 10 to 15 minutes a day in special time for the next week." Try to give some concrete examples of what child-led play might look like—blocks, reading, playing with cars or stuffed animals, coloring, sculpting with clay, playing at the park—depending on the resources and abilities of the family and the specific interests of the child. Remember that not all caregivers had positive models for what "play" looked like from their own childhoods. If you're following the principles of PCIT, these special time activities should be filled with praise and positive comments toward the child, and caregivers should avoid directing or criticizing during the activity.

Three Guiding Principles for Parents and Caregivers

It's 2014, and I'm leading a group for moms—facilitating tough conversations about behavior and discipline, friendships, acting out, school performance, and coping tools for their children. These women have been in a group with me for 3 years, and we meet every other Wednesday night. That's 24 meetings per year, a total of 72 sessions with a group of moms struggling together with guidance and support. They cry. They vent about their partners. They share overwhelm. They move through divorces and deaths and disappointments together. They bring curious questions and genuine love for each other. Their children get older, transitioning through major developmental milestones. In the beginning I lead, but after months, I'm simply there to gently guide discussions and reflection. It's not about perfect parenting. These moms struggle. They make mistakes. They have ruptures with their children and disagreements with each other about major parenting issues. But as we journey through motherhood together, I realize something magical is happening. They are co-parenting with me and they are parenting in a village of each other. A village is created where mistakes and questions are welcome and judgment is at bay. They amaze me.

What can be created between professionals and parents and then imparted from parents to children is what these women create and experience with this moms' group. These women are creating safe, stable, nurturing relationships (SSNRs) for each other and, as a result, for their children (R.J. talks about this in Chapter 6, Understanding Early Relational Health). What Garner and Yogman point out in the American Academy of Pediatrics (AAP) policy statement on preventing childhood toxic stress is that childhood adversity in small amounts (buffered by the type of help and support these moms received) leads to positive stress that builds resilience for children.[1] By experiencing a bit of stress, versus the absence of it, within the safety of SSNRs, these kids will learn to adapt to future adversity in a healthy manner. What is clear from the research is that children need at least one SSNR to form positive relational health and become resilient. The AAP policy statement points out that this type of relational health is a biological imperative.

Parenting is complex. We provide birthing classes, lactation consultation, and a bit of new parent and caregiver support through hospital systems. But as parents walk out of the hospital, car seat–bundled baby in hand, until there is a mishap, we don't offer parenting classes. We don't provide anticipatory support even though the next 18 years might throw some challenges their way as a parent. How is it that we provide hours of support for breathing in labor but no guidance as parents embark on this parenting journey?

So, when I began looking at interventions to mitigate trauma and build resilience, I had to dig deep into my experience as a psychologist working with thousands of families over 2 decades. Throughout my tenure as a psychologist, I've found there are components of parenting that transcend all others and that are critical to form secure attachment and long-term relational health. These are the guiding principles (adapted from the work of Ken Ginsburg and encouraged by the work of Andrew Garner) that I want physicians to be able to communicate about parenting above all else.[2,3] Here are some factors you might consider.

1. **Unconditional love is paramount.** Children require unconditional love. Resilience is built through caring relationships, and healthy development assumes that parents show unconditional love for their children. To be strong, children need security from a primary caregiver. Children who feel unloved, or loved conditionally, can carry these relationship patterns into their adult relationships and into parenting. Caregivers can reject behavior that a child exhibits but still love the child completely. In babies, this love is learned through a process of co-regulation and attunement (what we think of as "serve and return"). When babies know their needs will be met, it creates that foundation of trust. As children get older, I teach parents a fun game (I Love You Rituals) that allows their child to test this—check it out in Chapter 8, Revamping Anticipatory Guidance. *Unconditional love is a pathway to secure attachment, and secure attachment leads to resilience because of the enduring connection it provides.*

   > Go and love someone exactly as they are.
   >
   > And watch how they quickly transform into the greatest, truest version of themselves.
   >
   > When one feels seen and appreciated in their own essence, one is instantly empowered.
   >
   > —Anonymous

2. **Make expectations about family values clear.** Children regulate their behavior using expectations from the adults, experiences, and environments they encounter. Ginsburg points out that children live up or down to caregivers' expectations of family values and individual character strengths.[4] Expectations don't mean achievements but rather mean the qualities caregivers believe create good human beings. For instance, I often hear health care professionals setting goals around character traits (eg, hardworking, thoughtful, funny) with parents of young children. Rather than center on their children becoming good students or

excelling at school, pediatricians help parents focus on character traits such as grit or curiosity—features that lead to greater resilience versus outcome or achievements. Again, in Chapter 8, Revamping Anticipatory Guidance, we provide an example of a tool that emphasizes family strengths and enhances values that lead to greater resilience.

3. **Utilize parents and caregivers as coaches.** Caregivers are the primary models for their children, and they are in the best position to teach them about how to be resilient. Children watch their parents closely and will learn far more from what they do versus what they say. This means, as the AAP policy points out, that we must educate and encourage parents to model essential life skills—not only to provide SSNRs but also to model basic SE health so children can flourish.[1] The AAP encourages a multigenerational approach. The practice of this means leaning into family supports, caregivers as teachers, and extended family to provide models and broader support to children. Certainly, in our experience, this is a powerful way to address intergenerational trauma and intervene to create new experiences.

Do you teach these 3 principles to parents? It's an intervention in itself.

Note From R.J.

At the 12-month-visit, I usually talk about beginning discipline and the 4 parenting styles, based on what Amy's taught me. I draw 2 axes on the exam room paper, empathy on the horizontal and expectations on the vertical. The low expectation/low empathy quadrant I call "detached" parenting, followed by the high expectation/low empathy (militant), low expectation/high empathy (permissive), and high expectation/high empathy (loving and firm) quadrants. I talk through the 3 assumptions in relation to the parenting style embedded in each of these quadrants, how the parenting style impacts outcomes, and give parents a chance to reflect on how they were parented and what they want to do differently.

To take it a step further, I remind parents that no one is perfect. They will have days in each of those quadrants, and that's OK; it's where you spend the most time that matters. Relationships between caregivers and kids can be damaged, but they can also be repaired. When caregivers have a day that's less than ideal, they can talk it out with their kid. When they say to their child, "That didn't go the way I wanted, and I'm sorry," it not only helps repair the relationship but models how their kids can do relationship repair as well. This principle is sometimes called "good enough parenting"—the idea that no one is ever perfect as a caregiver, but we should always be doing our best. The goal is to be reliable as a caregiver and to have your child be well cared for. Ultimately, as a caregiver, it's more important how you are most of the time than how you are all of the time. The complete script is in Appendix Q.

Regarding principles 2 and 3 for parents and caregivers, much research supports parent education and parent coaching models in primary care. In addition to the research pointed out previously in Chapter 4, Building the Case for Resilience, Traub and Boynton-Jarrett point out that parent coaching models have been found to increase screening engagement and decrease emergency department visits.[5] Furthermore, the authors (and others such as Bethell and colleagues[6] as well as Winders and coworkers[7]) point out that children who are in medical homes fare better than children who are not when it comes to mitigating adversity and building resilience. In fact, family-centered care was shown itself to be a correlate to resilience.

In the AAP clinical report on early intervention, Individuals with Disabilities Education Act Part C services, and the medical home,[8] the authors point out that intervention services that utilize coaches and caregivers from the child's environment and partnering with families for comanagement of disabilities fare better. Features of family-centered medical homes naturally enhance the parent coaching model to support children by tailoring care to patients' needs, providing patient-centered care with cultural humility, and increasing access to care by using natural supports, the caregivers. As well, when physicians partner with parents, it underscores the value of medical homes by enhancing and collaborating care for the patient. Ultimately, this underscores the value of partnership that creates trust.

These 3 messages need to be reviewed, emphasized, and modeled throughout all developmental stages of a child's life and, therefore, throughout all visits where resiliency models are introduced. Garner and Saul point out that most important to this work is that children become caregivers who grow to value and build SSNRs because they've developed within them.[3] Without these 3 core principles being honored, the other components of creating resilience will not be as efficacious in their delivery. A longitudinal, 40-year study in the Isle of Wight demonstrated that parent-child interactions have a profound impact on resilience and that parental competence is critical for relationship quality.[9] So, it's imperative that physicians look for challenges to these 3 principles and address them whenever possible in a supportive, nonjudgmental way. Later, we will provide examples of how to pair resilience interventions with these core assumptions for parents.

Three Guiding Principles for Health Care Professionals

As I sit with a group of 25 primary care physicians during a conference, we immerse ourselves in principles of trauma-informed care and mitigating factors to build resilience and create buffering environments for children and families. One theme becomes crystal clear. A soft-spoken pediatrician clears his throat and says, "This is everything. What we're learning here [about relational health, connection with patients, trauma healing, and resilience building], this is *the most* important medicine." Another physician nods and says with a soft smile, "It's like we have to unlearn so much [from medical school and pressures of checking boxes in well-child visits] and just *be in* this work." Something is shifting in these dedicated souls as we discuss ways to create connection and focus on relational health as the way to transform primary care.

Garner and Yogman point out something similar in the AAP policy statement on preventing childhood toxic stress.[1] They indicate, "The use of trusted, supportive relationships within the [family-centered pediatric medical home] to promote the relational health of families is an emerging focal point for pediatric clinical research, and pediatric primary care is increasingly seen as a venue for fostering [SE] health." So, let's dive into the core assumptions that can drive that work in a trauma-responsive way (adapted from Blaustein and Kinniburgh).[10]

1. **Communicate with caregivers without judgment.** Patients and families must feel that professionals are communicating with them from a nonjudgmental stance. Caregivers often feel that their child is the primary target of intervention and may feel defensive when they realize you are attempting to both intervene on the child's behalf and support them as caregivers. Being in a space of nonjudgment allows you to align with the caregiver and create an ally.

   Research supports this premise. Caregivers who feel competent and are able to internalize the praise they receive for their decisions and actions as caregivers have been shown to be more resilient.[5] Garner and Saul point out that caregivers who feel that pediatricians listen to them and understand their concerns are more likely to build trust.[3] In the AAP policy statement, Garner and Yogman point out that a pediatrician's fostering of strong and respectful relationships with caregivers increases the likelihood that caregivers will trust the pediatrician's guidance and judgment, implement tools, and create parenting practices out of treatment strategies or tools suggested by the pediatrician.[1]

We might consider the intention of our messages and what outcomes we're hoping for. I truly think this will shift how we talk with caregivers about gaps between *what trauma is* and *what to do about trauma.* For instance, of course we want more positive outcomes, but if we focus solely on immediate answers, we might miss an opportunity to focus on a broader goal. Answers are easy, but how they are delivered is not. So, consider that while caregivers are hungry for help, the relationship and care from which the help is delivered is critically important. And for caregivers, while "tips and tricks" are great, if they don't understand that basic messages of unconditional regard and secure connections build trust with their children, then the behavioral change won't be long-lasting, nor will it have the desired outcome.

2. **Create collaborative, shared goals.** Remind patients and families that you have a shared goal with them by using "we" language. Instill in them that you want to help raise a healthy, resilient young person. Model this behavior through a connected, supportive relationship so that caregivers may feel that you are part of their support system. Again, this reminds the caregiver that you share healthy goals for their child with them, *and* it encourages caregivers to see you as a support for them, as well as their ally. Like with children, the more caregivers feel listened to and supported during daily experiences, the more likely they are to come to you during times of crisis.

   Savage-McGlynn and colleagues point out the most compelling rationale for this approach.[11] Their study showed that the best correlate of resilience at the age of 11 for a child was a mom's positive feelings about her ability to parent. In fact, the belief that she is doing "a good job" was associated with high resilience for her children.

3. **Provide support with caregivers present.** Intervention and training must happen within attachment systems or supportive dyads (eg, clinician to adult, clinician to child, caregiver to child). Remember, these kids go home to systems, primarily family systems. And, as Garner and Saul remind us, enhancing the dyad relationship provides a vehicle for building foundational resilience skills.[3] Modeling these safe, supportive, healthy interactions during appointments can underscore the importance of interactions between children and engaged, attuned adults.[12] Feldman supports this type of work as well, pointing out that research supports dyad connections and promotes biobehavioral synchrony.[13] Pediatricians are primed to model such behavior and encourage the attachment system.

What this means on a practical level is that if pediatricians want parents to engage in a process with them, one where they learn new tools and create positive experiences to promote resilience in children, they must approach parents with these 3 principles in mind at all times. All interactions between pediatricians and parents, and later between pediatricians and teens, carry these core assumptions about the relationship between clinician and parent. Parents have often experienced their own trauma or difficult relationship history. Creating an environment where they feel safe, talk openly, and feel that their child's pediatrician is part of a supportive team will elicit the outcome that leads to greater resilience for their child.

Note From R.J.

I hope that most of my patients experience an environment where they feel safe, and that's certainly what I strive for. Remember self-compassion, though—we're not always perfect. The system isn't currently designed to give us the time we need with patients, to access adequate resources for our families, or to support our being emotionally available 100% of the time as our patients deserve. Similar to good enough parenting, let's lay out an intention to provide "good enough pediatric-ing" to remember that we're all going to have days when we are less than ourselves. It's going to come down to how you are *most of the time* and whether you model good relationship repair with your patients when things don't go well.

Recently, I had another patient interaction that really got under my skin. There was a teen who had attempted suicide a few days prior. Our behavioral health consultant (or BHC…it's what we call our integrated behavioral health professionals) talked with the family to get things started in helping the family, and I scheduled an appointment (actually after hours to accommodate the family) to start the process of psychoeducation and safety planning. I thought it went well.

The next day, however, when Mom was talking with scheduling staff about getting a follow-up appointment with our BHC, none of the appointments worked because she "had activities planned." Honestly, it made me pretty mad. It didn't seem like Mom was prioritizing what I thought she should, and I struggled to suspend judgment and practice acceptance.

Later that day, I was still pretty irritable when I walked into a visit with a fourth-time mom. Partway through, I realized that my irritability was coming through. I decided to tell this mom what I was struggling with. Here's why.

- It's important to let patients know that when I'm not myself, it isn't about them. When we're rushed, upset, or otherwise distracted, it lets parents know, too, that we hold compassion for all our patients—and that I actually care deeply about the kids I help care for.

- It becomes a teachable moment. Mom and I talked about how she can express to her kids that they're her number one priority and how, starting at a young age, she can build that kind of consistent, predictable availability for her child. She also learned more about the deep compassion and concern that I hold for all my patients, and she knows that I extend that same concern to her family. I was also able to model (in my own fumbling way) the value of repairing relationships; after all, being irritable with a patient is essentially rupturing the relationship I have with that family. Being able to apologize to a caregiver (and their child) is a real-life example of showing how to repair that relationship.

- I am human. Knowing that means a lot to families. Expressing that makes me feel better and helps me let go of the things that are bugging me so I can take care of my patients with a clearer head.

We all have our struggles, so creating this universe where pediatricians are comfortable talking with patients and each other about how we're also struggling/adapting/learning/improving actually models connection, compassion, and relationship repair.

Having caregivers who are engaged and responsive, using primary preventions with targeted interventions, and encouraging relational health that buffers adversity and builds resilience are central to the emerging research on pediatric practice.

It's been pointed out that in order for that shift to occur, pediatricians should be afforded the following opportunities and training[1]:

- Sufficient time with patients and families
- Benefit of long-term continuity with patients and families
- Occasions to learn about interpersonal communication skills
- Communication enhanced by cultural humility and implicit bias training
- Skills to listen and understand parental/patient concerns and beliefs before making recommendations

Conclusions

We don't want resilience education and resilience intervention tools to feel like "one more thing" you add to already burdensome patient visits. The outline for resilience education is layered on types of anticipatory guidance you're already providing in your clinic, with a bit more focus and intention. The focus is shifting to specific tools that address childhood and caregiver adversity. A critical message is that, before we can utilize interventions to mitigate stress and adversity, we need guiding principles to communicate with caregivers that we want what they want for their children: emotionally healthy, well-adapted, supported children.

How we get there is a considerable task. *Why* we need to get there is clear.

Questions to Consider

1. What message feels most imperative to communicate to parents and caregivers as you embark on conversations around resilience? In other words, what are key elements that you feel are imperative to convey?

2. Are there other core principles for physicians or caregivers, not listed here, that you would build into your practice?

3. How are you already incorporating "we" goals and nonjudgmental language into other parts of your practice? Our guess is that you're already doing this!

References

1. Garner A, Yogman M; American Academy of Pediatrics Committee on Psychosocial Aspects of Child and Family Health, Section on Development and Behavioral Pediatrics, and Council on Early Childhood. Preventing childhood toxic stress: partnering with families and communities to promote relational health. *Pediatrics*. 2021;148(2):e2021052582 PMID: 34312296 doi: 10.1542/peds.2021-052582

2. Ginsburg KR, Jablow MM. *Building Resilience in Children and Teens: Giving Kids Roots and Wings*. 4th ed. American Academy of Pediatrics; 2020

3. Garner AS, Saul RA. *Thinking Developmentally: Nurturing Wellness in Childhood to Promote Lifelong Health*. American Academy of Pediatrics; 2018 doi: 10.1542/9781610021531

4. Ginsburg KR, Jablow MM. Building confidence. In: *Building Resilience in Children and Teens: Giving Kids Roots and Wings*. 4th ed. American Academy of Pediatrics; 2020:155–163

5. Traub F, Boynton-Jarrett R. Modifiable resilience factors to childhood adversity for clinical pediatric practice. *Pediatrics*. 2017;139(5):e20162569 PMID: 28557726 doi: 10.1542/peds.2016-2569

6. Bethell CD, Carle A, Hudziak J, et al. Methods to assess adverse childhood experiences of children and families: toward approaches to promote child well-being in policy and practice. *Acad Pediatr*. 2017;17(7)(suppl):S51–S69 PMID: 28865661 doi: 10.1016/j.acap.2017.04.161

7. Davis DW, Honaker SM, Jones VF, Williams PG, Stocker F, Martin E. Identification and management of behavioral/mental health problems in primary care pediatrics: perceived strengths, challenges, and new delivery models. *Clin Pediatr (Phila)*. 2012;51(10):978–982 PMID: 22514194 doi: 10.1177/0009922812441667

8. Adams RC, Tapia C, Murphy NA, et al; American Academy of Pediatrics Council on Children With Disabilities. Early intervention, IDEA Part C services, and the medical home: collaboration for best practice and best outcomes. *Pediatrics*. 2013;132(4):e1073–e1088 PMID: 24082001 doi: 10.1542/peds.2013-2305

9. Rutter M. Isle of Wight revisited: twenty-five years of child psychiatric epidemiology. *J Am Acad Child Adolesc Psychiatry*. 1989;28(5):633–653 PMID: 2676960 doi: 10.1097/00004583-198909000-00001

10. Blaustein ME, Kinniburgh KM. *Treating Traumatic Stress in Children and Adolescents: How to Foster Resilience Through Attachment, Self-Regulation, and Competency*. 2nd ed. Guilford Press; 2019

11. Savage-McGlynn E, Redshaw M, Heron J, et al. Mechanisms of resilience in children of mothers who self-report with depressive symptoms in the first postnatal year. *PLoS One*. 2015;10(11):e0142898 PMID: 26618860 doi: 10.1371/journal.pone.0142898

12. National Scientific Council on the Developing Child. Supportive relationships and active skill-building strengthen the foundations of resilience. Center on the Developing Child at Harvard working paper 13. 2015

13. Feldman R. Parent–infant synchrony: biological foundations and developmental outcomes. *Curr Dir Psychol Sci*. 2007;16(6):340–345 doi: 10.1111/j.1467-8721.2007.00532.x

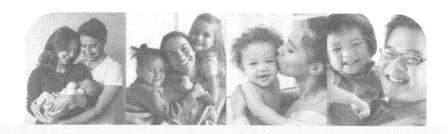

PART 2

Assessing Risks: Navigating Barriers to Safe, Stable, Nurturing Relationships

In this section, we're going to be discussing risks to safe, stable, nurturing relationships (SSNRs) that you'll need to be able to address as a vital component of taking relational health histories (RHHs) in our families. This starts with a fundamental understanding of early relational health (ERH; Chapter 6), followed by a review of common challenges that may get in the way of parents and caregivers being able to provide SSNRs to their children (Chapter 7).

In our view, the RHH is bread-and-butter pediatric care. As clinicians, we need go-to strategies to address barriers to ERH; this means we need to listen empathetically as we navigate sensitive subjects with our families, elicit their concerns, identify risks and strengths, and intervene or refer when necessary.

When approaching risks to SSNRs with families, you will need to have implemented some screening tools, both to assess the risks themselves and to evaluate any potential consequences of ruptured SSNRs. The latter primarily refers to screening tools for social-emotional health, which is likely going to be new work for your practice. They should be done universally with your patients but may need to additionally be used once a risk to SSNRs has been identified. When assessing risks—specifically caregiver depression/anxiety, social drivers of health, and parental/caregiver trauma histories—you will need some screening and assessment tools, as well as some new surveillance or history-taking questions. Some of them may already be part of your clinical care, whereas others may be new.

While the American Academy of Pediatrics does not endorse screening children for ACEs, the position on surveying parents and caregivers for ACEs is more nuanced. It is not specifically endorsed, but an understanding of parent and caregiver trauma history is recognized as a "promising practice" because of the correlations between those trauma histories and some key child outcomes.[1] Although my practice has been using the ACE survey with parents since 2013, assessing caregiver trauma histories can be done with intentional implementation of specific surveillance questions that we'll cover in Chapter 7, Supporting Caregivers to Strengthen Safe, Stable, Nurturing Relationships. Specific assessment tools and surveillance questions aren't mutually exclusive anyway: both can have an important role in our clinical care. Either way, understanding parent and caregiver trauma is a vital component of RHHs and should be addressed as another basic component of care.

Reference

1. Forkey H, Szilagyi M, Kelly ET, et al; American Academy of Pediatrics Council on Foster Care, Adoption, and Kinship Care; Council on Community Pediatrics; Council on Child Abuse and Neglect; and Committee on Psychosocial Aspects of Child and Family Health. Trauma-informed care. *Pediatrics*. 2021;148(2):e2021052580 PMID: 34312292

Chapter 6

Understanding Early Relational Health

R.J. Gillespie, MD, MHPE, FAAP

> *We are hardwired to connect with others, it's what gives purpose and meaning to our lives, and without it there is suffering.*
>
> **Brené Brown**

Years ago, I had a colleague say that he wanted to "specialize in infant mental health." It was a joke; he was implying that infant mental health (IMH) was a simple, maybe nonexistent, field and that it was easier than anything else we do in practice. After all, infants don't have thoughts; they're either awake or asleep, being fed or being changed. Simple, right?

Of course not.

When thinking about trauma and its effects on health and wellness, we spend a lot of time connecting trauma with early childhood. This is not only because the effects of trauma on the developing infant or toddler brain are potentially more powerful than traumas that occur later in life but also because resilience and reduction of the impact of trauma rely, at least in part, on strengthening the caregiver-child bond during those years.[1] Before considering implementation of trauma assessments and other components of the relational health history in practice, it's important for us to have a strong working knowledge of early relational health (ERH) and social-emotional (SE) health, including how to talk about ERH with families, assess for problems in the caregiver-child dynamic, and promote and repair ERH in practice. The resilience-based interventions in this book are based on the fundamental need to both promote and repair ERH, which is why we're including an understanding of ERH as a prerequisite skill for trauma assessments.

Although trauma can happen to children of any age, the adversities that our youngest patients face have the most profound impacts, because their brains are creating the foundational neural connections in response to their environments, including their relational environments. This discussion about ERH isn't meant to minimize the need to talk about trauma in other age-groups; it is to highlight the importance of the child's early relationships in forming safe, stable, nurturing relationships (SSNRs) throughout the life span, which ultimately buffer the effects of later traumas. In his book *Born for Love,* Dr Bruce Perry describes the comparison between 2 children with different trajectories: one with early trauma and later SSNRs versus another with early SSNRs and later trauma.[1] The second child fares far better, an outcome indicating the importance of ERH in a child's ability to develop resilience and withstand stress. In the early years, it's the parent or caregiver who provides the context in which a child's development is able to progress, including the achievement of SE skills, so it's important to include caregivers in your thought processes about development. We'll talk about barriers to relational health in Chapter 7, Supporting Caregivers to Strengthen Safe, Stable, Nurturing Relationships, but for now, your lens should be on the nature of the relationship between caregivers and their kids and how traumas of all types may impair the ability to maintain the requisite SSNR. Forkey, Griffin, and Szilagyi described the concept "If you see symptoms, think trauma; if you hear trauma, think symptoms."[2] Along these lines, think about the connection between trauma and SE health:

when you see disruptions in SE health, think trauma; when you hear trauma, think disruptions in SE health.

Note From Amy

I'm talking with Dawn Daum on my podcast, mother of 2 and self-reported childhood trauma survivor. I can feel my eyes welling with tears as she shares her story of entering motherhood. She was terrified of parenting and triggered by her children daily. But she had no words for what she was experiencing. She says that "moments that other mothers cherished filled me with fear and dread." Daily occurrences such as breastfeeding, diapering, bathing, and her baby's cries would send her anxiety through the roof. She began having flashbacks, headaches, back pain, and numbness in her body.

Because of the significant trauma she experienced beginning at a young age, when she became a mom, her unresolved experiences came crashing in. She tells me she was scared to tell her child's pediatrician, who never asked about how she grew up, because she looked like she "had it all together but was feeling crazy inside." And she was terrified that if she told her child's doctor, they would take her baby away from her. She knew she would never hurt or harm her baby, but she didn't know how to explain what was happening to her internally.

After meeting with a lactation consultant who told her that "everything looked great" and that breastfeeding was fine, Dawn began to seek out answers on the internet. There, she found refuge and relief. She found words like "triggering moments," "flashbacks," and "posttraumatic stress disorder." Only then was she able to label her trauma. She felt deep grief, sadness, and confusion that no medical professional had ever asked her about the early life experiences that might have been affecting her parenting. She also reflects, "I wonder if someone had asked my mom, if I would have had a different life experience as well."

Dawn's story is not unique. Many survivors of trauma are uncertain or afraid to discuss how their experiences impact child-rearing. But they also report that when they are asked about their experiences, provided resources and guidance, and reassured that they can change their trajectory, they experience great relief.

We know that parental trauma can result in lower scores on SE screening tools for young toddlers and that maternal depression can also negatively impact SE health.[3] In fact, the American Academy of Pediatrics (AAP) policy statement on peripartum mood disorders advises us to assess SE health in children of parents who experience depression because of the potential disruption of the SSNR between parent and child.[4] Studies have shown that there are specific vulnerable windows in which the impacts of caregiver depression may negatively impact kindergarten readiness, most notably between birth and 12 months and between 4 and 5 years of age.[5] It is reasonable to think that other disruptions in SSNRs, like caregiver trauma or social drivers of health (SDOH), should lead to a similar assessment of the child's SE health because they increase caregiver stress, may interfere with the caregiver's ability to bond with their child, and may also reduce the sense of safety within the household. We'll address these 3 barriers to ERH in Chapter 7, Supporting Caregivers to Strengthen Safe, Stable, Nurturing Relationships. Given the prevalence of these conditions in our practice, universal SE assessments are advised by the AAP, although the exact periodicity has not yet been determined.[6] For older children, universal assessments for behavioral and mental health serve a similar purpose: to identify disruptions in SE health in school-aged and adolescent patients.

In this chapter, we'll define what is meant by ERH and SE health, break down the steps for how we promote SE health in practice, discuss how to communicate about and assess SE health in practice, and set you up for understanding the resilience-based interventions that will help you promote ERH and repair disruptions in the dyadic relationship. We'll discuss specific tools for assessing ERH, so that you'll be in a better position to use them when addressing barriers to SSNRs that you identify in practice.

Defining Early Relational Health and Social-Emotional Health

Infant mental health, social-emotional health, and *early relational health* are all related concepts and often interchanged as terms, although they are distinct. Specifically, IMH is "the developing capacity of the child from birth to three years to experience, regulate, and express emotions; form close interpersonal relationships; and explore the environment and learn. Infant mental health is synonymous with healthy social and emotional development."[7]

Social-emotional health, while synonymous with IMH in infancy, expands in older children and adolescents to include the further development and mastery of emotional regulation skills. In that respect, IMH and SE health are describing what is going on in the infant's or child's life, whereas ERH factors the adult caregiver into the equation. This is an important distinction, because positive IMH can happen only in the context of an SSNR—sometimes called *foundational relationships*—with a supportive and engaged caregiver.

Early relational health refers to "the foundational relationships between a young child and their caregivers that advances physical health and development, social well-being, and resilience."[8,9] As such, ERH is meant to highlight the vital contribution of the SSNR between the caregiver and the child to emerging IMH or SE health, rather than focus on just the health and well-being of the infant or child alone. It's based on the attachment/attunement relationship between the caregiver and child and is the most important factor in buffering a child from adversity or trauma. Infant regulation is dependent on early co-regulation between the infant and caregiver, so the child's self-regulation can't develop well without that initial co-regulation with a caregiver. In other words, ERH highlights that SE health happens for an infant because of the context that the caregiver creates and provides, and good IMH is dependent on the early presence of SSNRs.

Attachment theory has emerged as the dominant model of human SE development, so it's important for clinicians to be able to observe attachment patterns in practice, describe attachment to parents and caregivers, and promote healthy attachment through specific interventions. Unfortunately, most of us didn't learn a lot about attachment theory in our training, so it's worth doing some outside reading on this fundamental concept. I tend to think about attachment as the relationship or bond between a child and their primary caregiver; attunement is (in the words of one of our more eloquent colleagues) how well the caregiver is "catching their baby's vibe"—that is, how well the caregiver is able to understand and respond to the infant's cues and use those cues to interpret the infant's physical and emotional needs. I use these simple definitions when discussing attachment and attunement with caregivers. For more information, there are plenty of thorough descriptions of attachment theory in the literature—which are a little beyond the scope of this book—but the important points are outlined in Forkey, Griffin, and Szilagyi's *Childhood Trauma and Resilience: A Practical Guide*[2] and in a great review article by Schore.[10] The big takeaways are the following:

- Attachment relationships between a child and caregiver facilitate the development of the brain's self-regulatory mechanisms.
- A child's attainment of self-regulation of their emotional state is a major and important developmental achievement.
- This achievement is dependent on the attachment relationship.

Therefore, the ability of a child to self-regulate is based on the strength and organization of the attachment relationship; this leads to future school success for children, as the strength of the attachment relationship has been positively associated with children's social and cognitive skills in kindergarten.[11] It's an important part of our job as clinicians who care for children to non-judgmentally assess and support this relationship in practice, both formally and informally, and intervene when needed.

The Process for Promoting Social-Emotional Health

According to *Bright Futures,* our role as clinicians who care for children includes establishing mental health and emotional well-being in our patients[12]; this is not just the absence of mental disorders but includes SE and behavioral health and *wellness.* Rather than just respond to mental health disruptions when they occur, we're called to actively promote SE and behavioral health and to implement interventions that build skills in patients and families. It's a tall order but an important one.

In fact, the AAP mental health algorithms propose a process for promoting SE health.[6] The steps are the following:

- Elicit concerns.
- Identify risk factors, including SDOH and medical risks.
- Conduct a functional assessment using validated instruments or screening tools.
- Make observations about the parent-child interactions.
- Identify strengths.
- Refer when necessary.

Over the course of the rest of the chapter, we'll work our way through these steps.

Eliciting Concerns

The first step in the workflow is to elicit concerns. On the surface, this seems obvious, but be sure to frame your questions in the context of SE health. I always ask a general question about any health-related concerns the parent may have but then try to follow up with questions about general development and SE development. It's fairly straightforward, but remember to keep the questions open-ended as much as possible. To me, there's a big difference between "Do you have any questions?" and "What questions do you have today?" The latter normalizes the culture that parents should have questions and are welcome to ask them. There are any number of ways to convey this message:

- What questions or concerns do you have today?
- What questions or concerns do you have about language, development, or learning?
- What questions or concerns do you have about your child's behavior (or how your child gets along with others)?

In survey research of caregivers about their family's well-child visits, it was found that over 90% of families left their well-child visits with important, unanswered questions.[13] I remember hearing that number and thinking, "Wow, that's not just some of us missing the boat, some of the time; that's all of us, most of the time." It comes down to not only giving caregivers the space and opportunity to ask whatever questions they may have but also helping guide them on what questions are in our domain to answer. For example, if a parent or guardian thinks their child's pediatrician deals only with physical health problems, it may not occur to them to ask questions about behavior, development, or social concerns. That's why we point this out specifically in our conversation prompts. By framing our opening questions differently, we signal to parents that behavior and SE development are part of our wheelhouse.

Identifying Risk Factors

When you think about ERH, risk factors are all the things that get in the way of SSNRs between infants and their caregivers. These factors—like social risks, caregiver depression, and, of course, caregiver and child trauma—can all cause disruptions in the child's SE health. We cover these pieces in depth in Chapter 7, Supporting Caregivers to Strengthen Safe, Stable, Nurturing Relationships, but it's important to think about the intersection of all the screening tools we do in practice to understand the connections between risk factors and ERH.

In their book *Thinking Developmentally,* Garner and Saul describe the ecobiodevelopmental model of health and wellness and how the environment in which a child develops is interrelated with their physiology.[14]

In practice, we translate that model into the surveillance, promotion, and screening efforts that we use to identify and mitigate biological, environmental, and developmental risk (**Figure 6-1**).

FIGURE 6-1.

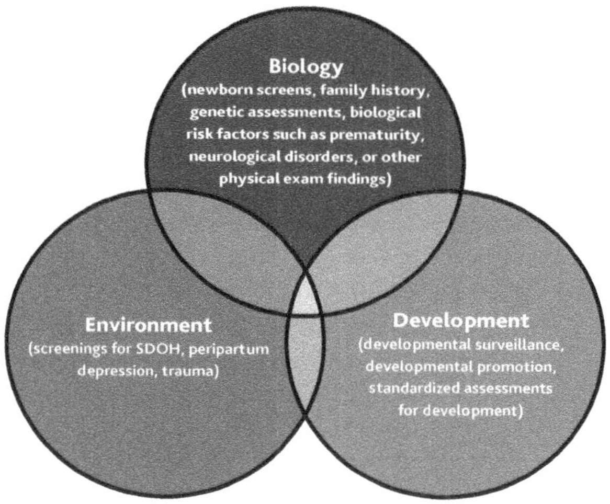

Translating the ecobiodevelopmental model into practice. SDOH indicates social drivers of health.

In my opinion, ERH sits at the intersection of these 3 different domains of risk. As mentioned in the Introduction, I think a lot of clinicians see all the screening tools we use in practice as independent data points, but it's much more meaningful to think about how the different screening tools intersect with each other, since our workflows are different depending on the patterns and combinations we see in a family. For example, you're going to have different workflows for a family where you see developmental risk along with caregiver trauma or social risks than with a family where there is developmental risk and prematurity, without those other environmental factors. In the latter case, referring for a specific therapy for development alone may be appropriate, whereas in the former cases, you'll need to consider other resources to support the family because addressing the developmental risk without addressing the underlying trauma would be insufficient.

As mentioned previously, when you see these risks—trauma, SDOH, peripartum depression— think about the consequences to SE health, and when you see disruptions in SE health, think about whether environmental risks may be part of the root cause.

Conducting a Functional Assessment With Validated Instruments

Universal SE screening has been recognized as clinically important, although it hasn't been widely implemented in pediatric practices except in programs designed to colocate specific services in practice, like HealthySteps (www.healthysteps.org). Although most general developmental tools like the Ages & Stages Questionnaires have sections for SE health, they are often the least sensitive and specific parts of the tool, which is why separate screening tools are advised. In the Introduction, we mentioned the 4 key questions for implementing screening tools:

- Why am I looking?
- What am I looking for?
- How will I find it?
- What will I do when I find it?

In the context of SE screening, we'll focus on the "how" part, which comes down to picking a tool and a periodicity (**Table 6-1**). I think it's important to think about tools that you use at all ages—not just in early childhood—because SE problems present throughout the life span of a child. After all, school-aged and adolescent patients still have the same SE tasks to master: forming relationships, regulating emotions, and exploring and learning; these just look different in each of those age-groups. The tools for older kids are typically the general behavioral health and mental health screeners that we use in the context of well-child visits.

Table 6-1. Screening Tools for Social-Emotional Health by Age-Group

Age-Group	Potential Tools
Infants/toddlers	Ages & Stages Questionnaires: Social-Emotional (ASQ:SE) Baby Pediatric Symptom Checklist (BPSC)[a] Brief Infant Toddler Social Emotional Assessment (BITSEA) Early Childhood Screening Assessment (ECSA) Preschool Pediatric Symptom Checklist (PPSC)[a] Welch Emotional Connection Screen (WECS)
School-aged children	Pediatric Symptom Checklist (PSC) Screen for Child Anxiety Related Disorders (SCARED)[b] Strengths & Difficulties Questionnaire (SDQ)
Adolescents	CRAFFT/Screening to Brief Intervention (S2BI) Patient Health Questionnaire (PHQ-9) Screen for Child Anxiety Related Disorders (SCARED)[b] Strengths & Difficulties Questionnaire (SDQ)

[a] BPSC and PPSC are embedded into the Survey of Well-being of Young Children (SWYC).

[b] Although the SCARED is typically used as a diagnostic tool for anxiety in school-aged children and adolescents, given the prevalence of anxiety in our population, the US Preventive Services Task Force has given universal anxiety screening of children older than 8 years a grade B recommendation; the SCARED is one of the few validated tools for this use.

Derived From Weitzman C, Wegner L; American Academy of Pediatrics Section on Developmental and Behavioral Pediatrics, Committee on Psychosocial Aspects of Child and Family Health, and Council on Early Childhood; Society for Developmental and Behavioral Pediatrics. Promoting optimal development: screening for behavioral and emotional problems. *Pediatrics.* 2015;135(2):384–395; and American Academy of Pediatrics Screening Technical Assistance and Resource Center. Screening Tool Finder. Accessed March 28, 2024. https://www.aap.org/en/patient-care/screening-technical-assistance-and-resource-center/screening-tool-finder.

These tools should be treated as universal, and the periodicity should be such that it fits well into your other screening tools. Remember the screening grid (Figure 2-1 from Chapter 2, Addressing Barriers)? Pull that back out and see what visits have space for SE screening. In my practice, we implemented SE screening with the Baby Pediatric Symptom Checklist and the Preschool Pediatric Symptom Checklist at 6 months, 15 months, and 4 years, since those visits were the easiest to fit an additional tool into. We do annual screening with the Pediatric Symptom Checklist for kids in the school-age group and universal depression and substance use screenings for adolescents. Most of these tools can be obtained through the AAP Screening Technical Assistance and Resource Center (www.aap.org/en/patient-care/screening-technical-assistance-and-resource-center).

Targeted screening can also be used if you identify trauma or other risk factors; the evaluation of a positive finding on peripartum depression screening should include an assessment of SE health in the infant. The same is true for trauma and the other SDOH.

Making Observations About Parent-Child Interactions and Identifying Strengths

Recently, the AAP did a learning collaborative called Addressing Social Health and Early Childhood Wellness with 6 states across the country and dozens of practices.[15] The purpose of the project was to improve implementation of maternal depression, SDOH, and SE screening tools and ensure referrals to necessary resources. Some of the feedback I heard from participating clinicians was that they implemented the SE screening tools, but oftentimes when the screening tool identified risk, families weren't convinced they needed to follow through with referrals that were made. Follow-through came down to whether or not families understood the context of the screening tool and the consequences of disruptions in SE health: when families don't have a good sense of what SE development means, they don't tend to take the results of the screening tools as seriously.

Before we can effectively implement formal screening for SE health, we have to be able to provide context to the family about what ERH means and its foundations in attachment theory. In my view, this is where it starts: with helping families understand what is meant by ERH, SE health, and resilience. After all, without providing that kind of context to our patients, how can any intervention work?

Using a strength-based approach, the simplest inroad is to make a positive observation about how the caregiver is interacting with the child and use that as a segue into discussing attachment and its importance for the child's development. In the algorithm we're following, it's when we make observations about the caregiver-child interaction and identify strengths; we then use the positive observations as ways to start conversations about ERH. As far as when: early and as often as possible. Some people call this intervention "catching the parent being good," where we make observations about interactions between caregivers and children that we want to reinforce.

"I love that you're talking to your baby during the exam to reassure her that you're here and that she's safe. Did you notice how she quieted to be able to pay attention to your voice?"

"That skin-to-skin time you're doing with your baby is amazing: Did you know that helps him learn how to soothe and calm himself when he's upset?"

"Look how she loves watching your face when you're holding her in your arms."

Note From Amy

When I was working with young mothers who were recovering from addiction and substance use, we worked on dyad interactions with their babies and toddlers. So many of them had experienced significant trauma and had not heard positive scripts, encouragement, or validation of how they parented. Encouraging comments, such as simply pointing out, "You're doing just what your baby needs right now," or "I think they like it when you talk and sing like that," or "You have such a beautiful way of consoling them. Let me see that again," had such a profound impression. It's important to note that when you support a caregiver's attunement and strengthen their attachment with their baby, you're having a critical impact on their child's development. Early relational health is the number one predictor of long-term relational health. Those early connections are everything!

From there, your next words can be a quick teaching script about attachment and ERH. In the FrameWorks Institute strategic brief *Building Relationships: Framing Early Relational Health*, the recommendation in this context is to use "foundational relationships" as a term to communicate the centrality of relationships on the child's development.[9] These conversations always feature the adult and the importance of the adult in the child's life. In these conversations, I talk about bids for attention, mirror neurons, how foundational relationships are the building blocks for future development, the still-face experiment, and even future kindergarten readiness. You don't have to do this work all at once; I use several different scripts for different visits to build on the concepts of SE development. See **Box 6-1** for some examples.

Obviously, these are the scripts that work for me. I tend to be informal in how I talk with my patients and families (as you can probably tell by how I wrote these); the point is to figure out what works for you and your style in terms of bringing up different subjects related to ERH. By using a strength-based approach to these conversations—recognizing something in the interaction that you like and want to reinforce—you have the opportunity to explain and promote SE health. By the way, those scripts are interventions in themselves.

I also try to keep ERH in mind in how I model interactions with infants and kids during the visit. It's a powerful message as a clinician to pick up a crying infant and model the 5 S's with families after an exam, which are swaddle, stomach/side position, shooshing, swinging, and sucking (all meant to mimic the environment in the womb); I do shooshing and swinging in particular, rather than just passing a fussy baby back to an exhausted new parent.[16] During exams, I talk to the baby about what I'm doing (eg, "I'm listening to your heart right now…your heart goes boom-boom, boom-boom, boom-boom"; "I'm going to look in your ears now") and reflect what the exam might feel like ("Did that tickle?" or "That feels funny, doesn't it?"). It seems simple, but remember that the impression you're making on the family can be a powerful example of how to soothe, engage, or distract a child; it's also a way of modeling the serve-and-return interaction where you respond to the infant's or toddler's signals with your comments and narrative.

In case it isn't obvious, talking about ERH with families will benefit the caregiver as well, particularly if you use the framework of identifying something the parent is doing well and reinforcing that behavior. It helps remind caregivers that they're doing so much more than just feeding and changing their babies; it gives purpose to their interactions. The challenge is helping caregivers find the time for positive and meaningful interactions with their children; some of that comes down to figuring out how to turn a mundane moment into an opportunity to bond and promote development. I love the Vroom app (www.vroom.org) because it's intended to teach parents and guardians exactly that: how to promote development during the everyday tasks they're having to get through. For example, when a caregiver is changing a diaper, they're at the right distance for eye contact with even a young infant, so taking a second to count toes, play "This Little Piggy," or sing a song to their baby helps build the attachment relationship at the same time that they're completing their chore. Another great resource for parents is The Greatest 8 initiative (https://thegreatest8.org), which gives parents and caregivers tips on how to promote relational skills throughout early childhood. If you implement the Ages & Stages Questionnaires: Social-Emotional as your primary tool for assessing SE health, there are corresponding newsletters and

Box 6-1.
Examples of Social-Emotional Scripts to Use With Parents

- "Did you know that human relationships are vital to our survival? The first relationship between an infant and their parent is the foundational relationship that forms the pattern for how all future relationships are made. It helps determine how children develop, learn, and grow. That's why I love how you're responding to your baby in such a loving and attentive way."

- "The way you talk and interact with your baby is important because your relationship is foundational for her future development. Did you know that at this age, when a baby watches her parents smiling and making faces, even if she doesn't make the same face back, her brain fires off as though she did. It's called *mirror neurons,* so when she has a chance to watch your face and how it moves, it helps build her brain and helps her develop."

- "I like how you reached for your baby when he started to cry. In relationships, we talk about bids for attention, including what happens when those bids are satisfied or not. For example, if you and your partner are sitting in the living room and one of you says, 'Hey, it's raining out,' that's a bid for attention. If the other says, 'It's supposed to be nice tomorrow,' then that bid for attention has been satisfied and the relationship is strengthened. On the other hand, if you say nothing at all, your partner will think that something's wrong or you're angry. Eventually, if bids aren't satisfied, the relationship gets weaker, and the other person might stop trying at all. Infants make bids too. Some of their bids are really obvious: they cry when they're hungry or need a new diaper, or they smile and point at something to get your attention. Other bids might be more subtle, like reaching toward a toy or cooing, but they're still bids your baby is trying to make. In those cases, they might be asking you 'What is this?' The more you recognize and respond to those bids, the stronger your relationship with your child becomes. For now, try to watch for those bids, and try to guess what your baby is telling you."

- "Have you ever heard of the still-face experiment? It's this study where they film a mom and her baby during an everyday interaction. At first, Mom and her baby are engaged in this lovely back-and-forth interaction. When the baby makes a bid for attention, like pointing at an object, Mom smiles and talks back to the baby. We call this kind of interaction 'serve and return'; it's like a tennis match going back and forth. Then the researcher asks Mom to just keep her face still and not respond to her baby's bids. Within a few minutes, the baby gets upset because Mom isn't responding anymore. This part is actually kind of hard to watch at first…but then Mom goes back to responding to her baby and all is well again. We can learn a couple of things from that: first, you are so important in helping your baby regulate her emotions. She's learning so much from watching you and interacting with you, even at this age. The serve-and-return interaction is the foundation of conversation, after all—one person says something and the other responds. The other thing is that when things don't go well—if you don't respond to all her bids for attention—there's a chance to repair the relationship. I figure it's not how you are all the time but how you are most of the time, so try to spend a little face-to-face time with her every day."

- "When I was a resident, we used to think about kindergarten readiness in terms of whether kids could tie their shoes and wipe their bottoms by themselves after going to the bathroom. At some point, we realized that knowing some letters and numbers might be helpful, but nowadays, we think about the fact that how a child is developing socially might be even more important than these other factors. Being successful in school really depends on being able to bond with a teacher and a peer group; if a child can do that, we can teach them anything else they need to know. Your relationship with your infant provides the foundation for those future attachment relationships, so the time you spend snuggling, rocking, talking, and reading with your baby will help them succeed in school later."

handouts (by age of the child) with ideas for stimulating SE health that caregivers can implement at home.

Refer When Necessary

Mental health referrals may be a part of the equation with disruptions in ERH, and there are many dyad therapies that help. These same therapies are evidence based as treatments for the sequelae of trauma if you've identified it in the course of your interactions with families. If you have integrated behavioral health clinicians into your practice, they can be a potential resource for helping families identified as at risk for SE delays. However, it's important to think beyond just mental health referrals and figure out other ways to support parents when needed. Home visitation programs are a great source of support for families, as are parent support groups, parent training programs, and community health workers, promotoras, or other peer navigators. Some of these programs that help with attachment are listed in **Box 6-2**. I think it's important to weigh parent and caregiver preferences—in other words, ask about their needs, priorities, capacity for engagement with resources, and cultural preferences—when making referrals and to try to target your referrals to mutually agreed-on goals between you and the family.

Box 6-2.
Programs That Support Early Relational Health

Positive Parenting/Parent Training Programs
- Triple P
- Conscious Discipline
- The Incredible Years
- SafeCare
- Chicago Parent Program

Dyad Therapies (evidence based for trauma treatment)
- Parent-Child Interaction Therapy (PCIT)
- Attachment and Biobehavioral Catch-up (ABC)
- Child-Parent Psychotherapy (CPP)
- Circle of Security

Parenting/Social Support Programs
- Nurse home visitation programs (Nurse-Family Partnership, Healthy Families)
- Family Check-Up
- Promoting First Relationships
- Child First

Conclusions

Early relational health is a fundamental concept to master before implementing trauma assessments in practice. This requires a good working knowledge of how to promote SE health in our patients and how to identify risks to and disruptions in the SSNRs that drive healthy development. By following the process outlined in this chapter, we have the opportunity to shine light on this vital component of family wellness. Remember: When you hear trauma, think disruptions in SE health; when you see disruptions in SE health, think trauma as a potential root cause. The implication of this reciprocal statement is that the same skills that we use to build

ERH as primary prevention against the effects of adversity can be used to help children and families heal in the context of trauma.

Upcoming chapters will continue to explain how we can effectively promote resilience in practice by focusing on ERH and SSNRs. The focus on resilience and promoting ERH is all about finding and supporting family strengths; and, as a bonus, shifting your focus to these strengths will actually make your clinical practice and interactions with families more fun and rewarding.

Questions to Consider

1. What are the scripts that you use to talk about ERH or SE health with families? What scripts do you still need to develop?

2. If you're not talking about ERH with your patients yet, in which visits can you pilot a script about ERH?

3. How are you currently assessing ERH and SE health in your practice? Are you using a specific screening tool? If not, do you need to implement one?

4. How do you currently link the different screening tools that you use in practice into a comprehensive picture of the family's health and wellness?

5. What resources do you have in your practice or in your community to support families with identified risks? Are they representative of the cultural and linguistic needs of your families?

References

1. Perry BD. *Born for Love: Why Empathy Is Essential—and Endangered.* Harper Paperbacks; 2011

2. Forkey HC, Griffin JL, Szilagyi M. *Childhood Trauma and Resilience: A Practical Guide.* American Academy of Pediatrics; 2021 doi: 10.1542/9781610025072

3. Folger AT, Putnam KT, Putnam FW, et al. Maternal interpersonal trauma and child social-emotional development: an intergenerational effect. *Paediatr Perinat Epidemiol.* 2017;31(2):99–107 PMID: 28140478 doi: 10.1111/ppe.12341

4. Earls MF, Yogman MW, Mattson G, et al; American Academy of Pediatrics Committee on Psychosocial Aspects of Child and Family Health. Incorporating recognition and management of perinatal depression into pediatric practice. *Pediatrics.* 2019;143(1):e20183259 PMID: 30559120 doi: 10.1542/peds.2018-3259

5. Wall-Wieler E, Roos LL, Gotlib IH. Maternal depression in early childhood and developmental vulnerability at school entry. *Pediatrics.* 2020;146(3):e20200794 PMID: 32817440 doi: 10.1542/peds.2020-0794

6. Weitzman C, Wegner L, Blum NJ, et al; American Academy of Pediatrics Section on Developmental and Behavioral Pediatrics, Committee on Psychosocial Aspects of Child and Family Health, and Council on Early Childhood; Society for Developmental and Behavioral Pediatrics. Promoting optimal development: screening for behavioral and emotional problems. *Pediatrics.* 2015;135(2):384–395 PMID: 25624375 doi: 10.1542/peds.2014-3716

7. Osofsky JD, Thomas K. What is infant mental health? *Zero Three J.* 2012;33(2):9

8. Center for the Study of Social Policy. Advancing early relational health: transforming child health care and early childhood system building. Accessed March 19, 2024. https://cssp.org/our-work/project/advancing-early-relational-health

9. FrameWorks Institute. *Building Relationships: Framing Early Relational Health.* FrameWorks Institute; 2020. Accessed March 19, 2024. https://cssp.org/resource/building-relationships-framing-early-relational-health

10. Schore AN. Back to basics: attachment, affect regulation, and the developing right brain: linking developmental neuroscience to pediatrics. *Pediatr Rev.* 2005;26(6):204–217 PMID: 15930328 doi: 10.1542/pir.26.6.204

11. Bernier A, Beauchamp MH, Cimon-Paquet C. From early relationships to preacademic knowledge: a sociocognitive developmental cascade to school readiness. *Child Dev.* 2020;91(1):e134–e145 PMID: 30295317 doi: 10.1111/cdev.13160

12. Hagan JF Jr, Shaw JS, Duncan PM, eds. *Bright Futures: Guidelines for Health Supervision of Infants, Children, and Adolescents.* 4th ed. American Academy of Pediatrics; 2017 doi: 10.1542/9781610020237

13. Schor EL. Rethinking well-child care. *Pediatrics.* 2004;114(1):210–216 PMID: 15231930 doi: 10.1542/peds.114.1.210

14. Garner AS, Saul RA. *Thinking Developmentally: Nurturing Wellness in Childhood to Promote Lifelong Health.* American Academy of Pediatrics; 2018 doi: 10.1542/9781610021531

15. Earls M, Heavrin M, Reilly E. Addressing Social Health and Early Childhood Wellness (ASHEW): a national learning collaborative to foster family resilience. *Pediatrics.* 2022;149(1):47

16. Karp H. *The Happiest Baby on the Block: The New Way to Calm Crying and Help Your Newborn Baby Sleep Longer.* Bantam Books; 2015

Supporting Caregivers to Strengthen Safe, Stable, Nurturing Relationships

R.J. Gillespie, MD, MHPE, FAAP

There is no such thing as a perfect parent. So, just be a real one.
Sue Atkins

When I'd been in practice for about 7 years, I had one of those patient encounters that keep you up at night, only this one kept eating away at me for years. It was actually a series of encounters with the same family, where I unknowingly watched the effects of a ruptured parent-child relationship progress, and I struggled with knowing how to help.

It began with a 6-month well-child visit. Up to this point, Mom had attended all the well-child visits alone because of Dad's work schedule. When I walked into the room, Mom laid her son on the exam table, pushed him all the way against the mirror on the wall, and sat back down. Already, I had warning sirens going off. I asked Mom if she had any questions, and her flat response was "No, should I?" As I sat on the exam table next to my patient, I was struck by how sweet and happy he was; throughout the visit, he used every trick in his playbook to get me to engage with him. He smiled, he cooed, he laughed, he stayed alert and watchful throughout the exam... The more I responded to his bids for attention, the more he ramped up his efforts to keep the interaction going. Through it all, Mom appeared disconnected.

It goes without saying that she was depressed. I asked how she was doing emotionally, and she talked openly about her depression but declined any offers of mental health resources or peer support groups. The last thing she wanted, in her own words, was to talk with other depressed moms. I gave her some contact information anyway, we concluded the visit, and she left.

At the 9-month visit, the boy was far more withdrawn. His developmental questionnaire showed some areas of risk, so I did another referral—this time for early intervention. They didn't go, even though I brought it up at subsequent visits, and I watched as my patient's development fell further and further behind. By the time he was 2, he spent the visit hiding in the corner, crying, and avoiding eye contact. It was like he just turned inward to shut the rest of the world out. Mom's depression had continued, so the referrals I made didn't go anywhere. In retrospect, it was just too hard for Mom to engage with any of the resources; eventually, I convinced Dad to start taking him for evaluations and therapy. Then, the family left my practice and moved out of town to follow a new job opportunity.

I may not have known the first thing about trauma back then, but it was obviously the effects of trauma that led to my patient's developmental unraveling. You don't even have to look at it retrospectively to see that. But knowing that my patient was suffering from the consequences of an untreated parental mental illness didn't help me prevent the outcome that was unfolding in front of me. To prevent the effects of adversity in our patients, we need to look at what gets in the way of parents and caregivers being able to provide the safe, stable, nurturing relationships (SSNRs) that kids need and then work on ways to "build the buffering" intrinsic in that caregiver-child relationship. In other words, addressing the things that get in the way of SSNRs for our families is a vital part of relational health histories (RHHs) for families and a major building block in our process of primary prevention against the effects of adversity. It's also an essential component of being a trauma-responsive practice. You should be prepared to assess these caregiver-level barriers to SSNRs and be ready to respond with empathy, some practice-based interventions, and whatever resources your community has to offer. Trauma that occurs in our patients is a consequence of ruptured, distressed, or distracted SSNRs, so it's a better preventive practice to try to take care of the things that cause those ruptures before the trauma occurs.

There are 3 main areas to consider here: caregiver and parental depression, social drivers of health (SDOH; or precipitants of toxic stress), and parental/caregiver trauma histories. These are often inextricably linked, of course, but for the moment, we'll discuss each as its own entity. Overall, I think it's helpful to think about the succinct framing provided by Garner and Saul: it's hard for a parent to be in relational mode when they're in survival mode.[1] It's also hard for caregivers to be in relational mode if they've had no appropriate models for how to do it or if they don't know the importance of it or what it entails.

Caregiver Depression and Anxiety

If you aren't screening for peripartum mood disorders (PMDs; ie, parental/caregiver depression and anxiety), start that before you embark on assessing the rest of RHHs in your practice.

Seriously, get a bookmark and come back to this page when you're done.

There are good reasons why the American Academy of Pediatrics (AAP) policy statement[2] encourages a focus on PMDs. First and foremost, PMDs get in the way of new parents' and caregivers' abilities to form SSNRs with their kids. If you haven't looked at the still-face experiment by Edward Tronick (we talked about it in our scripts in Chapter 6, Understanding Early Relational Health), it's worth looking up (www.gottman.com/blog/research-still-face-experiment). It's a simple illustration of the attachment/attunement relationship, which is dependent on a receptive and responsive caregiver in order to build the child's development.

Can you imagine how hard it is for a parent who is experiencing depression to maintain that receptivity and responsiveness to their infant's needs, when they're feeling exhausted and over-whelmed? We're advised by the policy statement on maternal depression to screen caregivers at every well-child visit in the first 6 months.[2] When my practice started screening for PMD in 2009, the focus was on maternal depression specifically—since most of the earlier studies on the effects of PMD on infants were conducted with mothers as the primary caregivers. Of course, not all families are the same; attachment and attunement between the child and primary care-giver are important regardless of the gender or gender identity of that primary caregiver. So, despite the language here, remember to think about assessing mood in all caregivers, not just new mothers.

Most pediatric practices I have worked with use the Edinburgh Postnatal Depression Scale (EPDS), which is meant as a screening tool for PMDs (not a diagnostic tool), but family medicine physicians often use the Patient Health Questionnaire (PHQ-9; a diagnostic tool) since the caregiver is also their patient. Either one works, but many pediatricians feel uncomfortable with a diagnostic tool since they aren't then going to treat the caregiver. In other words, the tool you use depends on your relationship with the parent as a practitioner; if you're treating the care-giver as well, it's fine to use the diagnostic tool. Of note, the EPDS captures peripartum anxiety as well as depression; if using the PHQ-9 as a screening tool for PMDs, you'll need another tool to screen for anxiety. Also of note, the Safe Environment for Every Kid (SEEK) and the Survey of Well-being of Young Children (SWYC) include questions about caregiver mood, which can

Note From Amy

To note, we should be screening for postpartum anxiety and depression, even if it's not clearly obvious in the caregivers. In other words, screen all caregivers, even those who do not "look" depressed or anxious. Many moms over-perform and underreport their symptoms. Moms with histories of trauma may hide their symptoms. And parents who look perfectly put together on the surface may be struggling with guilt, disconnection, and shame if they don't feel that they're bonding with their baby as they should. Often, being asked is a relief for new parents who might feel that no one else understands the pressures they're feeling or what it's like to have a new baby. Caregivers who've experienced intergenerational trauma may feel unequipped to deal with this new role. Osofsky and coworkers' research[3] showed that simply telling a mom, "You're doing a good job," could forecast later feelings of internal resilience and positive self-efficacy. This is a simple, validating phrase that you can use at any time in the course of your work with families—not just in the context of PMD screening but anytime you're reinforcing positive things that you're seeing in the caregiver-child interactions.

extend this assessment past the first 6 months after the child's birth. Although we are advised to screen both primary caregivers (not just birth mothers), that workflow is often challenging because oftentimes only one is in the office with the baby; if both caregivers are present, it's worth screening them both. If not, it's OK to inquire about the health and wellness of the caregiver who didn't make it to the appointment. It's good to spend some conversation time on how well the caregivers are doing on staying on the same page with their parenting decisions anyway.

One of the things you'll note about the EPDS is that the responses are anchored to the caregiver's baseline, since the responses start with "as much as I always could." If they were experiencing depression or anxiety before pregnancy, there's the potential to miss more long-standing challenges. I often follow up the questions on the EPDS with "Do you think you look happier on the outside than you feel on the inside?" to add to the depth of the conversation.

Be prepared to provide some referral resources for parents and caregivers who screen positive for depression or anxiety. At a minimum, you can refer Mom back to her OB-GYN or primary care clinician, if she's still insured and has access to that clinician. Postpartum Support International (PSI; www.postpartum.net) can provide mental health and peer support resources in every state in the country, as well as internationally; they have over 300 support coordinators that can help connect parents and guardians to local resources. My local PSI organization also provides support groups and resources for fathers experiencing depression and anxiety, so take a minute to see if yours does too. The AAP guidelines also support screening children whose caregivers experience depression with a tool to assess social-emotional (SE) health, which we talked about in Chapter 6, Understanding Early Relational Health.

The other, and more subtle, reason that we start with screening for caregiver depression is the cultural change that happens when you implement this workflow into practice. You are sending a clear signal to parents and guardians that you care about their health and wellness and that you are opening yourself up to helping support families beyond just responding to the specific physical health needs of the child. As with other sensitive types of assessment in practice, the goal of the screening is not the disclosure but the simple message that you care about caregivers. They'll open up when they're ready. Starting with screening for PMDs—and successfully providing resources to families—will make the next conversations about SDOH and caregiver trauma easier, since you've already communicated a commitment to partnership with your families. It's a gentle, non-shaming way to enter into psychoeducation about the connection between the caregiver's health and the child's development, particularly if you are able to provide the tangible support they need.

It's worth thinking about how you address caregiver mental health beyond the newborn period. As we mentioned, child exposure to parental depression is particularly impactful for kindergarten readiness in the first year but also between ages 4 and 5 years[4]—not typical ages at which we screen unless using the SWYC or SEEK as previously mentioned. Furthermore, substance use disorders (SUDs) can have similar impacts on relational health; although there aren't a lot of commonly used screening tools for SUD in caregivers, the SEEK[5] does include questions about both caregiver depression and SUD, along with other precipitants of toxic stress.

Social Drivers of Health

I once had a family of a child with special health needs come in for a long-overdue well-child visit. In reviewing the chart before the visit, I noticed a lot of letters from the child's specialists and therapists stating that the patient had missed the vast majority of his appointments over the past year. When I walked into the room, the patient's older sister was the one bringing him into the appointment. She was in her early 20s and had an overwhelmed and exhausted look about her. In our talking through the events since the last well-child visit, it came out that their mother had been struggling with housing insecurity—Mom and her 2 sons had been bouncing between friends' couches and their car as their only shelter—and finally the patient and his brother had come to live with their older sister. Before I had much of a chance to ask about all the missed appointments, she looked me squarely in the eye and said, "I know all those appointments are important, but right now we're struggling to get food on the table."

Putting aside for a minute how awesome it was that the sister trusted me enough to open up and ask for help, it really enhances our ability to provide care for families if we understand the context of their daily lives to better know where they are coming from. A lot of clinicians think about patients being "compliant" or "noncompliant" with our advice, but suffice it to say that when patients can't or don't follow our recommendations, there's usually a good reason why. If you think back to Maslow's hierarchy (introduced in Chapter 1, The ACE Debate and Ethical Considerations), the family's most basic needs have to be supported before they can actualize to become grounded and mindful, let alone amazing, parents. When caregivers are under stress, they aren't as available to provide SSNRs for their children; again, it's hard to be in relational mode when you're in survival mode. If you consider that one recognized resilience factor is engaging the support of others,[6] the simple process of hearing a family and providing a needed resource will reinforce help-seeking behavior—and thereby build resilience—and goes a long way toward building your relationship with the family.

Of course, there are both positive and negative SDOH; we're primarily talking about the negative ones—including, but not limited, to food and housing insecurity, unemployment or underemployment, and transportation problems—which are often referred to as "precipitants of toxic stress." Although evidence supporting the use of SDOH assessment tools is fairly limited,[7] some models like the SEEK (https://seekwellbeing.org) have been shown to reduce rates of child abuse,[5] making implementation of primary care programs to address SDOH a promising preventive practice.

Thinking back to the screening grid we talked about in an earlier chapter (Chapter 2, Addressing Barriers), adding SDOH assessment tools can seem burdensome, particularly if the tools are long. When choosing a tool, think about the burden on the parent or caregiver if they're being asked to complete a lot of paperwork during a visit; many practices choose to start with food insecurity screening as the first SDOH tool they implement because it's short and simple. The Hunger Vital Sign, which consists of 2 questions (**Box 7-1**), has been recommended for implementation at every visit by the AAP and the Food Research & Action Center (FRAC). Food insecurity also gets in the way of adequate nutrition for our families. It's a little more complex than just telling kids they need to eat their broccoli; we have to make sure they have access to broccoli in the first place. If you aren't doing this now, there is a great toolkit from FRAC and the AAP called *Screen and Intervene* (https://frac.org/aaptoolkit) that walks you through how to get a simple food insecurity screening process moving in your office, including key resources that you'll want to have at your fingertips for referrals.

Box 7-1.
The Hunger Vital Sign

Within the past 12 months we worried whether our food would run out before we got money to buy more.

    Often true/Sometimes true/Never true

Within the past 12 months the food we bought just didn't last and we didn't have money to get more.

    Often true/Sometimes true/Never true

Reproduced with permission from Hager ER, Quigg AM, Black MM, et al. Development and validity of a 2-item screen to identify families at risk for food insecurity. *Pediatrics.* 2010;126(1):e26–e32.

Another relatively simple foray into SDOH screening is asking about diaper insecurity. Research has shown a correlation between caregiver depression and difficulties obtaining needed supplies like diapers,[8] so asking some simple questions about diaper insecurity can help open up the idea that you are willing and able to help with this. There is sadly a correlation between diaper insecurity and corporal punishment[9]; imagine the stress of having an uncomfortable infant or toddler who is fussy because of a dirty diaper (and probably a severe diaper rash) and how that plays out in a caregiver under stress. We added a simple question to assess diaper insecurity (along with The Hunger Vital Sign questions) to the PMD screening tool we use to start assessing some of the SDOH early in the child's life. A common example of a diaper insecurity question is "Do you ever feel that you do not have enough diapers to change them as often as you would like?"

As with screening for peripartum depression, when you start to examine SDOH in practice, you subtly shift the culture of your practice by letting families know you care about the context of the family and your office is a safe place to talk about sensitive issues. It makes subsequent conversations about trauma histories feel like less of a shock to parents and caregivers. Some of the commonly used SDOH tools are listed in **Table 7-1**. They can also be found on the AAP Screening Technical Assistance and Resource Center website (www.aap.org/en/patient-care/screening-technical-assistance-and-resource-center/screening-tool-finder).

Parent and Caregiver Trauma Histories

In 2013, my practice made the bold and controversial decision to start assessing parental ACEs; as I've mentioned, this was before we were aware of a lot of the debate about ACE assessments and before the AAP became clear about its position on ACE surveys of children. It started with one of my partners and me; she had just completed a sabbatical with developmental and behavioral pediatricians and mental health clinicians, trying to understand the root source for a couple of patients who had experienced terrible outcomes based on their trauma histories. I had just returned from a meeting with the AAP Medical Home for Children Exposed to Violence Project Advisory Committee—not as an expert in trauma but as someone with background in medical home implementation. It was where I first learned about the ACEs study, and I was all in with the idea of implementing something real and impactful in practice. Through these 2 experiences,

Table 7-1. Common Social Drivers of Health Tools

Tool	No. of Items	Estimated Time to Complete, min
Health Leads	10	3
The Hunger Vital Sign	2	>1
IHELLP: Income, Transportation, Housing, Education, Legal Status, Literacy, and Personal Safety	11–24	5
PRAPARE: Protocol for Responding to and Assessing Patients' Assets, Risks, and Experiences	17–21	9
SEEK: Safe Environment for Every Kid	15	2
SWYC: Survey of Well-being of Young Children (Survey includes development, caregiver depression, and social drivers.)	10–17	5–10
WE CARE: Well Child Care, Evaluation, Community Resources, Advocacy, Referral, and Education	6	>5

we simultaneously learned about the ACEs study, along with the 2012 AAP policy statement describing the role of the pediatrician in addressing toxic stress.[10] We felt like we needed to do something, but waiting until ACEs already happened to our patients felt sorely inadequate. We're pediatricians, so we wanted to focus on prevention.

In the years since our implementation, we've modified our approach many times—adding questions to our assessment tool, enhancing how we talk about resilience, and asking parents what resources they would be most interested in. It was initially a terrifying idea: What was going to happen? Would we be able to manage the conversations? All the barriers to screening that we identified earlier came to our minds. But we soldiered on with the hope that we would be changing parenting patterns—breaking the cycle of intergenerational transmission of trauma—by destigmatizing the issue, committing to radical acceptance of our patients, and promising a partnership toward teaching a better way to raise children. Since then, we've continued to expand our focus to not only addressing past caregiver traumas and how they show up in parenting but also how to promote early relational health with the brief, practice-based interventions you'll learn more about in subsequent chapters.

As pediatricians, we must start with how we support parents and guardians. It's a bit of a paradigm shift for many of us, given that we were trained that the child is our primary patient, but the obvious counterpoint is that children grow and develop in the context of a family. There is a lot of conversation in the literature about the role of SSNRs and PCEs in mitigating or buffering the effects of toxic stress.[11] As we discussed in the Introduction, the primary difference between tolerable and toxic stress is whether or not the experiences were buffered by a loving caregiver (see Table 1 in the Introduction).[12] We need caregivers to be healthy and resilient if we are to have any hope that they can model those skills for their children. To me, that's the fundamental reason we started our focus on parents and guardians and their trauma histories—not only to better support all caregivers but also to help prepare caregivers who have experienced trauma for how they provide an SSNR to their children. In many cases, it's not immediately obvious to a parent or caregiver who has experienced adversity how they're supposed to help their children. There are certainly many lessons to be learned in how parental supports can be incorporated into our toolbox for addressing toxic stress from a clinical perspective.

Why Caregiver Trauma and Toxic Stress Matter

Assessing parental stress and trauma is a controversial approach for all the same reasons that universal ACE screening is controversial, which were described in Chapter 1, The ACE Debate and Ethical Considerations. The ACE questions are not standardized for this use. There is a paucity of evidence-based interventions for families. The ACE score isn't predictive of physical or mental health outcomes (or parenting abilities) at an individual level. The ACE score in isolation overly focuses on deficits and doesn't take into account the buffering effects of resilience and PCEs. The ACEs don't capture all potential traumas that could affect a family.

In fact, one of the earliest parent responses we got filled in this gap pretty articulately. The father who completed the tool had an ACE score of 1—parental separation. His comment was that the survey "simplified what life was really like living with a single mother." Captured within that comment is an overlay of the poverty and social isolation he experienced, along with bullying for his socioeconomic status. Framing the problem as "parental separation" was potentially minimizing, *but* it opened a conversation that helped the father really express his deepest hurts. Whether you choose to take the road of a full assessment tool or simply ask about how a parent was raised, inquiring into this topic can provide crucial information about how to support the family. In fact, when it comes to parental RHHs, I don't believe an assessment tool is the only way to approach the information; empathetic questions about strengths and challenges about their past will suffice. For example, you can ask the following questions:

- Can you tell me how you were raised? What do you want to repeat with your kids, and what do you want to do differently?

- Did anything scary or upsetting happen in your childhood? How do you think that affects your parenting now?

- Can you tell me a little bit about your childhood? How was it overall?

- What did you learn from your parents that you want to bring to your parenting experience? What do you want to do differently?

To illustrate why parental stress and trauma histories matter for pediatricians, let's start with some examples from the literature that forged the pathway for the clinical work my practice has undertaken.

The first is a study that showed that the more ACEs a parent has, the more ACEs their child will eventually experience.[13] This isn't to imply that ACEs are inherited in a linear way; for example, someone who was physically abused doesn't necessarily inflict physical abuse themselves. But that same parent who experienced physical abuse may have challenges with their own relationships, suffer from mental health problems, or experience SUDs, which then may affect their children. In fact, review of the literature shows that there is a direct association of parental ACEs and the emotional availability of parents with their own children; parents exposed to ACEs also likely engage in maladaptive parenting because their own ACEs resulted in "insensitive and inconsistent caregiving that led to the development of internal models of others as unreliable."[14] Other psychology literature asserts that parenting styles are at least in part learned—that if a parent experienced harsh parenting styles, they are more likely to engage in harsh parenting styles themselves.[15] This is partly due to modeling; after all, our biggest examples of how to be a parent came from how our parents treated us. Also, when we are under stress, we tend to revert to what we know—that is, what was modeled to us as children. If that model was positive and affirming, all the better, and we can reinforce those strengths with the parent in our office. On the other hand, if that upbringing was a difficult or challenging experience, it behooves us to know that information so we can invest more time and effort into coaching our families with infants in how to do better (or at least "good enough") parenting.

Note From Amy

In training physicians, I use the term "early and often" or "100 little conversations," encouraging them to talk often, over the course of many well-child visits, about developmental themes such as parenting styles, SE health, and relational health. The first time you discuss these topics, parents may be reluctant to discuss or disclose difficulties. But if you continue to talk about these factors, they'll know it's both important and acceptable to use you as a guide and resource. There are so many physicians who tell me that it was the 3rd, 10th, or 12th time they'd talked with a parent about a tough topic when, finally, the parent confided that they needed help or support.

Neuroplasticity studies out of the University of Denver have shown that new parents experience the development of new gray matter in the first 6 months after a child's birth, both in the amygdala (the emotional center) and the frontal cortex (the logical/thinking center).[16,17] These areas develop together unless the parent is experiencing major stressors after the child's birth—food or housing insecurity, domestic violence, or others—in which case the amygdala develops new growth but the frontal cortex doesn't. The researchers propose that this leaves these new parents with an emotionally reactive brain without the physiological ability to regulate those emotions, which could potentially lead to harsh parenting styles. This highlights why the precipitants of toxic stress (or the SDOH) must be addressed in primary care practices. If parents aren't able to meet their own basic safety needs, they aren't able to engage in functions that are higher on Maslow's hierarchy, like providing positive experiences for their kids.

Studies that examine kindergarten readiness and childhood adversity demonstrate that kids who experience 3 or more ACEs have worse outcomes when it comes to kindergarten readiness, with both worse literacy and numeracy and higher rates of behavioral problems.[18] Pause on that for a minute: *kids who have 3 or more ACEs before the age of 5 years.* The fact is, a lot of the ACEs our kids experience are happening when they're pretty young. One family mapping study showed that 32.2% of preschoolers were exposed to at least 1 ACE, 15.4% were exposed to 2 ACEs, and 8.4% were exposed to 3 or more ACEs.[19] Another prevalence study showed that 26.3% of kids between 2 and 4 years of age had been exposed to a traumatic event.[20] These ACEs are happening to very young children who don't have the developmental capacity to buffer the effects of these experiences with functional coping strategies. Notably, kindergarten readiness scores are roughly correlated with eventual high school graduation, meaning that those early experiences can predict long-term school (and, therefore, life) success.[21]

A number of studies have looked at parental ACEs and specific health outcomes for kids. For example, parental ACEs have been correlated with higher developmental risk for kids—in terms of both their overall development and, specifically, their SE development.[22,23] Other studies have associated parental ACEs with child behavioral problems,[24] where parental ACEs were associated with higher scores on the Pediatric Behavior Index, higher rates of attention problems, and higher rates of internalizing disorders. Another study correlated parents' ACEs with risk for poor overall health status and higher rates of asthma.[25] Parental ACEs are also correlated with missing well-child visits in the first 2 years, with each additional ACE resulting in a 12% increased risk in missing well-child visits.[26] While this didn't result in missing immunizations, presumably kids were at risk of missing opportunities for anticipatory guidance, developmental promotion, and the on-time administration of developmental screening tools, meaning a delay in identifying those kids at risk and timely referrals to services.

All that is to say, parents' and caregivers' histories matter a great deal. If we're going to be successful in bending the curve on the prevalence of ACEs among our patients, it's a reasonable area to explore in the context of taking RHHs. It's often said that if something is predictable, it becomes preventable; but to predict it, we really have to ask about it and know about it in one manner or another, in order to understand potential risks and explore those with the family. Again, that doesn't require a formal assessment tool like we use, but you have to be aware of where parents are coming from to be able to understand how to support and build SSNRs. You've probably already figured out that we see caregiver stress on a daily basis; how it presents in practice might not be explicit, but it's often intuitive. It's the parent who blows up at the front desk. It's the parent who shows up exhausted and disheveled with kids climbing up the exam room walls. It's the anxious parent who is always asking a million questions in the visit. The mnemonic FRAYED describes the manifestations of stress that we see in our patients (**Box 7-2**). They're the same symptoms we may see in their parents.

Box 7-2.
FRAYED Mnemonic

- **Frets and Fears**
- **Regulation difficulty**
- **Attachment challenges**
- **Yelling, Yawning, and Yucky feelings**
- **Educational and developmental delays**
- **Defeated (hopeless), Dissociating, or Depressed Feelings**

From Forkey HC, Griffin JL, Szilagyi M. How trauma can manifest in children and teens. In: *Childhood Trauma and Resilience: A Practical Guide*. American Academy of Pediatrics; 2021:73–87.

What this means is that we don't necessarily need a screening tool to understand that a parent or guardian is experiencing stress. It certainly helps, but there's a role for surveillance as well. Without the use of a screening tool, we can always ask parents about their support network. We can ask open-ended questions about how the caregiver was raised and how that influences their parenting style or skills now. We can approach the parent or guardian whom we might typically (and inappropriately) label as "difficult" or "challenging" with curiosity and compassion, understanding that the FRAYED symptoms we see are usually the manifestation of some underlying stress rather than a personal attack. In all the years I've been asking about caregiver trauma histories through conversations or assessment tools, the almost universal reaction from a caregiver is relief. If they have experienced trauma, they have carried fear and worry in the backs of their minds—worried that they will repeat the same cycle, worried that they will be judged for their pasts, worried that no one will help and partner with them to create new cycles of healthier parenting. Besides, if they're focused on that big of a worry, they probably aren't mentally able to hear much of anything else we're saying in our visits.

Before I knew the first thing about parent and caregiver trauma or even trauma in general, I (of course) saw it firsthand, even though I didn't recognize it as such. But with one mom, I was able to recognize it for what it was, unlike the hundreds of times I'd missed it before that. It was back when we had paper charts, and I was surprised to see all the phone notes that were attached to one particular patient's paper chart—sometimes representing over a dozen calls to our advice nurses a day. The subject of the calls was always something seemingly benign or even inane: questions about formula volumes, how to burp the child, a single pink dot that showed up on the baby's face, the baby pooping only once that day. Pages upon pages, hundreds of little pink phone note slips, and the child was just over a year old. In my not-yet–trauma-informed brain, I thought, "What's wrong with this mom?"

It became pretty clear that this was a mom who worried—perhaps more than what I considered "reasonable." So, I decided to ask her if everything was OK and if she was worried that there was something more serious going on with her child. She sighed and explained to me that she'd had many miscarriages before she finally gave birth to her daughter. All her worries and past losses were piled on this infant, despite the fact that the baby was developing beautifully and completely healthy. At that time, we referred to this as a "vulnerable child,"[27] when the parent perceived health or developmental vulnerability that wasn't actually there. It was the classic frameshift to "What happened to you, and how can I help?" that helped illuminate a significant parental stressor and helped me navigate future visits. It's also noteworthy that this type of trauma, pregnancy loss, is not one of the original ACEs, but it still represented a significant stressor for this mother. It highlighted the value of surveillance and open-ended questions as part of my inquiries about caregiver trauma.

Asking Mom about her traumas may or may not have changed her in that moment, but it changed me and my perceptions about her—strengthening a sense of empathy for her experiences. It helped me better navigate future visits with her and improve how I reassured her when other worries surfaced. Talk about an aha moment.

A funny, yet wonderful, thing happens when you start addressing parents' trauma in your clinical visits with compassion and empathy: they open up. It's not really surprising when you think about it; by asking about their childhood traumas or their current challenges, you've presented yourself as someone who cares, someone who can be that trusted partner and bridge to services as families navigate their own personal land mines. Before implementing our caregiver ACE assessments, I had exactly zero caregivers spontaneously open up to me about domestic violence. Although we've never formally screened for intimate partner violence, I've had spontaneous disclosures from moms in my office at least a dozen times since we started asking the ACE questions. I've also had conversations about stresses in their relationships, financial worries, family losses and ruptured support systems, food insecurity, and a myriad of other fears that were inhibiting their abilities to nurture their kids. In every case, the fear raised by the caregiver was far more important to address than my usual anticipatory guidance checklist (I mean, honestly, imagine having a parent disclose domestic violence and then shifting the conversation back to being sure the car seat is still facing backward), and in all cases, I managed to find a resource to help support the family in addressing their specific needs.

Conclusions

Being a trauma-responsive practice means addressing the things that get in the way of parents and guardians providing SSNRs to their children. Implementing caregiver depression and SDOH screening, inquiring about caregiver trauma histories, and figuring out how to connect families to appropriate resources are basic components of the care we give as primary care practitioners. After all, if we want to promote SSNRs to mitigate the effects of ACEs experienced by the next generation, we have to start with supporting parents and understanding their perspectives and needs. It can feel like a lot, but remember that you aren't doing all this work within a single visit. Like Amy said, it's more like 100 little conversations. Nor are you doing all of this alone; there are resources and referrals you can implement to help.

By way of an epilogue to the little guy I told you about in the beginning of this chapter: Several years after the family had moved out of my practice's geographic area, I was surprised to see the mom on my roster of families I rounded for in the maternity ward one morning. She had been transferred in from the rural hospital to give birth to her second child and coincidentally got me as the on-call pediatrician. When I walked into the room, her face lit up.

"I'm so glad to see you," she said. "I've wanted to tell you how well my son is doing. We got him into a bunch of therapies and he's really thriving. And I've been doing a lot better too. Thank you for everything you did for us while we lived here."

You may not always know how your advice, recommendations, or supports are going to land— but plant the seed anyway. When you focus on trying to support caregivers and families, they feel it, and that can be healing in and of itself.

Questions to Consider

1. Have you adequately implemented assessment tools for PMDs in your practice, including a workflow for appropriate referrals and follow-up to those referrals?

2. Do you need to consider implementation of an SDOH assessment tool as part of your trauma-informed practice? What needs do you see in your patient population that you can address first?

3. Can you line up resources for the things you need to start screening for?

4. How do you understand caregiver experiences and perspectives, including how trauma might show up in their parenting responses and decisions? How would implementing a surveillance question related to caregivers' trauma as a part of taking RHHs work in your practice setting?

5. What processes would best help you support relational health and build the buffering within your families?

References

1. Garner AS, Saul RA. *Thinking Developmentally: Nurturing Wellness in Childhood to Promote Lifelong Health.* American Academy of Pediatrics; 2018 doi: 10.1542/9781610021531

2. Earls MF, Yogman MW, Mattson G, et al; American Academy of Pediatrics Committee on Psychosocial Aspects of Child and Family Health. Incorporating recognition and management of perinatal depression into pediatric practice. *Pediatrics.* 2019;143(1):e20183259 PMID: 30559120 doi: 10.1542/peds.2018-3259

3. Osofsky JD, Osofsky HJ, Frazer AL, et al. The importance of adverse childhood experiences during the perinatal period. *Am Psychol.* 2021;76(2):350–363 PMID: 33734800 doi: 10.1037/amp0000770

4. Wall-Wieler E, Roos LL, Gotlib IH. Maternal depression in early childhood and developmental vulnerability at school entry. *Pediatrics.* 2020;146(3):e20200794 PMID: 32817440 doi: 10.1542/peds.2020-0794

5. Dubowitz H, Lane WG, Semiatin JN, Magder LS. The SEEK model of pediatric primary care: can child maltreatment be prevented in a low-risk population? *Acad Pediatr.* 2012;12(4):259–268 PMID: 22658954 doi: 10.1016/j.acap.2012.03.005

6. Riopel L. Resilience examples: what key skills make you resilient? Positive Psychology. January 20, 2019. Accessed March 20, 2024. https://positivepsychology.com/resilience-skills

7. Sokol R, Austin A, Chandler C, et al. Screening children for social determinants of health: a systematic review. *Pediatrics.* 2019;144(4):e20191622 PMID: 31548335 doi: 10.1542/peds.2019-1622

8. Austin AE, Smith MV. Examining material hardship in mothers: associations of diaper need and food insufficiency with maternal depressive symptoms. *Health Equity.* 2017;1(1):127–133 PMID: 29082357 doi: 10.1089/heq.2016.0023

9. Chung EK, McCollum KF, Elo IT, Lee HJ, Culhane JF. Maternal depressive symptoms and infant health practices among low-income women. *Pediatrics.* 2004;113(6):e523–e529 PMID: 15173532 doi: 10.1542/peds.113.6.e523

10. Garner AS, Shonkoff JP, Siegel BS, et al; American Academy of Pediatrics Committee on Psychosocial Aspects of Child and Family Health; Committee on Early Childhood, Adoption, and Dependent Care; and Section on Developmental and Behavioral Pediatrics. Early childhood adversity, toxic stress, and the role of the pediatrician: translating developmental science into lifelong health. *Pediatrics.* 2012;129(1):e224–e231 PMID: 22201148 doi: 10.1542/peds.2011-2662

11. Bethell C, Jones J, Gombojav N, Linkenbach J, Sege R. Positive childhood experiences and adult mental and relational health in a statewide sample: associations across adverse childhood experiences levels. *JAMA Pediatr.* 2019;173(11):e193007 PMID: 31498386 doi: 10.1001/jamapediatrics.2019.3007

12. Center on the Developing Child at Harvard. Toxic stress. Accessed March 20, 2024. https://developingchild.harvard.edu/science/key-concepts/toxic-stress

13. Randell KA, O'Malley D, Dowd MD. Association of parental adverse childhood experiences and current child adversity. *JAMA Pediatr.* 2015;169(8):786–787 PMID: 26030177 doi: 10.1001/jamapediatrics.2015.0269

14. Rowell T, Neal-Barnett A. A systematic review of the effect of parental adverse childhood experiences on parenting and child psychopathology. *J Child Adolesc Trauma.* 2021;15(1):167–180 PMID: 35222782 doi: 10.1007/s40653-021-00400-x

15. Lomanowska A, Boivin M, Hertzman C, Fleming A. Parenting begets parenting: a neurobiological perspective on early adversity and the transmission of parenting styles across generations. *Neuroscience.* 2015;342:120–139 PMID: 26386294 doi: 10.1016/j.neuroscience.2015.09.029

16. Kim P, Evans GW, Angstadt M, et al. Effects of childhood poverty and chronic stress on emotion regulatory brain function in adulthood. *Proc Natl Acad Sci U S A.* 2013;110(46):18442-7

17. Kim P. The parental brain: how parenthood shapes the adult brain. Life Course Research Network webinar. April 1, 2016. Accessed October 31, 2023. http://www.lcrn.net/the-parental-brain-how-parenthood-shapes-the-adult-brain

18. Jimenez ME, Wade R Jr, Lin Y, Morrow LM, Reichman NE. Adverse experiences in early childhood and kindergarten outcomes. *Pediatrics.* 2016;137(2):e20151839 PMID: 26768347 doi: 10.1542/peds.2015-1839

19. Whiteside-Mansell L, Aitken M, McKelvey L. Adverse childhood experiences: family map-ACEs and child health in pre-school. *Pediatrics.* 2019;144(2):45

20. Briggs-Gowan MJ, Ford JD, Fraleigh L, McCarthy K, Carter AS. Prevalence of exposure to potentially traumatic events in a healthy birth cohort of very young children in the northeastern United States. *J Trauma Stress.* 2010;23(6):725–733 PMID: 21171133 doi: 10.1002/jts.20593

21. Fitzpatrick C, Boers E, Pagani LS. Kindergarten readiness, later health, and social costs. *Pediatrics.* 2020;146(6):e20200978 PMID: 33139455 doi: 10.1542/peds.2020-0978

22. Folger AT, Eismann EA, Stephenson NB, et al. Parental adverse childhood experiences and offspring development at 2 years of age. *Pediatrics.* 2018;141(4):e20172826 PMID: 29563236 doi: 10.1542/peds.2017-2826

23. Folger AT, Putnam KT, Putnam FW, et al. Maternal interpersonal trauma and child social-emotional development: an inter-generational effect. *Paediatr and Perinatal Epidemiol.* 2017;31(2):99–107

24. Schickedanz A, Halfon N, Sastry N, Chung PJ. Parents' adverse childhood experiences and their children's behavioral health problems. *Pediatrics.* 2018;142(2):e20180023 PMID: 29987168 doi: 10.1542/peds.2018-0023

25. Lê-Scherban F, Wang X, Boyle-Steed KH, Pachter LM. Intergenerational associations of parent adverse childhood experiences and child health outcomes. *Pediatrics.* 2018;141(6):e20174274 PMID: 29784755 doi: 10.1542/peds.2017-4274

26. Eismann EA, Folger AT, Stephenson NB, et al. Parental adverse childhood experiences and pediatric healthcare use by 2 years of age. *J Pediatr.* 2019;211:146–151 PMID: 31079855 doi: 10.1016/j.jpeds.2019.04.025

27. Schmitz K. Vulnerable child syndrome. *Pediatr Rev.* 2019;40(6):313–315 PMID: 31152106 doi: 10.1542/pir.2017-0243

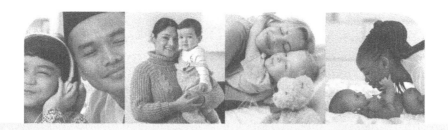

PART 3

Building Caregiver-Child Relationships: Finding 100 Little Conversations to Build Connection

By this point in the book, you've already been introduced to some of the interventions that promote early relational health; in this section, we'll be going more in depth into those interventions. As we discussed in the book Introduction, the primary difference between tolerable and toxic stress is the presence or absence of the support of a nurturing caregiver over the course of time. The presence of safe, stable, nurturing relationships (SSNRs) in a child's life mitigates the effects of toxic stress by providing the support needed to contextualize and recover from traumatic events, so using these interventions to build SSNRs for the families in our practice is a primary prevention against the long-term effects of traumatic experiences. Because the interventions are designed to be trauma informed and developmentally relevant, they're also useful for children and families that have directly experienced traumas and are working on their healing journeys.

We'll start by discussing anticipatory guidance, a mainstay of primary care pediatrics—but also a potentially missed opportunity to provide 100 little doses of relational health promotion. Hopefully, it'll give you a new and revitalized way to address common counseling themes in your practice. We'll then discuss how to design and implement your own interventions to complement the ones we've provided and give you an opportunity to think of what you might want to create for your own patients.

One of the outcomes of becoming a trauma-informed and trauma-responsive practitioner is that you'll start to build a reputation for your work within the caregiver community. This means that families may seek you out when their children have already experienced complex trauma. If you've successfully changed the culture of your practice by signaling to caregivers that you are open to conversations about tough subjects, you'll likely get some spontaneous disclosures of family and child trauma as well. One of my colleagues described kids who have experienced trauma as needing developmental promotion times 10; Chapter 10, Supporting Families That Have Experienced Trauma, addresses how to give enhanced support to families that have disclosed such traumas to you. In these cases, you'll want to deploy some safety planning and practice-based care coordination services in addition to amplifying your resilience-building efforts to provide them even more relational health promotion.

In the last chapter of this section, we'll provide you with a table that pulls everything together. It's the comprehensive curriculum of what resilience-based intervention or anticipatory guidance areas we recommend be covered at each of the well-child visits in the first 6 years after birth. We've also included the screening or assessment tools that will help you assess the risks to relational health that we previously covered in Chapter 7, Supporting Caregivers to Strengthen Safe, Stable, Nurturing Relationships. It's essentially a roadmap to how to do a longitudinal relational health history for a family, integrate the different screening tools that we implement in practice, and prioritize which developmentally appropriate interventions support families at different stages of their parenting journeys.

To help frame the overall table, we've aligned the assessments and interventions with some of the priority areas advised by Bright Futures. Obviously, the sequence is what has worked for R.J. in his clinical practice—and was guided strongly by Amy's advice and wisdom—but it's not meant to be prescriptive. You may already have ideas for how to build resilience in your families—or you may come up with some from Amy's chapter on designing and using resilience-based efficacious interventions (Chapter 9)—so you can supplement the curriculum with ideas that work for you in your own practice.

Chapter 8

Revamping Anticipatory Guidance

R.J. Gillespie, MD, MHPE, FAAP

Don't let yourself become so concerned with raising a good kid that
you forget you already have one.
Glennon Doyle

Anticipatory guidance is a mainstay of the pediatric well-child visit. You've been doing this your entire career, using the same teaching scripts (probably ones you developed years ago), every well-child visit, day in and day out.

It gets a little dull, doesn't it?

Believe me, it does for our patients as well—if it's the same information for the same family, again and again, child after child. Sitting across from a sixth-time mom at her child's 2-year appointment, I started my anticipatory guidance conversation with my usual "Let's talk about safety"…at which point she slumped in her chair and waved her hand as if to say, "Let's get on with it"—visibly tuning out. I ended up pausing, swinging the computer around so she could see my checklist, and asking her what she wanted to talk about instead. I calculated that if I talked about car seats at each of her kids' well-child visits between birth and age 2, then over the years, she'd heard the same boring messages from me at least 60 different times. It was an important reminder to me to spend time figuring out the caregiver's agenda, understanding each family's experience, and focusing on the patient and family in front of me instead of forcing my own agenda in a mindless manner.

The way many of us were trained to do anticipatory guidance is a rote checklist of a dozen different safety topics at each well-child visit. Often, we're pressed for time, given the mere minutes we have to complete each visit, which can turn anticipatory guidance into a rapid-fire, one-way information flow from us to the family. If we aren't inquiring about existing routines and structures that already work for the family, then our anticipatory guidance is not particularly strengths based; at its worst, it may be perceived as paternalistic and condescending. As it stands, the typical anticipatory guidance process is a missed opportunity to build connection with our patients and their caregivers and to build relational health within our families. As discussed in the mid-1980s by Barbara Korsch, MD, anticipatory guidance is often a missed opportunity to truly connect with our families: "when communication flows in only one direction…, education is relatively ineffective…. The physician must consider not only what the patient needs to know, but also what he or she wants to know."[1]

When we approach anticipatory guidance with a resilience lens, a few tweaks to our teaching scripts can become a dozen different interventions to promote relational health without sacrificing much time. Think of the 100 little conversations about relational health promotion that Amy mentioned. If we make an effort to match our advice with the family's goals, needs, and priorities, then we're also accomplishing a win with our relationships with our patients and families, and we have a better chance of influencing positive parenting practices and outcomes. In fact, children living in a family whose provider always listens well and provides needed advice are more likely to live in a household that practices resilience activities and protective routines.[2]

Keep the concepts of motivational interviewing (MI) in mind when providing anticipatory guidance; this comes down to eliciting concerns, understanding barriers to health promotion, and gauging motivation to change before launching into our teaching scripts.

Good anticipatory guidance—touching on a lot of the same subjects you already talk about in practice—can be a preventive strategy for trauma and toxic stress. Shaking up what you're already doing, with a focus on how to infuse anticipatory guidance with both relational health and trauma perspectives, will make your conversations a bit more rewarding (and a little less like nagging). Done effectively, a lot of our anticipatory guidance—meant to prevent ill health and enhance safety—can also be used to promote healthy mental and emotional development and to mitigate the effects of toxic stress.

Most of what we cover in this chapter are primary prevention strategies that should be applied universally to help build resilience; they are also important concepts to highlight for parents or patients who have experienced trauma. Up next, in Chapter 9, Designing and Using Efficacious Interventions to Support Early Relational Health and Heal Trauma, we'll show you some new skills to help build relational health, effectively adding new skills to your toolbox. It has been proposed that there are 7 main pillars to addressing stress, toxic stress, and ACEs: sleep, nutrition, exercise, getting out in nature, mindfulness, good mental health, and positive relationships.[3] While they have been proposed as treatment strategies to address toxic stress and trauma, for primary care we propose that these are good, basic suggestions and can be transformed to complement 100 little doses of relational health promotion, in combination with other approaches and education. Like many practicing pediatricians, I've been talking about some of these since residency—although I wasn't specifically trained on how to address others, like teaching mindfulness or building positive relationships. If you consider that one of the hallmarks of addressing stressors in children is to return to routines and structures as quickly as possible, these routines and structures have to be present *before* a major stressor so a child experiencing stress can return to them. That's where our anticipatory guidance can help: these pillars of stress management can also become preventive strategies for promoting optimal health, development, and well-being. However, it's important for primary care clinicians to remember that these pillars of stress health may help with minor symptoms of mental distress, like mild depression or anxiety, but if a person has experienced complex trauma, these pillars are, alone, insufficient. The patient and caregiver are going to need more than their pediatrician telling them to get a good night's sleep and a hike in the woods; they're going to need to do some challenging work with a therapist that engages in evidence-based therapeutic modalities. We'll touch on strategies for these patients later.

Meanwhile, let's break down these pillars of stress health, their role in prevention, and how to incorporate them in your anticipatory guidance. I'm going to add in another couple of preventive pillars, trauma education and positive parenting, since understanding trauma can be an intervention in itself, and positive parenting is part of the foundation of good caregiver-child relational health. Although a comprehensive review of the literature in each of these subjects is beyond the scope of this book, we'll provide you with some practical tips to effectively get started.

Note From Amy

This is an important differentiation in the area of trauma. While all the preventive strategies mentioned *do* help promote wellness and can mitigate some symptoms of complex stress, they are not the antidote. There are efficacious treatments for complex stress, which we'll talk about later. But for now, imagine you're a teenager who's survived sexual abuse. If your pediatrician suggests eating better or going for walks in nature, your symptoms of posttraumatic stress disorder such as frequent waking, nightmares, avoidance of public spaces, or ritualized behaviors to reduce anxiety will feel significantly minimized. Harm can actually be done, and, at a minimum, you will feel misunderstood and unheard.

Healthy Relationships

As Amy mentioned in Chapter 4, Building the Case for Resilience, one of Ken Ginsburg's list of 7 Cs of resilience is Connection.[4] Healthy relationships matter for buffering stressful events and preventing a tolerable stressor from becoming a toxic stressor. It's important to think beyond the caregiver-child relationship and assess whether or not the caregivers have healthy relationships (with each other and with a broader support network) and whether or not the child has positive role models outside the immediate family and connection with a peer group. When you think about the list of PCEs, they include "having two or more non-parent adults who take a genuine interest in you," "enjoying participating in community traditions," and "feeling supported by friends."[5] These statements highlight the importance of a larger support network for both the child and their caregivers—and emphasize the old adage that it "takes a village to raise a child"; if parents and caregivers are able to access a larger support network, it can also help directly reduce their stress. When I talk with caregivers about self-care, I point out that a caregiver's efforts in maintaining their relationships and support networks have a dual benefit—not only what the healthy relationships and the support network do for the caregiver but also what they're modeling for their child by maintaining those relationships.

Since your patient's relational health is dependent on the time that caregivers and children spend together in positive interactions, ask about those positive events and celebrate them. A simple intervention for building family connections and routines is to ask about what they do for fun together as a family, which helps the family recognize the importance of the time they spend with each other: "What are 3 routines or family celebrations you like to do together?" Help the family list out some of these routines and rituals, family values, and activities that they love to share.

When I talk with parents and caregivers about PCEs (which I do at the 4-month visit as part of my psychoeducation about trauma and resilience), I ask them to look at the list of PCEs and then talk about which ones they're most excited to have happen for their child. I think it's helpful to educate families about PCEs, but it's more helpful to have them start setting some intentions about making sure they happen. It also helps caregivers reflect back on what they enjoyed in their own childhoods and gives them clarity about their values and what they most want to replicate for their kids. Plus, it's a fun conversation—hearing about the value caregivers put on their relationships with siblings and cousins, the good group of friends they had in high school, the hobbies they learned from their own caregivers, or being free to express their feelings, for example, helps you get to know the family better and gives life to their own wishes for their children.

Here's another intervention from Amy that specifically focuses on building family relationships.

I Love You Rituals/I Love You No Matter What!

In every encounter I've had with caregivers, in every keynote I've ever delivered to caregivers, at every visit I've had with families, talking about unconditional love and I Love You Rituals[6] is tricky. We can get stuck there for a while. Are you curious as to why? The short answer is that most adults did not experience unconditional love as children. They experienced love and relationships with many conditions. In his book *Unconditional Parenting*,[7] Alfie Kohn points out the deleterious effects of love withdrawals. Big picture, our goal in teaching brief interventions is to create positive childhood mental health, boost relational health, and increase connection between caregivers and children.

I'd like to introduce you to a tool that gets right to the heart of the matter. Here's the script I offer pediatricians. It's built off Becky Bailey's I Love You Rituals and expanded to my own intervention to discuss the importance of unconditional love.

I Love You No Matter What! A Resilience Intervention to Build Unconditional Love and Create Secure Attachment and Connection

All children question our relationship with them at times. It's a normal part of building a secure attachment—feeling safe enough to make mistakes and wonder, "Is there anything I could do that would make my caregiver stop loving me?" It's normal for kids to test boundaries, push limits, and test the strength of their bond with us. And it's our job to remind children that, no matter the mistakes they make, they're loved unconditionally.

I know, for some of us, this feels truly hard. If you didn't grow up experiencing unconditional love, this might feel hard. Or it might bring up *big* feelings. That's normal too. The more you build a connected relationship with your child, the more you're allowing yourself to heal too.

Here's a script that might help!

While you're playing with your child, or putting them to bed, or simply driving in the car, try this:

Caregiver: Did you know there's *nothing* you could ever do that I would stop loving you?

Child: Nothing? *Or,* I bet there is! *Or,* I know that. *Or,* Are you sure?

Caregiver: Try me!

Child: What if I...

Caregiver: *No matter what your child says, your job is to respond with these words:* If you did X, I might be Y *(confused, sad, worried, etc),* but I would *never* stop loving you.

Or: Even if you did X, I would still love you!

Or: How you behave and how much I love you are different.

Your child will begin to truly test limits. They'll find the trickiest, perhaps most activating, issue for you and push boundaries. Your job is to remain steadfast. Does that mean there won't be a natural consequence? No, of course not. Does it mean you won't have your own feelings about your child's behavior? Of course you will! Does it mean you can't be disappointed? No. Your child's job is to test limits and push boundaries. That's normal! It's your job as a caregiver to remind them that their relationship with you is *separate* from the love you have for them.

In other words, it's normal for our kids to mess up and misbehave. And it's critical that we remind them they're lovable, no matter what. When we separate relationships from behaviors, we're reassuring our child that they have a strong bond with us.

I've had parents tell me that if just one adult had modeled this type of love for them growing up, their life would now be different. And my response is always "You can do this now for your children!"

Trauma Education

One of the chief modifiable resilience factors in primary care identified by Traub and Boynton-Jarrett is enhancing a patient's or family's understanding of trauma.[8] This means figuring out a simple, patient-centered way to explain trauma by developing a short teaching script to use with your families that may help build resilience. It can be one of the natural outcomes of using an assessment tool to explore caregiver trauma in practice, as the tool itself should be accompanied by a conversation about trauma, the effects of toxic stress, and resilience. Ideally, it will also help parents and caregivers who have experienced trauma understand why they may be having strong reactions to their child's behavior and set them on a course of more mindful parenting. Dan Siegel and Mary Hartzell's book *Parenting From the Inside Out*[9] is a great resource to further explore how our own childhood baggage may show up in parenting experiences. Every patient and family deserves this information about trauma, which is why we're adding it to the key preventive strategies for mitigating the effects of toxic stress in practice. This is probably a bit new if you're just starting with relational health histories, but as we discussed in Chapter 7, Supporting Caregivers to Strengthen Safe, Stable, Nurturing Relationships, it's an important practice change to consider.

When we talk about trauma and its effects on our bodies and minds, and how trauma may activate behavioral and physiological responses in each of us, we offer an explanation that helps patients and families understand their own reactions in a way that is physiological, rather than as some sort of shameful character flaw. Our fight/flight/freeze/faint response is natural and normal. It doesn't represent a defect in our brains; it's meant to be there because it protects us from actual danger. We just need to know how to differentiate real danger from the ghosts of past traumas and why those may be resurfacing at weird times. Talking about the physiology of stress gives people an opportunity to start to think about how they might make different choices in how they respond to that natural, normal function of our brain. When we ask parents what resources they are most interested in, more information about trauma and its effects is in the top 3.[10] In their quest to be better caregivers, the simple translation of this request is "Help me understand what's going on in my body or my child's body."

Note From Amy

I was seeing a family where the dad had experienced complex trauma as a child. He'd been beaten, emotionally abused, and neglected for a large portion of his childhood. As a father, he was trying to break cycles of violence and trauma, but he still struggled to regulate himself, often screaming at his 2 young boys.

When they came to see me, we talked about anger and that we all have a fight-or-flight response. We used Siegel's hand model of the brain to understand that when we get upset, we "flip our lid" and don't always make the best decisions (the full script for Flipping Your Lid is in Appendix O). With these 2 young boys, aged 5 and 7 years, they began to understand their dad's anger and their own fear of him. We externalized Dad's anger and called it "the angry bear" because the boys described

Dad as big, loud, and growly. We also talked about how Dad's brain got triggered, because of how he grew up, and how the boys got triggered too, when Dad was angry. Understanding *why* everyone was mad or worried created a *lot* of empathy.

We labeled the brain like we would any other body part; the boys loved talking about how they would "lose their executive brain" because they were in their "reptile brain" when Dad was big or scary. And Dad was able to talk with the boys about how he was "all feelings in his limbic brain" when he felt overwhelmed. We practiced ways to interact, take breaks, label feelings when the lid was flipped, and regroup.

After a few visits, the boys came in to tell me this story: "Dr Amy, we broke a dish in the bathroom this weekend. Our dad heard it crashing down and then we heard his loud footsteps coming down the hall." I asked the boys how they felt in that moment. The youngest of the 2 raised his hand and said, "Well, I lost my prefrontal cortex…," and then proceeded to tell me that when his dad entered the bathroom, instead of screaming, he got down on their level and softly said, "What happened? How can we clean this up together?" I asked my young clients how this felt, and the young boy responded again, "Well, my prefrontal cortex, it just went right back down and I felt safe again and hugged my dad." Trauma education is healing.

●

With the assessment tool that I use to inquire about caregiver trauma in my practice, I always pause to talk about the purpose of the tool before I open it up to look at the answers. This lead-in is independent of—and complementary to—the cover letter that accompanies our tool. My scripts are below; to me, it's an important moment to use the assessment tool as a teachable moment, regardless of the answers given by the caregiver. Discussing trauma as a universal experience helps reduce the shame that is often associated with having that as part of your history. When you start to connect the caregiver's past experiences with their current child-rearing challenges, it's also an opportunity to introduce the concept of "good enough parenting"—that everyone makes mistakes, but we're in a position to learn from them, repair the relationship with the child, and do better in the future.

To be clear, you can initiate the conversations around trauma without using an assessment tool; as we've discussed, that can be as simple as asking the caregiver, "Tell me a little bit about how you were raised," "What are some of the things you most want to achieve with your parenting experience," or "Is there anything you experienced as a child that you use in your parenting style today? Is there anything you try to avoid doing?" With surveillance questions, you can precede the conversation with some of the same scripting about why you think talking about trauma is important. As I mentioned, I use these scripts to open the conversation before looking at the results of our survey; the lead-in is an important teachable moment, helps open up the conversation, and is an opportunity to display compassion and build a relationship with the family that a piece of paper just doesn't provide. Consider kicking off with a simple question: "What do you know about how trauma and adversity affect us? Would you like to learn more?"

Here are a couple of scripts I've used over the years.

> "We've learned a lot about how stresses in our childhood can affect us. People who have a lot of traumatic experiences in their childhood *may* have more challenges with their physical and mental wellness as adults. It also *might* make it harder to make decisions about how to be a parent. That said, we know that building resilience—the ability to bounce back and grow from traumatic experiences—can happen at any time in your life and is something we can help you work on together. I ask you these questions about your past because that might help me know how to best guide you when you ask me about your parenting challenges. I'm the only person who will see what you've disclosed here. Anytime you want or need to talk about stressful things going on with your family, I'm here to help you."

"I've just asked you some really personal questions, huh? The way I see it, most of what we learn about parenting comes from how our parents were with us; after all, they're our biggest role models for how we parent our own children. If that was a challenging experience, then I'd like to be able to help you figure out how to parent differently if you need to. Knowing about your past experiences also helps me know how to better help you if you're ever struggling with your parenting. More importantly, we know that providing positive experiences for your family will help make your child strong throughout their life, so we want to help figure out how to make sure those positive experiences happen."

After using one of these scripts, if the caregivers have questions, I answer those before going on to look at their responses. In the course of these conversations, I've had several parents take back the tool and up-score their results—which means the conversation helped give them a better understanding of the assessment tool that our cover letter didn't provide. It means that for every patient who has received the tool from me, they've also received some basic information about trauma and toxic stress. That is an intervention by itself.

As we've stated, part of the education you're providing to your caregivers and families should include information about PCEs as well as about trauma itself. I tell parents that the PCEs are actually stronger in determining lifelong outcomes than ACEs; in fact, the research shows that people who have high ACE scores and a lot of PCEs actually have better mental health outcomes than people who have neither ACEs nor PCEs.[5] In my view, if we want to promote PCEs, parents have to know what those things actually are; I then ask parents which of the PCEs they're most excited to have happen for their child, so they can start setting some intentions about what they want their child to experience. Planning for PCEs means they're more likely to happen, and the presence of PCEs is an important strategy to optimize development and help ensure positive outcomes for that child's life.

There are some more sample scripts in Appendix A that will help you start framing the teaching script you'll use in practice. For a teaching script to be effective, though, it should be comfortable for you to discuss and should fit in with your communication and practice style—so modify it as you see fit.

Family Strengths and Connection

Note From Amy

Let's talk about a really positive tool we can teach parents that highlights family strengths and the importance of connection. The Family Strengths Inventory,[11] which is where this tool originates, encourages families to consider factors that create routine and celebrations and highlight strengths they have as a family. It provides an opportunity for a fun discussion about "what we're doing well and right that builds resilience" and "what we want to build on." It's a refreshing conversation for so many families.

Following are a few factors that the clinician can review with the family:

Routines and rituals: We have routines we can count on and rituals we honor.

Communication: We respect each other's thoughts and opinions.

Mutual respect: We respect each other as individuals.

Value of member strengths: We each have inherent strengths that we contribute to the whole.

Recognizing/celebrating successes in our family: We notice when we've had accomplishments and celebrate those with each other.

Celebrating our culture: We have a strong sense of culture and/or ethnicity that we celebrate.

Shared family goals/family loyalty: We know our common goals and values as a family, and we express loyalty to each other.

Managing crises together: We manage crises fairly well and stick together through tough times.

Spiritual well-being of family: We have a sense of spirituality, religion, or belief that our family practices together.

Do you see how these are similar to words regarding PCEs?[5] And this is what I encourage pediatricians to consider: When we identify strengths of a child or family, we give them knowledge of the traits they already embody and help them use those strengths and build new ones. I encourage clinicians to ask families about these strengths, observe them when they're present, name them for the family, and help families set goals toward new ones.

When we encourage families to celebrate their strengths and recognize positive characteristics, even during difficult times, it helps them build more positive experiences to mitigate adversity. When families celebrate current strengths, and make a plan to improve or increase others, it builds resilience in relationships.

Sleep and Caregiver Self-Care

Sleep is definitely impacted by trauma and disrupted in cases of depression and anxiety, but it is also critical for good mental functioning and, therefore, a component of optimizing outcomes, including for children who have experienced trauma. In one study, sleep was an independent factor in the rates of delinquent behaviors in teens with roughly equal numbers of traumas: those teens who were sleep deprived in addition to having ACEs were more likely to exhibit delinquent behaviors than the teens with ACEs but good sleep.[12] I think we've all experienced how much harder it is to make good decisions after a bad night's sleep, so think about sleep from the perspective of both the child and the caregiver; after all, if a child isn't sleeping, neither is the caregiver. In practice, it's most important to educate our patients and parents about the role of sleep in good mental health functioning and counsel them on sleep hygiene and bedtime routines. More often than not, in my experience, sleep hygiene comes down to getting screens out of bedrooms (I tell my patients about sleep association—that if they watch TV, scroll the internet, or play video games from their bed, they're basically training their brain to stay awake when they get in bed) and turning screens off an hour or so before bed.

The bedtime routine is a resilience-building activity that communicates safety and structure to kids, so it's something we should be doing as a basic counseling point as well. In longitudinal studies of what makes kids successful in school, there are a couple of basic things that impact school readiness and cognitive abilities: being read to regularly and having a bedtime routine[13-15] (particularly when combined into a "language-based bedtime routine"). That seems so basic, but if you think about a family that doesn't do those things, there's probably a fairly unstructured living situation (maybe chaotic because of social drivers that disrupt the ability to maintain good routines), so when you drop a kid from that kind of situation into a highly structured school environment, it's not what they're used to, and it's harder for them to thrive. That's why self-care and household routines are part of the modifiable resilience factors in pediatrics that were identified by Traub and Boynton-Jarrett[8] and are an area that we can generally be more effective in teaching.

Besides, a bedtime routine is often the time when parents actually get to spend some one-on-one time with their kids, so it can and should be a time for relationship building. Consider starting off with questions like "How's it going with establishing or maintaining a bedtime routine? What routines work for you? Are you able to get some reading into that routine? How does your child respond to that routine?"

As I've mentioned, it's important to consider caregiver rest as well, particularly for new parents who are always sleep deprived and tired. When I talk about caregiver rest (see **Box 8-1** for a resilience-building spiel involving a baseball analogy that I use at every newborn visit—thanks, Amy!), I highlight to parents the importance of taking care of themselves not only for what it does for them but also because by taking care of themselves, they are modeling the importance of good self-care routines to their kids. Caregivers always seem to appreciate the conversation, because in spite of their exhaustion, they prioritize care of their child over any form of self-care, and they often need to give themselves permission for engaging in their own care routines. I've had countless conversations with parents who abandoned all their best self-care routines when they had kids, but it's transformative to help problem-solve ways that parents can continue their favorite routines—particularly if we can help them involve or include their young children in those routines (again, think about modeling). The bottom line is that a rested caregiver will make better parenting decisions. Part of the message within the parental self-care intervention on the next page is that we should normalize the need for parents and caregivers to reach out to others for help. Maintaining their support network includes utilizing that network for support.

Box 8-1.
Parental Self-Care: The Baseball Analogy

Start the intervention by drawing a baseball diamond on a piece of paper (I use the exam table paper). I usually then say to parents that if they've ever been to a Little League game, they've seen a kid hit the ball and run wherever they feel like, but pros know you have to hit the bases in the right order to be successful.

First base: taking care of yourself. I think a lot of people see self-care as being selfish, but it's not true. When it comes to parenting, you need to be rested, fed, and cared for in order to take care of anyone else. Part of this is about creating boundaries for yourself, but a big part of this is what you're modeling for your kid—that it's important to take care of yourself and your body.

Second base: taking care of the people who care for you. This includes your support network, but it also includes your primary relationship. I once had a family come in for their child's 5-year well-child visit, and the parents were bickering with each other, in a way where you could tell they didn't like each other very much. I asked when they last went on a date; it was before Mom got pregnant. So, they had gone 6 years without any relationship maintenance. They lasted about 6 more months before they divorced. That's not particularly good for anyone. Again, think about what you're modeling for your child here—that caring for your relationships is important. Also, remember that your support network, the people who care for you, should be there to offer help you when you need it. You and your children will benefit from having access to a "village" to help raise your kids.

Third base: taking care of your dependents. It probably feels odd to put that last, doesn't it? Right now, you're doing the Little League thing where you're running to third base first, and that's OK. But I want you to think about how you can start putting the bases back in order over the next few weeks—finding little ways to take care of yourselves and each other every day.

Nutrition

According to research, healthy diets rich in fruits and vegetables have anti-inflammatory effects that may help counter some of the proinflammatory effects of toxic stress, which make them a promising practice in prevention.[16] I think we have all felt physical differences in our bodies after we've downed half a pizza versus a healthy meal of lean protein and vegetables. I try to point that exact scenario out to teens who are going out for sports, because for an athlete, it's easy to relate our dietary choices to how our body feels and, indirectly, to how we end up feeling about ourselves when our body feels poorly.

But...

When was the last time you went to the grocery store and bought an apple that cost $1.50? A single piece of fruit isn't going to cut it for me personally when it comes to curbing my appetite, but what if that's the only $1.50 you have to spend on food for that meal? Wouldn't you rather get a cheap, high-calorie food to fill you up?

We can't reasonably counsel about healthy foods and good nutrition without first understanding and addressing barriers to obtaining healthy foods. Before the COVID-19 pandemic, 1 in 7 children was living in a food-insecure household; during the pandemic, that number jumped to about 1 in 4.[17] That means that one of your preventive measures for addressing toxic stress has to be screening for food insecurity. We talked about this in Chapter 7, Supporting Caregivers to Strengthen Safe, Stable, Nurturing Relationships, because food insecurity is an important thing that gets in the way of safe, stable, nurturing relationships (SSNRs).

Perhaps more importantly, when talking about nutrition, make sure you discuss mealtime routines. From the perspective of trauma-responsive care, it's more important that the family have mealtime routines and that they eat together as often as they're able, regardless of what they're eating. And really, this applies to whichever meals and frequency they're able to do—depending on work schedules that may get in the way of the "traditional" nightly dinners together. Most family rituals and traditions (holidays, birthdays, celebrations, and vacations) revolve at least in part around food, and usually not the healthiest of foods. That's OK. These moments are positive experiences; it builds relationships when families sit down, turn off their screens, and eat a meal together—even if it's talking and laughing over an order of fries at a fast-food restaurant. Consider starting with a kickoff question like "What opportunities do you have as a family to eat together? What do you talk about?"

I also talk about conversation starters that can be used at dinnertime. When the family reflects together on the day, it provides an opportunity to not only practice gratitude for things that went well (practicing gratitude is a common positive psychology intervention) but also problem-solve challenges that each family member may have experienced. My goddaughter's family does "highs and lows" (some people refer to it as "roses and thorns"), where everyone in the family talks about something that went well in their day and something that didn't go so well. It not only gives parents an opportunity to connect and hear about their child's day but also gives the family a chance to collaborate on problem-solving skills as they reflect together on the "lows" of the day and how to address them in the future. Mealtime routines can be an important opportunity for caregivers to provide consistent, predictable availability to their kids, which ultimately helps promote healthy outcomes for kids and families.

Note From Amy

I love talking about mealtimes with families. It offers so many opportunities to learn about family culture and encourage routine. I can learn about cultural foods, rituals, how families celebrate, what conversations are happening, and who is literally at the table. But most importantly, I encourage families to eat together—regardless of whether it's a meal from scratch or quick fast food because families are busy. Taking time to eat is a way to connect and support those SSNRs.

Exercise and Getting Out in Nature

The effects of exercise on physical and mental health are well-documented. Even if you never achieve the "runner's high" of an endorphin release after vigorous exercise, you probably know how much calmer you feel from getting even a little exercise or movement every day. Spending time in nature can release similar feel-good hormones, so both exercise and getting out in nature can be preventive factors in addressing the effects of stress. Essentially, physical activity helps people metabolize big emotions. We've been telling our patients to get more exercise since day 1, so this should be a slam dunk, right?

Guess what? Our patients aren't hearing us.

Part of it is that when we simply tell people to exercise, it comes off as nagging and gets lost in all the other messages, unless we take it a little more slowly and methodically. As I said in the beginning of the chapter, our anticipatory guidance topics often feel like a rapid-fire checklist of everything that a patient or family is supposed to be doing, but bear in mind that people remember only a handful of things we talk about in a visit.[18] It's hard to sort out how exercise or getting into nature helps with stress and trauma if we don't spell it out and make that cognitive connection for the family. After all, if it were that easy to get the recommended amount of exercise, people would already be doing it. It's better to use an MI approach where you assess what's getting in the way of getting good exercise, their readiness to change, and their interests and capabilities.

Consider starting with a kickoff question like "What opportunities do you have to move your body on a regular basis?" or "What kind of physical activity do you like to do?" It's important to start with positive experiences with exercise or movement, since an exercise that is enjoyed is more likely to be repeated and thus sustained. Remember, though, that there are real barriers to families getting the exercise that we have doggedly recommended our entire careers. Not all families live in an area where exercising is safe or where open spaces like parks or nature trails are accessible. Many schools have either cut or significantly decreased physical education, which used to be a major opportunity for some kids to play outside. Furthermore, some patients and families find the word *exercise* to be shaming; we're constantly bombarded with images from the fitness industry about what an "ideal" physique should look like, which can be traumatizing in and of itself. It has been suggested that we consider abandoning the word *exercise* in our counseling and instead talk about *movement*. This simple change in language helps emphasize that any kind of physical activity, like putting on some music and dancing, is valued and that you don't have to run a marathon to be achieving specific fitness goals.

Note From Amy

Remember, many parents and caregivers grew up in families where exercise was not valued. Or, parents think that exercise means many minutes or hours of sweating. Ultimately, we don't know unless we ask about challenges and barriers to exercise. Encourage families to dance, stretch, walk, or play outdoor games. Ask questions about messages of health and movement; those are a great conversation starter. I often ask, "What kind of physical activity are you engaging in that brings you joy?" It stimulates a different kind of conversation, and I hear wonderful stories about gardening, dancing, kayaking, and family hikes.

Once you've assessed barriers and motivation to change, you can pull out your quality improvement (QI) skills and help the patient set a SMART (**S**pecific, **M**easurable, **A**ttainable, **R**ealistic, and **T**imely or time-specific) goal. I'm a big believer in micro-goals. When a patient sets a goal like "I'm going to lose 30 pounds by summer," it's pretty unreasonable to expect that it'll work, because it's just too big and overwhelming, and there isn't a clear path to getting there. As soon as there's a setback, it's easy to give up. Setting a more reasonable goal, like losing a pound in the next week or incorporating movement into the day 3 times this week, breaks the goal down into more manageable pieces; then it doesn't feel like as much of a failure if you don't achieve the end goal straight away. At the end of a week, the patient or family can reassess what went right or wrong and try again the next week. This approach can be a great way to help patients start with something like movement or exercise.

As with any QI process, the idea with SMART goals is to start with a small test of change, see what worked and what didn't, and then build from there. Some examples would be "I'm going to walk for 15 minutes a day, for 5 days this week"; "I'm going to dance in my room for 10 minutes a day"; or "I'm going to go to the gym twice this week." If the patient is starting at zero exercise, these are reasonable goals to start off with. Once the patient has a few weeks of success under their belt, they can modify or increase the goal as they feel comfortable.

Bonus: If you get the caregiver and the child to move, exercise, or get into nature together, you're building relational health at the same time! I'm not a big fan of video games for a lot of reasons (mostly because they're often used in isolation by our kids, which gets in the way of time spent in social connection), but in some cases, a movement-based video game may be the safest or most comfortable movement our families can do. If patients and their caregivers engage in a movement-based game together, it creates a sense of fun and helps with developing relational health.

Mindfulness

Another easy one, right? Again, if it were easy, our patients would already be doing it. There's not a lot of question about the effects of mindfulness on physical and mental health, but mindfulness is a discipline and has to be applied appropriately for it to be useful. For a practicing clinician, it's a good idea to have some specific, quick mindfulness techniques you can teach a caregiver or patient in the course of a visit. That means having either some specific resources or a quick teaching technique under your belt. It's another opportunity to build 2-generational skills as well, if the caregiver and child practice mindfulness skills together, so encourage your caregivers to model mindfulness skills to their kids. Consider kicking off with this question for the caregiver: "How do you keep yourself calm and in control when faced with a challenge?"

In the day-to-day life of a family, it can be as simple as having the caregiver call out a big feeling, state what they're going to do about it, and then invite the child to participate: "I'm feeling really frustrated right now. I'm going to take some deep breaths to calm down… Do you want to do them with me?" or "I'm angry right now. Should we go for a walk together and get some fresh air?" This actually models both resilience and relationship building at the same time.

The tricky thing about mindfulness techniques is that they don't work that well if you wait until the moment of crisis, when the child is lost in a big emotion, to pull out the mindfulness skills. When a toddler is in a full-scale tantrum, they aren't hearing us when we ask them to take deep breaths. You have to practice the skills when everything is calm to expect the child to access them during a big emotion. I often recommend that my patients take a few deep breaths together as a family as they're sitting down for a meal; that way, the breathing exercise is part of the muscle memory of the child when they need to access it during a moment of crisis. Plus, it helps the whole family let go of whatever was preoccupying them during the day and be present for their time together. Again, engage the caregivers to encourage them to model the skill through parallel process, which builds relational health if it's a shared activity.

Breathing exercises are among the most universally applied mindfulness techniques, and there are several simple ones that can be taught during a visit:

- **Falloff breathing:** Have the child/parent take in a deep breath, then suck in a little bit more air, and then huff out all at once in a big sigh. Repeat.
- **Square breathing:** Have the child/parent take in a breath for 3 to 4 seconds, hold it for 3 to 4 seconds, and exhale for 3 to 4 seconds. Repeat 5 to 10 times. Incidentally, there's an app for that (Tactical Breather).
- **Belly breathing:** Have the child lie on their back and place a small toy, stuffed animal, or ball on their belly. Have them take in a deep breath, calmly enough to keep the object on their belly. And if they laugh at the attempt—hey, they're still calming down.

These are just a few simple techniques, but there are many more. Pick a favorite, and be ready to teach it during a visit. The key for mindfulness techniques is practice as well as having the parent co-regulate with the kid, which not only models the technique but helps the parent calm down as well.

For older kids, or kids who would be capable of a longer meditative practice, I'm a fan of Mind Yeti (www.mindyeti.com), an internet-based program with a series of guided meditations for kids from about 4 years through 11 years of age. It's based in good developmental science and very popular with preschool and school-aged kids. Meditations are divided into *calm, focus,* and *connect* categories, among others, so they're helpful for a wide range of behavioral goals. For teens, I often have them look up 5-, 10-, 15-, or 20-minute body scans on YouTube—they're free and simple to use and walk kids (and adults) through a simple body scan that they can adapt to how much time they have to spend on the practice.

Good Caregiver Mental Health

Of course, we want our patients to experience good mental health. But just as importantly, we want their caregivers to experience good mental health. Living in a household with a family member who experiences mental illness is an ACE, after all. Think about shifting your opening greeting. "How are you?" is so often answered with a rote "I'm fine" that it becomes a conversational non sequitur. "How are you feeling?" or "How are you doing emotionally?" is a simple shift in language that reminds the parent that we care about their experiences and not just how their child is doing. Get more specific with "How's parenting going for you?" or one of my favorites from a colleague at The Trauma Healing Project: "They say there are 4 challenges in parenting: exhaustion, confusion, guilt, and isolation. Which one is taking up the most space for you?" You can flip that to the positive by asking about the 4 rewards of parenting: joy, wonder, gratitude, and love. It's a deeper and more meaningful question than "Hey, how are you?"

Note From Amy

I like to ask kids or parents to define mental health—often, they confuse mental health with mental illness. It's a great starting point because we all need to work on our mental health. It takes down barriers by asking curious questions like "How does your family talk about feelings?" "How did you learn about mental health?" or "Did you know you can love your kids and not like parenting all the time?" Often, finding a space of validation gets parents talking about their own family of origin—and now you're in the business of breaking some of the cycles of intergenerational trauma.

As we discussed in Chapter 7, Supporting Caregivers to Strengthen Safe, Stable, Nurturing Relationships, the American Academy of Pediatrics (AAP) endorses universal screening for postpartum mood disorders at every well-child visit in the first 6 months, and when screenings are positive, we should use a social-emotional screening tool to assess the development of the child.[19] If you aren't currently addressing postpartum depression and anxiety in practice, you need to backtrack and implement that before doing any trauma assessments in practice.

Here's why. Caregiver depression and anxiety are important because of the potential effects on the infant, including whether or not a caregiver who experiences these conditions is able to meaningfully respond to their infant's cues and to appropriately and meaningfully attach to their baby. But beyond that, asking about depression or anxiety—and caregiver wellness in general—creates a culture change where families know you care about their health and wellness, and that makes it easier to talk about trauma when the time comes. I've had plenty of experiences where a caregiver, having been screened in my office, calls back later to say, "The doctor asked me if I was depressed and I said no, but now I think I am and need some help."

Mission accomplished.

Again, the bottom line is that attending to caregiver mental health is a preventive strategy for interrupting the cycle of trauma in our patients. Simply acknowledging that having a newborn is challenging can sometimes reassure a new parent or caregiver that they are not alone. Maternal depression is often called "the smiling depression" because new moms want to be good moms, and they often feel like depression or anxiety is unnatural, so they keep it to themselves. Society is filled with messages that parenting is a magical and uplifting and positive experience for everyone, so depression isn't part of the equation, right? If you don't ask the questions, destigmatize the issue, and make an offer to connect to resources, you just don't know which parents are hiding their true feelings from you. Imagine how isolating that is.

Positive Parenting

In the 2012 AAP policy statement on the role of the pediatrician in addressing toxic stress in practice, one of the key recommendations is to support positive parenting skills with our families.[20] It's also one of the modifiable resilience factors that we keep referring back to, so it belongs squarely in your toolbox of preventive strategies.[8] It turns out that when caregivers who have experienced trauma are asked what resources they are most interested in, support groups and learning about parenting skills top the list.[10] Discussing positive parenting techniques is well within our wheelhouse as primary care clinicians, and you probably already have some interventions in this area. Remember to frame positive parenting in the context of building and supporting relationships between caregivers and children; in fact, it's important for caregivers to understand that the concept of "discipline" is about teaching and learning, not about punishment.

There are a lot of resources out there for learning positive parenting techniques (there's a book from the AAP[21] that helps with this if you need an idea about where to start, and the Centers for Disease Control and Prevention has age-specific tip sheets on their website[22]), so it's beyond the scope of this book to teach a complete course in positive parenting, but the literature reveals common themes in terms of what positive parenting means. These include parents showing lots of love and affection for the child (you don't have to love the behavior that's being addressed, but always love the child), keeping expectations high for the child's behavior but appropriate to the child's age and developmental stage, and modeling the behaviors they want to see in their kids.[4] It should go without saying that corporal punishment should be avoided, and although spanking as a punishment has been decreasing in recent years, studies have shown that 25 % of parents have spanked a child before the age of 6 months.[23] It's not enough to counsel parents to stop spanking their kids; we have to also give them options for what to do instead. Following the 3 principles of parenting that we discussed in Chapter 5, Guiding Principles of Resilience Education, I often talk about how important modeling behaviors are to caregivers—particularly those who have experienced trauma. Oftentimes these caregivers are doing their best to avoid spanking in their efforts to break patterns of intergenerational trauma, so they feel that yelling is at least better than what was done to them. If we're following the idea that kids learn more from what they see us do than what they hear us say[4] (ie, what we model to them), then these parenting strategies may, in fact, be a mixed message for kids. I explain that yelling at a kid to get them to calm down might be confusing and that it's important to be sure that our behaviors as caregivers show kids what we want to see in them.

Note From Amy

Often, when I'm speaking with parents, I'm asked, "If there's only one piece of advice for parenting, what would you give?" My answer, resoundingly, is *"Love your child unconditionally."* When a child knows you're a safe harbor, regardless of the behavior—because let's face it, kids are going to mess up—they feel safe and secure in the relationship. They'll come to you with more information and reach out for support. Unconditional love is a core assumption of positive parenting. It's foundational.

As a primary care clinician, you already know a lot about child development, so remember to frame behavior in terms of the developmental stage the child is navigating. You've probably heard caregivers refer to their child with all sorts of negative adjectives that the child isn't capable of being: selfish, stubborn, mean spirited (I even had a mom of a newborn tell me in all seriousness that her baby was already "spoiled" the day after birth). Helping caregivers understand the developmental context of the behavior will not only help normalize the behavior but also make the solution more obvious. I love the phrase from Collaborative & Proactive Solutions that "kids do well when they can,"[24] which implies that if they aren't doing well, there's usually a lagging skill we need to help them build, such as the ability to self-soothe, to name an emotion, or to master another developmental task. It's just up to us to interpret what that lagging skill might be. As a sidenote, that phrase also extends to parents and caregivers—they do well when they can; when we provide them with skills to help soothe and nurture their child, set appropriate limits, and understand child development, their skills will also improve. This shift in thinking when responding to a child's behavior is often phrased as "instead of getting furious, get curious."

In all my well-child visits, my first question after addressing the caregiver's concerns is "Do you have any concerns about language, development, or learning?" followed by "Any concerns about behavior or how your child gets along with others?" When there are concerns about behavior, my most rudimentary explanation starts with the A-B-C of behavior: the *antecedent* (what happened right before the behavior), the *behavior* itself, and the *consequence* (what happened right afterward). Encourage caregivers to think about what they saw as though they were watching a movie of the event from a bird's-eye view. For the antecedent, was the child hungry or tired? Was the child trying to get attention in another way, but that bid for attention wasn't satisfied? Was the child told no to something they wanted? Did something remind the child of a scary or upsetting event? For the consequence, what did the child get out of the behavior? Were they given food to "quiet them down"? Did they finally get the attention they wanted (albeit negative attention)? The key to understanding the behavior usually lies in understanding these steps from an objective point of view.

This process of helping reframe behavior is particularly poignant if a caregiver has experienced trauma, as they may not have had positive parenting models to work from, may not understand the developmental context for their child's behavior, or may feel triggered by certain behaviors they see in their children. One mother in my practice was relaying how frustrated she was with her 4-year-old son's behavior; whenever she would try to correct his behavior, he would giggle. As she was describing his response to her parenting attempts, she was getting visibly angry—red faced, with the veins in her neck starting to pop out. When we explored what the behavior meant to her, it came out that she had grown up with a lot of verbal abuse and yelling; so to her, a child laughing at her discipline attempts felt humiliating. I helped reframe the behavior ("Do you think maybe he's laughing because he's embarrassed?"), her shoulders relaxed, and she said, "Oh, I never thought of that… He always apologizes right after he giggles." We were then able to talk through how to frame his behavior based on his developmental stage and how to keep herself centered as she's correcting behaviors.

Looking Beyond the Behavior

Note From Amy

This is one of my favorite tools to teach caregivers because there are so many epiphanies. It's also such a nice link to parenting styles because it really encourages caregivers to think about the lesson they're wanting the child to learn based on an unmet need or expressed communication via behavior. Here's how I frame it.

"Hazel, I noticed you have several concerns about Luca's behavior. Let's write 3 of them down. We're going to take a piece of paper and fold it down the middle. On the left side, we're going to write down your concerns about difficult behaviors. I hear you saying that Luca is having a lot of tantrums, hits his little brother, and won't clean up his room when asked."

Difficult Behaviors	
Crying/throwing tantrums	
Hitting his brother	
Refusing to clean his room	

"OK, what if I told you that behind every behavior is either an unmet need or a skill that your child simply hasn't yet learned? What if we agreed that behavior is simply a way of communicating this? How might we look beyond the behavior?"

Then, I begin to problem-solve with the parent and brainstorm other reasons this behavior might be happening. Take a look.

Behaviors as a Form of Communication	Unmet Need or Skill They're Learning
Crying/throwing tantrums	• Not sure how to express his feelings with words • Feels jealous of his little brother • Tired, hungry, or overwhelmed
Hitting his brother	• Turn taking • Coping with jealousy • Using words to problem-solve • Talking instead of hitting/hurting • Is around other people at home who hit
Refusing to clean his room	• It's overwhelming. • He's not sure where to start. • He feels like it's a punishment.

When we talk about behaviors this way, you can see the light bulb go on in caregivers' heads. "Oh, I never thought of it that way; that makes total sense" is often the response I hear from them. After we go through this brief problem-solving exercise, I encourage them to "respond" to the right side versus "reacting" to the left side. For instance, I might suggest that Hazel say, "Luca, I want you to clean your room because, in our house, it's helpful to find things if they're picked up. It's part of helping each other out too. Should we make a list of where to start?" or "Luca, when you hit your brother, it's scary for him. Instead, if you're frustrated with him, come and get me and I'll help. Or you can wait until he's done playing with that toy and then have a turn."

My experience is that so many caregivers were punished or shamed or simply don't understand other ways to look at behavior. Once they have the reframing and look at behavior through a different lens, they feel much more competent.

Following are a few other positive parenting principles I've picked up over the years and teach to my families on a regular basis:

- **The 5:1 ratio:** Kids thrive on attention from us. Although they'd prefer to have positive attention, they'll take what they can get. If we believe the equation that *behavior + attention = more behavior,* it's in our best interest to reinforce the desired behaviors as much as possible. The challenge for parents: for every 1 time they have to correct a behavior in their child, they should try to praise a desired behavior 5 times. It's a lot of math, but it means we're focusing on reinforcing desired behaviors far more than having to correct difficult behaviors. Make sure the praise is as specific as possible (eg, not just "You're being so good" but "I like how you're waiting so patiently").

- **Time-ins (or special time):** Caregivers often get caught up in the chores and routines that parenting brings, so it's important to try to spend time playing with children every day. This may seem basic, but for some caregivers who have experienced trauma, they may not have ideas about how to play if they didn't experience that themselves. For infants, the caregiver provides the context for the interaction; for older children, the child provides the context when they're developmentally ready and able. Based on Parent-Child Interactive Therapy, the child can choose the activity, and the caregiver's job is just to put everything else aside and play—commenting on what the child is doing but not criticizing or directing the play themselves, just narrating what they're seeing. If the child does something the caregiver doesn't like (like throwing a toy), the caregiver just goes quiet until the child goes back to the activity that was getting the narration (and attention) from them. If you tell caregivers to start with a simple SMART goal (5 minutes a day, every day this week), they usually find that they're having fun and enjoying their child, so they do more and more. If your practice has implemented a Reach Out and Read (ROR) program (https://reachoutandread.org), remember to frame daily reading as helping beyond simple language and literacy; it is an attachment/relationship-building activity as well. If you haven't implemented ROR, do so. It's an important universal resilience-promoting intervention that all families benefit from and a great way to teach emotional language. Remember, too, that time-ins are necessary at all ages; they evolve into time for meaningful conversations with preteens and adolescents. What you're building is the idea of consistent, predictable availability of the caregiver, which strengthens resilience.

- **Loving touches:** Did you know that studies show toddlers who get 30 hugs a day have fewer tantrums? Don't you think every parent or guardian of a toddler wants to know that? Human beings regulate through physical touch; that's why infants do well when we talk about skin-to-skin time, why we want a hug from a loved one when something upsetting happens, and why kids' behavior transforms when they get physical affection from their caregivers. It's a simple thing to counsel but more powerful if you help explain why that physical touch is so important. Sidenote: Even teens need physical touch from us, but if they're too prickly to be hugged in front of their friends (you've heard the "Ewww, Mom!" exclamations from them too), then high fives or fist bumps will suffice as well.

- **The Three R's:** This comes from Dr Bruce Perry's work and is short for "regulate, relate, reason."[25] It's part of the Flipping Your Lid intervention (see the full script in Appendix O). The main intervention here is helping caregivers understand that in the middle of a tantrum, kids aren't able to receive a correction in their behavior until the big emotion is dealt with first. The sequence of the Three R's is to essentially parallel the development of the brain (ie, brainstem/breathing first, amygdala/relationships and connections second, frontal cortex/thinking third). In this model, we help the child regulate their body first, which can be as simple as having a caregiver state the emotion they're witnessing ("It looks like you're sad"), or sit calmly with the child as they experience their emotion, and then help the child calm down through loving touch, deep breathing, or other modeling. The caregiver can relate to the child by reflecting on the feeling they experienced, based on the child's developmental stage. Then, and only then, can they go back to the reason for the correction in the first place.

I pull these principles together in my script about how to handle tantrums in the toddler years (**Box 8-2**). I think that tantrums are often activating for caregivers who have experienced

---

Box 8-2.
Normalizing Tantrums

Start with some probing questions about whether the caregiver is seeing tantrums, how they're handling the outbursts, and whether that's been effective. If the family is receptive to hear advice on the subject, I use the following script:

"First, it's important to remember that people regulate through physical touch. In fact, toddlers who get 30 hugs a day have fewer tantrums. Think about how good it feels when you get a hug during a bad day: physical touch helps calm a lot of big feelings for you and your child.

Second, we talk about trying to 'keep the mind in mind.'[26] In other words, what is your child feeling in that moment? Are they trying to express something but don't have the skills? Kids usually understand a lot more than they can say at this age, which is frustrating from their perspective. As adults, we often don't understand the reason for the strength of the emotions our kids are feeling, so it helps to try to see it from their perspective. Breaking a crayon may not be a big deal to us, because we know we can still use a broken crayon, or get a new one, but it might actually be the worst thing that's happened to your child that day, and they haven't yet learned what they can do about it. That perspective of 'keeping the mind in mind' will help you better understand what's going on so you can keep yourself calm in the middle of an outburst.

Third, show them how you handle your big feelings. For example, when you're mad or frustrated, say so, and tell your child what you're going to do about it. Invite them to do the calming activity with you, if you're comfortable. If your child is in the middle of a tantrum, show them what a calm body and calm breathing look like, so they can start to mirror those.

Finally, I think it's important to name the big feelings you're seeing, so your child starts learning the vocabulary for what they're feeling. If you get in that habit now, they'll eventually start recognizing the feelings and be able to use the words to tell you what they're experiencing. For now, they need to know the words. Later, when they tell you what they're feeling, you can help them problem-solve their big feelings."

If there's time, I expand on the Three R's that we talked about and why this works in a child's brain. It's a good model to weave into the script to help parents understand the rationale behind the sequence.

---

trauma in particular; if they experienced a lot of yelling or hitting in their childhood, having a yelling or hitting toddler may remind them of their own past. Helping them recontextualize the behavior will help them to maintain their own sense of calm during the behavior—given their better understanding of what they're witnessing—and will lead to a more positive outcome for the interaction.

As I mentioned, there are a lot of resources for positive parenting, so find other "tips and tricks" that work for you. Remember that positive parenting along with building parenting skills is a prevention strategy, and it's the skill or resource that caregivers want more than anything else.

Conclusions

Anticipatory guidance, when done with the family's goals, needs, and challenges in mind, can be a powerful tool in the primary prevention against the effects of trauma. Using our teaching scripts as opportunities to build relational health is a way to revamp our anticipatory guidance to benefit patients and families.

Hopefully, at this point you've realized you have a lot more tools in your toolbox than you thought. A lot of the prevention strategies we've discussed are foundational aspects of physical health, and you've been counseling about them for years, just not in the context of trauma prevention and resilience building. Supporting parents and caregivers should be a key component of your practice as well, but remember that building healthy and resilient caregivers will make it a lot easier for them to teach their kids those same skills. Maybe the tools we've discussed needed a bit of a recalibration to make them into trauma prevention strategies, but you are already good at these things. These pointers should help make you even better.

Questions to Consider

1. What is your favorite anticipatory guidance script? How do your patients and families respond to that script, and why? Does that script serve to build relational health? If not, how can it be made more explicitly focused on building SSNRs?

2. How will you explain trauma, the neurobiology of trauma, and the effects of toxic stress to your families in the context of universal education? Does your teaching script include messages of hope: that trauma, toxic stress, and ACEs are not our destiny and that we're in a position to do better?

3. Are there specific skills you want to enhance to ensure that you can counsel parents effectively, like building out teaching scripts on positive parenting techniques or a specific mindfulness technique that you can teach?

4. What interventions are you currently using in your anticipatory guidance scripts to help build relational health in your families? How consistently are you doing these scripts? What new scripts are you most excited to implement?

References

1. Korsch BM. What do patients and parents want to know? what do they need to know? *Pediatrics*. 1984;74(5):917–919 PMID: 6493893 doi: 10.1542/peds.74.5.917
2. Bethell CD, Davis MB, Gombojav N, Stumbo S, Powers K. *Issue Brief: A National and Across-State Profile on Adverse Childhood Experiences Among U.S. Children and Possibilities to Heal and Thrive.* Johns Hopkins Bloomberg School of Public Health; 2017. Accessed March 20, 2024. https://www.cahmi.org/docs/default-source/resources/issue-brief-a-national-and-across-state-profile-on-adverse-childhood-experiences-among-children-and-possibilities-to-heal-and-thrive-(2017).pdf?sfvrsn = 18ba657f_0
3. Center for Youth Wellness. Stress Health. Accessed March 20, 2024. https://www.stresshealth.org
4. Ginsburg KR, Jablow MM. *Building Resilience in Children and Teens: Giving Kids Roots and Wings.* 4th ed. American Academy of Pediatrics; 2020

5. Bethell C, Jones J, Gombojav N, Linkenbach J, Sege R. Positive childhood experiences and adult mental and relational health in a statewide sample: associations across adverse childhood experiences levels. *JAMA Pediatr.* 2019;173(11):e193007 PMID: 31498386 doi: 10.1001/jamapediatrics.2019.3007

6. Bailey BA. *I Love You Rituals.* HarperCollins; 2000

7. Kohn A. *Unconditional Parenting: Moving From Rewards and Punishments to Love and Reason.* Atria Publishing; 2006

8. Traub F, Boynton-Jarrett R. Modifiable resilience factors to childhood adversity for clinical pediatric practice. *Pediatrics.* 2017;139(5):e20162569 PMID: 28557726 doi: 10.1542/peds.2016-2569

9. Siegel DJ, Hartzell M. *Parenting From the Inside Out: How a Deeper Self-Understanding Can Help You Raise Children Who Thrive.* 10th anniversary ed. TarcherPerigee; 2014

10. Gillespie RJ, Folger AT. Feasibility of assessing parental ACEs in pediatric primary care: implications for practice-based implementation. *J Child Adolesc Trauma.* 2017;10(3):249–256 doi: 10.1007/s40653-017-0138-z

11. DeFrain JD, Stinnett N. *Creating a Strong Family: American Family Strengths Inventory; A Teaching Tool for Generating a Discussion on the Qualities That Make a Family Strong.* University of Nebraska–Lincoln Extension, Institute of Agriculture and Natural Resources; 2008. Accessed March 20, 2024. https://extensionpublications.unl.edu/assets/pdf/g1881.pdf

12. Hambrick EP, Rubens SL, Brawner TW, Taussig HN. Do sleep problems mediate the link between adverse childhood experiences and delinquency in preadolescent children in foster care? *J Child Psychol Psychiatry.* 2018;59(2):140–149 PMID: 28862324 doi: 10.1111/jcpp.12802

13. Kitsaras G, Goodwin M, Allan J, Kelly MP, Pretty IA. Bedtime routines child wellbeing & development. *BMC Public Health.* 2018;18(1):386 PMID: 29562892 doi: 10.1186/s12889-018-5290-3

14. Hale L, Berger LM, LeBourgeois MK, Brooks-Gunn J. A longitudinal study of preschoolers' language-based bedtime routines, sleep duration, and well-being. *J Fam Psychol.* 2011;25(3):423–433 PMID: 21517173 doi: 10.1037/a0023564

15. Kelly Y, Kelly J, Sacker A. Time for bed: associations with cognitive performance in 7-year-old children: a longitudinal population-based study. *J Epidemiol Community Health.* 2013;67(11):926–931 PMID: 23835763 doi: 10.1136/jech-2012-202024

16. Gilgoff R, Singh L, Koita K, Gentile B, Marques SS. Adverse childhood experiences, outcomes, and interventions. *Pediatr Clin North Am.* 2020;67(2):259–273 PMID: 32122559 doi: 10.1016/j.pcl.2019.12.001

17. American Academy of Pediatrics, Food Research & Action Center. *Screen and Intervene: A Toolkit for Pediatricians to Address Food Insecurity.* 2021. Accessed March 20, 2024. https://frac.org/aaptoolkit

18. Kessels RP. Patients' memory for medical information. *J R Soc Med.* 2003;96(5):219–222 PMID: 12724430 doi: 10.1177/014107680309600504

19. Earls MF, Yogman MW, Mattson G, et al; American Academy of Pediatrics Committee on Psychosocial Aspects of Child and Family Health. Incorporating recognition and management of perinatal depression into pediatric practice. *Pediatrics.* 2019;143(1):e20183259 PMID: 30559120 doi: 10.1542/peds.2018-3259

20. Garner AS, Shonkoff JP, Siegel BS, et al; American Academy of Pediatrics Committee on Psychosocial Aspects of Child and Family Health; Committee on Early Childhood, Adoption, and Dependent Care; and Section on Developmental and Behavioral Pediatrics. Early childhood adversity, toxic stress, and the role of the pediatrician: translating developmental science into lifelong health. *Pediatrics.* 2012;129(1):e224–e231 PMID: 22201148 doi: 10.1542/peds.2011-2662

21. Jones CW. *High Five Discipline: Positive Parenting for Happy, Healthy, Well-Behaved Kids.* American Academy of Pediatrics; 2022

22. Centers for Disease Control and Prevention. Positive parenting tips. Accessed March 20, 2024. https://www.cdc.gov/ncbddd/childdevelopment/positiveparenting/index.html

23. Gershoff ET, Grogan-Kaylor A. Spanking and child outcomes: old controversies and new meta-analyses. *J Fam Psychol.* 2016;30(4):453–469 PMID: 27055181 doi: 10.1037/fam0000191

24. Greene R. Collaborative & Proactive Solutions. Accessed March 20, 2024. https://www.cpsconnection.com/ross-greene

25. Perry B. The Three R's: reaching the learning brain. Restorative Practices Whanganui. Accessed March 20, 2024. https://restorativepracticeswhanganui.co.nz/wp-content/uploads/2018/06/3-Rs-reaching-the-learning-brain-Dr-Bruce-Perry.jpg

26. Forkey HC, Griffin JL, Szilagyi M. Attachment. In: *Childhood Trauma and Resilience: A Practical Guide.* American Academy of Pediatrics; 2021:19–31

Designing and Using Efficacious Interventions to Support Early Relational Health and Heal Trauma

Amy King, PhD

As I sat with pediatricians in our small pilot group, they were pining for practical ways to address trauma. They grew comfortable with the idea that they were a catalyst for healing and providing education and awareness regarding complex trauma. They got keen in identifying how trauma presented, sitting with trauma disclosures, empowering caregivers, and providing them with knowledge about resilience building. But what was missing was practical interventions, tools, and next steps. After all, if a child has chronic asthma, you don't solely provide education about asthma; you also support caregivers and guide them toward resources. You tell them what to *do* to address the problem and show them *how*. So, that's what we set out to do.

Up to this point, we have made the case (hopefully!) that discussing resilience and its features during a patient encounter is, in itself, an intervention. One of the previously mentioned pediatricians I worked with, Dr Erika Meyer, once told me that she often does not have time in a patient encounter to talk about a specific resilience intervention. But she's aware of components of resilience, mostly from the work of Ken Ginsburg (we talked about Ginsburg's work in Chapter 4, Building the Case for Resilience). So, if she's short on time, she'll pick *just one* of the 7 Cs and point out what the parent or caregiver is doing well. That, in and of itself, is an intervention. Osofsky and coworkers reported that simply telling a mom that she was doing a good job was the best correlate to resilience for that mom later in a child's life.[1] In fact, in our work, we developed posters for all pediatric exam rooms with Ginsburg's 7 Cs (**Box 9-1**) to promote interaction, remind clinicians about components that build resilience, and offer a jumping-off point for discussion (R.J. mentions how he uses this poster in Chapter 4, Building the Case for Resilience).

Box 9-1.
Ginsburg's 7 Cs

- **Connection:** Arguably the most important of the 7 Cs, Connection is the relationships that children and caregivers have to family, friends, and community supports.
- **Character:** How children are seen by others and how they know themselves.
- **Coping:** The ability to manage struggles and respond to environment or personal cues.
- **Competence:** A sense that a child has handled a situation effectively.
- **Confidence:** The belief the child has about their own abilities.
- **Control:** A child's sense that they can control an outcome or response.
- **Contribution:** Ways in which children give back to their world, their family, and their community.

Derived from Ginsburg KR, Jablow MM. Ingredients of resilience: 7 crucial Cs. In: *Building Resilience in Children and Teens: Giving Kids Roots and Wings.* 4th ed. American Academy of Pediatrics; 2020:39–48.

We've discussed why resilience education is important in pediatric settings, and we've described understandable barriers and apprehension. We've also created a bridge of understanding between what trauma is and how we begin to mitigate the trauma our patients experience. We've talked about a formula to guide efficacious interventions. As we move into the next part of our work, we're moving beyond universal tools to more pointed interventions that can be used to decrease stress or create a healthier trajectory for a child and/or caregiver. What I am often confronted by when I collaborate with pediatricians is a paucity of practical tools that they can use to build buffering resources and relationships that aren't cumbersome. They are not sure how to take what we know from the academic literature, best practices, and efficacious interventions and then create a tool that can be used in a primary care setting within 3 to 5 minutes. But they want to, so together, we collaborated on just that. To be clear, these supportive tools and interventions could be used at any well-child visit or patient encounter as a type of anticipatory guidance. And they should be used with any patient where there is a concern about adversity or trauma. The goal is to address relational and social-emotional (SE) health as a way to mitigate trauma and adversity.

A Formula for Designing Resilience Interventions

As we outlined in Chapter 5, Guiding Principles of Resilience Education, I've found the following formula to be successful for creating interventions that build resilience:

1. **Identify** the significant tasks at each developmental or transitional stage. You already do this through developmental screeners, for example.
   - Examples here include brain development, play, attachment, and attunement for infants; independence and autonomy for teens; or sense of self for latency-aged children. These are just some examples; see **Table 9-1** for more.

2. **Notice** when significant tasks are not being met or healthy development has gone awry. Think about this like another way of developmental surveillance, from an SE lens.
   - Examples here include a baby experiencing insecure attachment, a mom not providing emotional engagement with her baby, or a mom experiencing depression. In later years, it may be a child with poor coping tools or a teen with no sense of purpose or goals for later in life.

3. **Combine** efficacious interventions with caregiver guidance and education to support the caregiver and meet developmental tasks for the child.
   - For instance, if you've identified that a baby and caregiver are struggling to attach, or a caregiver is struggling to meet the emotional needs of their baby, you might begin to look at efficacious tools and interventions to course correct. One possible intervention would be providing education about the importance of brain development and attachment; recommendations for books and videos are helpful, as are direct observations of the interactions between the caregiver and baby. Importantly, you want to support the caregiver, without judgment, about ways to observe and attune to the baby's needs.

4. Provide **interventions** known to mitigate trauma and build buffering mechanisms through resilience, relational health, and caregiver engagement.
   - We want to restore hope for the caregiver and family and build buffering mechanisms that we know will build resilience and well-being, when possible. Interventions should keep core tenets of trauma-informed care in mind: realize the widespread impact of trauma on families, recognize the symptoms of trauma when they're present, respond by integrating trauma-informed practices (see more on this in Chapter 3, Getting Your Organization

Ready: Creating Compassionate Pediatric Practices) into the care you provide, and resist actively re-traumatizing the patient.[2] In other words, we want to provide support that moves our lens from "What's wrong with you?" or other language that is shaming or blaming toward "What happened in your past, and how can I help support you?"

Table 9-1. Important Developmental Tasks That Boost Resilience and Well-Being

Age, y	Developmental Tasks
Birth–2	Co-regulation, brain development, attachment, attunement, play
2–5	Social-emotional development, positive discipline, family strengths, connection, play
6–10	Regulation and coping, family strengths and connections, positive mental health, character
11–14	Positive mental health, sense of self, peer relationships, problem-solving
15–18	Positive mental health, autonomy, peer and partner relationships, sense of future, self-worth

In this chapter, we will review a few examples of resilience interventions that I've designed and that I teach in practices. But I'm sure you can think of more as we go along.

Resilience Intervention Formula in Action

Let's take a look at the 4 steps we just described in action.

During the first 18 months after a child's birth, attachment, co-regulation, and attunement are examples of features that promote healthy development and lead to resilience. If a caregiver lacks skills in attuning with their baby, has never experienced secure attachment, has a history of intergenerational trauma around discipline and parenting, or lacks resources to support child development, attachment and connection could be jeopardized (Step 1).

You may see this often in your office. A caregiver who appears to be distracted comes in for a visit. Her baby sits in a carrier while she scrolls on her phone. While the baby makes bids for her attention—cooing, fussing, rubbing her eyes, or flailing—Mom appears to take little note. The baby escalates and then Mom is seen reacting in what appears to be an overwhelmed (almost exasperated) manner, picking up the baby and hastily saying, "What now? I just fed you." Maybe she props a bottle. Maybe she quickly changes a diaper. And then she settles the baby back into the carrier. She's *not* a "bad mom." She's a mom who may have never been taught or modeled how to attune to and anticipate her baby's needs. She may have never received that type of attention herself. And you realize that if she does not receive some support and encouragement about ways to address attachment and meet the emotional needs of her baby, the cycle of unmet needs from caregivers to babies that you feel you're witnessing may repeat itself (Step 2). At best, you're guessing the baby could develop an organized, yet insecure, attachment. More so, you're worried that the baby is potentially at risk for maltreatment if Mom feels frustrated, disconnected, and underprepared.

But you want to build strong, supportive, attuned engagement between the mom and her baby. You want to support them. You've asked questions about trauma and adversities that this mom has faced. You've listened with curiosity. You've suspended judgment about her parenting and offered encouragement. You know that how you intervene with this mom and her baby may be the first step to breaking cycles of insecure attachment and, possibly, child maltreatment (Step 3). She trusts you as the professional. So, you begin with small steps—efficacious steps that mitigate trauma and build resilience (Step 4).

Conversation Starters

When I'm working with physicians, I call these small moments "having a script in your back pocket" or "conversation starters" (see Appendix A). They're the little points of education you use throughout your clinical day. You already do this! Think about your script for helmet safety, healthy foods, or checking in about how school is going. Developing scripts on ways to mitigate trauma will become second nature too. Until you develop your own, borrow some or ask other colleagues how they're talking about ways to build resilience. Here's one example, for a pediatrician talking with a new mom at her baby's 4-month well-child visit.

> **Pediatrician:** Stacey, I really like how you picked up Sara when she was fussy. Did you notice that she stopped crying right away?
>
> **Stacey:** Yeah, she fusses a lot. She's pretty fussy. [*Stacey has put Sara back into the carrier. Sara seems more consoled but is still making bids for Mom's attention and care.*]
>
> **Pediatrician:** I get it. Babies can be pretty demanding. There are around-the-clock demands for sure.
>
> **Stacey:** Yeah, and I have no help. Her dad bailed and I had to move in with my mom, and she's no help either. She said it's my fault I got knocked up.
>
> **Pediatrician:** That's a pretty awful and unhelpful statement to hear from someone. I would feel angry and sad if my mother said that to me. Being a new mom can be pretty lonely as it is. But I noticed when I looked at your relationship history form that you had some tough experiences growing up.
>
> **Stacey:** I don't want to talk about that. I just want to be a good mom for Sara.
>
> **Pediatrician:** I know you do. *(Just saying this is trauma responsive!)* Did you know that when you respond to Sara like you did just now, you're being a good mom? When you pick her up and hold her, it helps her feel safe. You can't spoil Sara. When you notice what she needs by watching her, you learn a little bit about her and she learns about you. Over time, if you pay attention to her cues, she'll learn she can count on you, and that can actually help her grow up and be healthy.
>
> **Stacey:** How do I know it's a cue? What are those, anyway? What if I miss them? What if I mess her up?
>
> **Pediatrician:** You don't have to be perfect. Let's watch Sara together for a minute—we'll see what signals she gives that she needs you. If you try to respond, you can't mess it up. You and Sara will figure out, together, what she needs. Sometimes, she'll just want to be held and feel close to you. And each time we see each other, I can show you some more ways to help Sara and you have a great relationship where she will be strong and build resilience.

Sometimes, guidance and education are straightforward. In their book *Thinking Developmentally*, Garner and Saul describe how we can use developmental science to boost resilience, nurture relationships, and create safe, stable interactions with primary caregivers.[3] This brief interaction between Stacey and her baby is one example of how we might use developmental themes to boost resilience and provide patient/caregiver education. Take a look at Appendix M for more sample scripts for encounters like Stacey and Sara's.

An Intervention to Support the Primary Caregiver

At times, caregivers need more than education and support. You might notice that, without intervention, a family is on a trajectory to poor outcomes that increase concern and need for surveillance, such as child maltreatment, disorganized attachment, continued cycles of abuse, or developmental delays. That requires a more focused approach for the primary caregiver, the child, or both.

In this section, we'll describe several ways we might step in with efficacious interventions that provide buffering mechanisms and boost resilience by supporting safe, stable, nurturing relationships and therefore mitigate trauma and stress. The examples are not exhaustive, but we hope they provide guidance and inspiration for implementing resilience interventions in your practice. To reiterate, some interventions can be used at any visit, and for some children and families, they're necessary to provide information and support that may buffer adversity.

Connection, as Ginsburg points out, is the primary way we build resilience. When we're babies, this connection happens through our primary attachment figure.[4] But when that person is overwhelmed, overstressed, and lacking connection themselves, it can place a great deal of stress on both the caregiver and the baby.

It's important to support the primary caregiver in babies' lives. Here's one way to do so.

CIRCLES OF SUPPORT

Circles of Support is a resilience-building intervention that I have had the good fortune of teaching to hundreds of health care professionals, and it seems to be a favorite among them.

I developed Circles of Support using adapted work from the Indiana Institute on Disability and Community and the work of Robert Perske titled *Circle of Friends*. Circles of Support builds on the knowledge and importance of connection as key to relational health. Many studies point us to the importance of caregivers being supported to build children who are resilient and can identify safe, stable, nurturing people in their lives. This tool was created as a way to map relationships in a primary care setting. It can be used for new parents or caregivers of young children. Then, as the child grows, they can work with the pediatrician to complete their own circles of support. Take a look at **Figure 9-1**, and then we'll describe how it works.

FIGURE 9-1.

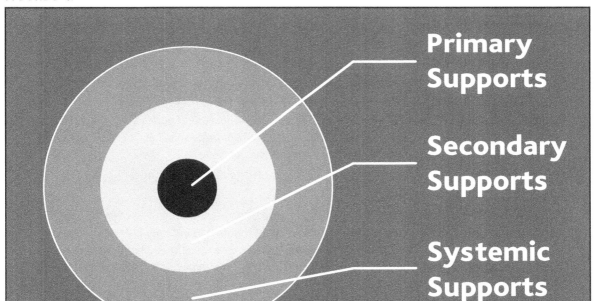

Circles of Support.
© Amy King, PhD, LLC.

Primary supports: This circle usually comprises the core people in a person's life—the ones the person most trusts and goes to for support, advice, encouragement, and confidential listening. Most children and adults can identify 2 to 3 people within this circle.

> Scripting: *We all need go-to people in our lives. Who are the people you call, day or night, even at 2:00 am, if you're overwhelmed? If you're stressed, depressed, suicidal, scared, or in crisis, tell me 2 or 3 people you rely on who'll be there for you.*

Secondary supports: This circle comprises other supportive people in a person's life—the ones the person would turn to if the core group was not available to meet their needs. It's like the "second team" or "backup" helpers. Often, these are people within a system the person belongs to, such as work, school, neighborhoods, or other social groups. Most people can identify 3 to 5 people from their secondary circle.

> Scripting: *Now I want you to think of your backup people. Who might you call if someone from your primary circle isn't available? For instance, I see you have "X" in your primary circle. If they weren't available, who would you call or reach out to? Maybe these are people you wouldn't call right away at 2 in the morning, but these are definitely people you know would be there for you if you reached out.*

Systemic supports: This outer circle is usually systems that the person interacts with or people who are paid to be in that person's life. Pediatricians, teachers, and systems such as schools, religious organizations, and community centers may fall within this circle. Often, there are other systems the family *must* have in their lives, such as court-appointed therapy, human services, or case workers. Such systems can provide structure, oversight, and guidance. These are supportive people but not necessarily ones the person would go to for comfort or close relationships.

> Scripting: *OK, finally, I want you to think of other supportive people or groups in your life. People who provide you support or information or do helpful things for you or your family. Often, these are people whose job is to be in your life, such as me, your teachers, places of worship, etc. Who are these people?*

Secondary circle push: If the primary circle is empty or the individuals within it are unhealthy for or unavailable to that person, there must be an intervention. A *secondary circle push* happens by inviting people from the secondary circle into the primary circle. If you've identified that there are unhealthy people in a caregiver's or patient's primary circle, don't shame/blame the person or point that out; simply encourage more helpful people in that person's life.

> Scripting: *I noticed your primary circle doesn't have anyone within it. Or, I noticed that you could use some more supports outside your primary circle; we all can use more people. I wonder how it would feel to invite someone into your primary circle from your middle circle?*

Note: Most people feel nervous or uneasy about burdening others or feeling rejected. Be sure to address this fear with reassurance.

> Scripting: *I know asking for help can be hard. Do you have "X's" phone number? Have you thought of asking them for help? We could even create a little script together about how to ask. Or, I could sit with you while you call. Or, I can call with/for you. What I know is that most people want to help and don't even know when others are struggling. I'm sure that's the same for "X." I'm sure they would want to help you. Let's try together.*

Remember, although "systems" is the label for the tertiary circle of support, systems may be on any level of the circles and are often critical supports to have in place. Don't forget to encourage a push for systems as well. Food boxes, suicide helplines, utility companies, domestic violence shelters, and counseling centers are examples of systems you can add to a person's circle.

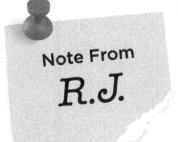

Note From R.J.

In case you didn't notice, Circles of Support is an extremely helpful intervention for a couple of different clinical contexts. You can think about this as a preventive, universal intervention for all new caregivers, since caregiving nowadays can be pretty isolating. It seems that more often than not, young caregivers have moved away from extended family to follow school or career goals, so spending some time looking at support networks is an important intervention. Another context in which it's useful is peripartum mood disorders, where reminding parents and caregivers of their support networks can help them navigate times of isolation or even crisis. It's also useful for teens who experience depression and anxiety, although I usually embed it within a pair of related interventions for teens.

In their book, Forkey, Griffin, and Szilagyi talk about "triangle training," which is essentially psychoeducation about mental functioning based on principles of cognitive behavioral therapy (CBT) and is the first part of helping patients understand depression or anxiety. In the triangle, thoughts, behaviors, and feelings are depicted as interrelated corners. They affect each other, for better or for worse. When one of the corners of the triangle is out of balance (with depression it's usually feelings, and with anxiety it's thoughts), the 2 choices are to fix the thing that's out of balance or to change one of the other points on the triangle to influence the other 2. Ultimately, it's always easiest to change your behaviors and expect that to influence thoughts and feelings. Replacing negative behaviors (eg, isolating yourself in your room, skipping school) with positive behaviors (eg, engaging in hobbies, getting exercise, meditating, having fun with friends) is referred to as *behavioral activation*, which is the first intervention.

I then tell patients that CBT therapists talk about depression as involving 3 downward spirals: The first is that when you're in a bad mood, you do less of your hobbies and activities, which puts you in a worse mood, which makes you do less of your hobbies and activities, and so on. The next 2 downward spirals are the same, except with negative thoughts and social interactions instead of hobbies and activities. To get out of depression, you have to break one or more of those cycles, which reinforces the importance of behavioral activation since changing thought patterns is more challenging. Then I can talk about Circles of Support as a way of supporting patients to break another of the 3 downward spirals (fewer social interactions); this is the second intervention.

I never expect to take the place of a mental health clinician, but nowadays, there are months-long waiting lists in our area. I recently had one patient who was experiencing suicidal ideation who was told there was an 8-month wait to see a mental health professional! I didn't feel comfortable sending her out into the world without something to do in the meantime to mitigate the immediate danger and to set her on a path to help her heal. My primary goal in these situations is simply to help patients start on their path toward improvement. Personally, I've seen measurable improvements in a patient's Patient Health Questionnaire scores with just a few weeks of behavioral activation and increased social interactions...and it is, in fact, an evidence-based treatment for depression.[5]

One important qualitative note: In the 20 + years I've used the Circles of Support in my practice and trained countless professionals, it's one of the most highly used and transformational tools. As well, it not only helps the patient or caregiver understand the importance of connections in their lives but underscores the connection between the pediatrician and the patient. This type of listening and relationship mapping is truly healing.

Sometimes, supporting Mom transforms how she's able to take care of her baby without exhaustion and overwhelm. Sometimes, dads need encouragement to ask for help and support. Yet, there are times when a more pointed, efficacious intervention is needed to boost development and build resilience.

Here are 2 more specific interventions that pediatricians love.

An Intervention for Babies and Toddlers

Think about Stacey and her interactions with Sara. Just small gestures toward enhanced interactions between them could mean the difference between unmet developmental outcomes and healthy trajectories. In their work, Gillespie and Folger[6] showed that as a mother's identified adversities increased, so did the risk of her baby failing to achieve developmental milestones. So, if we think developmentally, as Garner and Saul advocate, how do we get that baby and caregiver back on track?

In Stacey's example, she needed some intervention focused on ways to respond to her baby's cues. Here's how we might go about this.

BECOMING A BABY OBSERVER

While in office, point out to caregivers when and how they attune to their baby. Greater attunement promotes attachment, which ultimately prevents poor health outcomes. However, most caregivers don't know that these interactions are so critical. Some caregivers do them without effort, whereas others need quite a bit of guidance. Pointing out these critical moments between babies/toddlers and caregivers promotes Competence, Connection, and Confidence (3 of the 7 Cs) in caregivers.

Following are some things you can say to point out important interactions you may observe during visits:

- Look at how your baby is smiling at you.
- Wow, he was crying and you knew just what he needed.
- Look at those eyes—she's really tracking your voice.
- I really like how you're holding him: he's facing you, and that helps him feel safe.
- You really understand when and why your baby needs sleep.
- Did you know you can hold/nurse/rock your baby while we give vaccines? This will help comfort your baby.
- You have great ideas about ways to connect and play with your baby!
- I notice that your toddler really watches you. She's really interested in your emotional state, that is, your feelings. That's great!

In Appendix M, you'll find a worksheet that you can provide to caregivers with ideas and cues to watch for and talk with you about at your next well-child visit.

An Intervention to Mitigate Harm and Boost Emotional Intelligence

Remember the example from the book's Introduction about the pediatrician who was using the resilience intervention Yolky Feelings at all his 6-year-old well-child exams? It's a great tool to help caregivers and kids reflect on what's truly going on behind anger. And as a bonus, when we can teach kids to express primary feelings of sadness, worry, or confusion rather than anger (and all the acting-out behavior that comes with it), we increase emotional intelligence and mitigate possible harm that can occur when children feel angry or act violently. Now that's some cool stuff! Here's how it works.

YOLKY FEELINGS

Sometimes, processing feelings is difficult for children because they lack the proper terminology to sort through the complex feelings they have inside. Also, children (like adults) mistake secondary feelings as primary feelings, which often leaves them feeling misunderstood or corrected or lands them on the receiving end of discipline.

Primary feelings: Primary feelings are just that: the core feeling of what's going on inside of us. They best exemplify what is happening and, if labeled properly, most often lead to help.

Sadness, worry, and confusion are 3 primary feelings; they may also be called by synonyms (eg, *blue, anxious, misunderstood*). Other feelings children often list include boredom, disappointment, and loneliness. But for the purpose of the exercise, we try to stick with primary feelings.

Secondary feelings: Secondary feelings are still *very real* feelings, but they often mask our primary feelings. Examples of secondary feelings include anger, upset, annoyance, jealousy, "being mad," and contempt. Secondary feelings often lead to fights, discipline, and defensiveness. They rarely get us the help we need.

The Yolky Feelings exercise is meant to help children sort through their emotions and identify primary feelings so they can get the help they desire. Here's the script we utilize while drawing a picture of an egg, cracked open.

> "Sometimes, when you're sad or worried or confused, it comes out as anger. *(Give an example here of when this has happened to you or the child.)* When your feelings come out as yelling, screaming, or pushing, it's hard for you to get the help you need. In fact, I bet sometimes you might even get anger in return, or, worse yet, punishment for your behavior.
>
> You see, the inside of this egg [*pointing to the yolk*]—the squishy, yolky part—is what contains our 'yolky feelings.' These feelings are *sad, worried,* and *confused.* The outside of the egg and the part surrounding the yolk contain protective feelings—just like the egg whites protect the yolk from getting broken. Our 'egg white feelings' protect our yolky feelings. These feelings are *anger* and *mad (or any synonym for those).*
>
> When we express anger, the helpers in our lives can't lend us the support we need. If I'm screaming or yelling, many people will scream or yell back at me, right? But if instead, I think about my yolky feeling and identify how I felt on the inside, I will get more help. Let's try it."

Here's an example of a Yolky Feelings interaction between a pediatrician and child.

First, I draw a picture of an egg and a yolk, write down all the feelings, and give it to the child; they can take it home with them when we're finished.

> **Pediatrician:** Remember when your mom mentioned that you'd crumpled up your homework and thrown it at her? How were you feeling then?
>
> **Child:** Mad!
>
> **Pediatrician:** I bet you were. And I wonder if you were feeling any of these other yolky feelings as well?
>
> **Child:** Well, I was really confused because I didn't understand my homework.
>
> **Pediatrician:** Sure, I get confused too.
>
> **Child:** And I was worried because my teacher said if we don't get our homework done, we have to stay in from recess and I don't want to miss recess.
>
> **Pediatrician:** Ah, I see. What would it be like if you had told your mom about feeling confused and worried? Do you think she would have helped you?
>
> **Child:** Yes, but instead I got sent to my room because I was mad.
>
> **Pediatrician:** Right. I want you to get the help you need. And yolky feelings help adults know 2 important things: how you're feeling on the inside and how to help. Way to go!

Efficacious Resilience Interventions: Supporting Caregivers, Mitigating Trauma, and Boosting Resilience

Some caregivers and families will benefit from universal education and support—what we identify as general precautions. Those are discussed in Chapter 8, Revamping Anticipatory Guidance. And some caregivers and families require specific therapists and specialized intervention, often in outpatient settings. But there are many dyads and families that need more than education but not necessarily specialized care. These types of interventions, as shown in this chapter, can begin to address stress and trauma during patient encounters. When we identify caregivers and children who, without more pointed intervention and support, will experience a cascade of failed developmental milestones, poor relationship outcomes, and, worse, continued intergenerational trauma, pediatricians are in a prime space to intervene. The interventions we refer to do not replace specialty, outpatient mental health care. But they can bridge the gap for much-needed services and provide greater competence to the caregiver to support their child who is struggling or the caregiver relationship when it seems jeopardized.

These efficacious, trauma-informed interventions have been shown to both bolster resilience and address stress and trauma in families. Moreover, pediatricians who learn them feel more competent and less burned out, and their patients are more satisfied with their care.[7]

You can do this. Your patients will benefit, and you will feel more competent and resilient as well. There is no other professional in a child's life more primed for this type of acute, resilience-building work than pediatricians. You've got this!

Questions to Consider

1. Having read this chapter, perhaps you already use interventions or scripts to build relational health and, therefore, resilience. What comes to mind?

2. Having read this chapter, do you feel more confident in intervening to support relational health through resilience-building interventions? Why or why not? If not, what would help give you that confidence?

3. Do you know how to identify and triage caregivers who need any of the following?

    a. Education and support

    b. Referrals for specialized counseling

    c. In-office interventions to boost resilience

4. What approach or intervention might you try first?

References

1. Osofsky JD, Osofsky HJ, Frazer AL, et al. The importance of adverse childhood experiences during the perinatal period. *Am Psychol.* 2021;76(2):350–363 PMID: 33734800 doi: 10.1037/amp0000770

2. Substance Abuse and Mental Health Services Administration. *SAMHSA's Concept of Trauma and Guidance for a Trauma-Informed Approach.* HHS publication (SMA) 14-4884. Substance Abuse and Mental Health Services Administration; 2014

3. Garner AS, Saul RA. *Thinking Developmentally: Nurturing Wellness in Childhood to Promote Lifelong Health.* American Academy of Pediatrics; 2018 doi: 10.1542/9781610021531

4. Ginsburg KR, Jablow MM. *Building Resilience in Children and Teens: Giving Kids Roots and Wings.* 4th ed. American Academy of Pediatrics; 2020

5. Sturmey P. Behavioral activation is an evidence-based treatment for depression. *Behav Modif.* 2009;33(6):818–829 PMID: 19933444 doi: 10.1177/0145445509350094

6. Gillespie RJ, Folger AT. Feasibility of assessing parental ACEs in pediatric primary care: implications for practice-based implementation. *J Child Adolesc Trauma.* 2017;10(3):249–256 doi: 10.1007/s40653-017-0138-z

7. Moshofsky D, Stoeber A, Rumsey D. Targeting adverse childhood experiences by promoting resilience through anticipatory guidance: a quality project. Poster presented at: American Academy of Pediatrics National Conference and Exhibition; September 16–19, 2017; Chicago, IL

Supporting Families That Have Experienced Trauma

R.J. Gillespie, MD, MHPE, FAAP

Healing doesn't mean the damage never existed. It means the damage no longer controls your life.

Akshay Dubey

One of the natural consequences of taking relational health histories, specifically ones that address trauma histories, is that parents and caregivers become more comfortable with seeking your help and advice. This often leads to spontaneous disclosures of traumas and stressors that have happened to their children; you'll also hear a lot more disclosures if you're specifically listening for and responding to stressful events with compassion. I think this is partly because you've changed the culture of your office by normalizing these conversations, which helps destigmatize them, and partly because you've built a trusting relationship with your families. It also becomes part of your reputation in the community of families—that you are the kind of person who is willing to listen, suspend judgment, and help.

I recently had a family come into my care that illustrated this point. Mom reported to me that her son, who was 5 years old, witnessed the murder of his older brother. He had also been severely physically abused while in his father's custody, with visible scars from that abuse across his face and ears. The prior pediatrician had been working on getting him in for an autism evaluation because he wasn't speaking and was having "explosive" behavior, although once Mom was given sole custody, his speech was starting to improve and his behaviors were becoming less frequent. He wasn't currently connected with any sort of mental or behavioral health support. Mom made a comment along the lines of "I've heard you're the guy who can help."

This history all came to light in the first 5 minutes I was in the exam room with the family. Unfortunately (but not uncommonly), our time had been scheduled as a 10-minute "to meet" visit, so I had to think and act fairly quickly.

Step 1: Breathe, and make myself fully present for the visit. Trying to corral the visit to "save time" by forcing my own solutions on the family rarely works for me (you've probably had the same experience). It's always easier to take a motivational interviewing approach, to hear what the family has to say, and to use the family's information and perspective to determine what the family actually needs. It's helpful to communicate compassion with body language as well, so lean in, set aside the laptop, and listen (more on this in Chapter 12, The Art of Listening).

Step 2: Assess Mom's priorities for the visit, ensure that the family is physically safe, and assess what strengths and assets are present.

Step 3: Make an interim plan. The key word here is *interim*. I'm not going to solve everything in a single visit, nor will I solve it alone. Part of this plan is to offer my partnership in getting whatever services the family needs (Remember the HELLPPP mnemonic from Chapter 2, Addressing Barriers?). Part of it is lining up what's going to happen in this visit, deciding who is responsible for each of the to-do items in the interim plan, and then scheduling a follow-up to continue helping the family on their journey toward healing.

At the end of this process, Mom was reassured that we had a specific plan of action, and I was able to convey both compassion and partnership with the family. Remember that statistic from *Compassionomics,* that it takes only 40 seconds to convey all the benefits of compassion?[1] Obviously, we still have work to do to keep this kid on his path toward healing, but in our relatively short initial encounter, we were already off to a great start.

If a child has experienced trauma, you'll need to pull out all the stops in providing care for that family. This is particularly true for foster families, where most of the children placed into foster or kinship care have experienced some pretty awful things. As we discussed in the Introduction, I think it's important to take a medical home approach in these cases, as you would for any patient with complex needs. The same care coordination workflows that are used for kids with complex medical conditions should be used for patients and families that experience trauma. That includes creating a system for tracking patients who need additional care and services, making referrals and tracking them, developing a safety plan, and creating a written shared care plan when appropriate.

A comprehensive guide to medical home implementation, care coordination, and shared care plans can be found through the American Academy of Pediatrics (AAP) National Resource Center for Patient/Family-Centered Medical Home (www.aap.org/en/practice-management/medical-home). This chapter will focus on how to implement these components in the context of trauma. It's a lot, and you're going to have to figure out how to drum up resources for some of this. In our practice, we've negotiated per-member, per-month funding in some of our insurance contracts to help support care coordination services. Other practices have used grant funding to add ancillary staff for care coordination or peer navigation to their practices. Additionally, in our state, certifying as a medical home has resulted in enhanced payments that allow for some of these services. Engage your administrative team to help seek out these opportunities.

Patient Tracking, Documentation, and Decision Support

Once you've identified a patient or family as having experienced trauma, you will need to come up with a way to identify that family for future visits so you can continue to offer appropriate care. Your electronic health record (EHR) system may support this, but with trauma, there are particular confidentiality issues you'll want to keep in mind. For me, that means avoiding the use of problem lists as a way of identifying patients who have experienced trauma, because the problem list is visible on any records transfer or release of information, as well as printed into after-visit summaries. This may violate the principles of autonomy that we mentioned earlier, in allowing patients and families to decide how this information is released or shared.

There are several different ways to identify a patient within your EHR as one who needs additional care or support. The patient photo part of the banner is a feature our practice never used, so we upload graphics that indicate different patient needs. For example, one says "care coordination" for our medically complex patients; there are others to note things like when a patient is transgender. Most health records have pop-up features that will allow you to keep notes to yourself of particular care needs or gaps. Another option we've used is to create a confidential history field within visit templates where a clinician can write details about a patient that don't get printed in the visit note. These notes appear the next time a visit template is opened and can be added to over time. Any of these methods can be used to remind you that you are working with a patient or family that has experienced trauma at the time of the visit. Tracking patients through a registry or separate spreadsheet is also an option; care coordinators often keep lists like these to proactively track when contacts with the patient are due or to close the loop on any outstanding referrals.

Decision support refers to the reminders that are built within a visit template to remind you about what is due during that encounter or how to handle certain results that are obtained. We include a note about which resilience interventions are recommended for each of the visits and include conversation prompts for the visit where we conduct our trauma assessment. In our 4-month visit template, when we typically assess caregiver trauma, we added the 3 questions from Chapter 2, Addressing Barriers, to help clinicians remember how to guide conversations about trauma disclosures:

1. Do any of these experiences still bother you now?

2. Of those experiences that no longer bother you, how did you get to the point that they don't bother you anymore?

3. How do you think these experiences affect your parenting now?

Some of our assessment tool documentation templates also include information about scoring or what to do with the results, such as referring to the care coordinator or to Help Me Grow (www.helpmegrow.org). These types of decision supports help the clinician do the right thing during the visit and help remind clinicians how to manage the patient's ongoing care.

Safety Planning and Shared Care Plans

Basic safety planning consists of 4 components:

1. Assessment of child/family safety

2. Assets, resources, and resiliencies in the family—including coping and self-management strategies and an assessment of support networks

3. Follow-up tools for assessing mental health or social-emotional (SE) development in patients as needed; in other words, assessing for symptoms caused by the traumatic event

4. Connecting with appropriate resources

In medical home models, a shared care plan is a document that is cowritten by the clinical team and the family. In cases of trauma, this written plan should include a summary of resources and strategies to address each of these steps in safety planning. In the first step, we help the patient or family know when they need help and understand that help is available; this may be challenging for patients, since their experiences of trauma may mean they're not used to getting help in the first place. This line of questions includes identifying both physical and emotional safety for the patient or family. In cases where physical safety is threatened, your most immediate priority is addressing how to get the patient to a safe place. I have the list of domestic violence resources on my laptop, organized by county, in case of immediate safety concerns. These scenarios often trigger mandatory reporting by clinicians (**Box 10-1**); be sure you know the laws in your area about your legal responsibilities.

Note From Amy

There are many reasons that patients may not have disclosed trauma before or received intervention or support. Part of being a trauma-informed clinic means looking through the lens of "I wonder what happened here?" and "How can I help?" Communicating to the family, especially parents, the positive intention that *all families* want to be healthy and *all parents* want their children to be happy and well-adjusted is an important beginning to creating safety plans and coordinating care. We can convey this using language such as "We know you're doing your best; here are some ways we can work together to ensure your child is getting all the help they need" or "Let's work together to be sure that your goals and wants for your child, to be healthy and happy, are met successfully. We can help and work together as a team."

●

Assessing Safety

Since shared care plans are supposed to be patient and family centered, I usually start the conversation by asking the patient or caregiver about their own physical safety needs. This usually begins with the simple question "Are you safe?" and moves on to "What do you think you need to be safe?" This often applies to disclosures about intimate partner violence, which may trigger a report to child protective services (**Box 10-1**); be transparent with the family about your responsibilities and their role in the reporting process.

Box 10-1.
Mandatory Reporting

It will happen. It's never easy. That said, it's an important part of keeping patients and even parents and caregivers safe. If you've been transparent about this issue when you introduced your trauma assessment to the patient and family, it helps minimize the degree of surprise.

As you know, mandatory reporting laws are in place to protect children and families. It may help to explain to the caregiver that they may be the only person who can keep their child safe from the person responsible for the violence or abuse, so coming forward is the caregiver's best way of providing safety for their child. You can also explain that our role is to help protect children, even if we're not 100% certain that abuse is happening. The caregiver should understand that the process of reporting is to help start the next steps in the evaluation of their child's health and to help access additional resources and supports for the family.

If the caregiver feels comfortable with it, you can even encourage them to make the report themselves, with you in your office. This isn't intended to absolve you of your responsibility as a mandatory reporter, but making the report together with the caregiver may serve to reinforce their role in keeping their child safe. It empowers caregivers to get themselves out of a potentially harmful situation and gives them a sense of choice in a time of trauma.

Emotional safety usually applies to patients who experience symptoms of mental illness, like anxiety or depression, and is assessed by asking a question like "What are your warning signs that you're starting to have a problem?"—the answer to which can include behaviors, thoughts, or feelings (Remember the cognitive triangle from my note in Chapter 9, Designing and Using Efficacious Interventions to Support Early Relational Health and Heal Trauma?). You can then probe about what they do when they are experiencing their warning signs. When talking with caregivers about their own trauma histories and how those may show up in their parenting, you can ask similar questions about what the caregiver feels would be warning signs for them, how they know when they're feeling overwhelmed with their parenting, and what would be most helpful for them in terms of resources and supports.

Part of a safety assessment includes helping parents recognize when symptoms may represent manifestations of trauma. It's not always self-evident to caregivers when an explosive behavior, emotional withdrawal, or somatic symptom may represent how a child is revealing that they're under stress. While I've turned to open-ended questions to assess if a somatic symptom might be a manifestation of stress ("Has anything scary or upsetting happened to your child?" is my go-to), sometimes directed questions are helpful in uncovering what's precipitating a behavior.

The AAP Trauma Guide series[2] provide some examples:

- "You have told me that your child is having some problems with aggression, acting out, attention, and sleep. Just as fever means the body is dealing with an infection, when these behaviors happen, they may mean that the brain and body are responding to a stress or threat. Do you have any concerns that your child is being exposed to a threat or feeling stressed?"

- "The behaviors you describe and the trouble she is having with school and learning are often warning signs that the brain is trying to manage stress or threat. Sometimes children respond this way if they are being harmed, or if they saw others they care about being harmed. Do you know if your child saw or witnessed violence at school, with friends, or at home?"

Note From Amy

My experience with parents is that validating and explaining symptoms of trauma can prove quite helpful. I remember talking with a foster mom about the child in her home. We discussed behaviors such as food hoarding, hypervigilance, and protectiveness of the child's younger sibling. The behaviors were confusing to the foster parent: she commented, "I don't know why she's acting this way; we have plenty of food and I'll take care of them. They're safe here."

I offered, "Isn't it incredible how we learn to protect ourselves and take care of people we love, even when we're stressed? I think she's just letting you know she's not sure how to trust you quite yet. She's not positive about food or caregiving because her most trusted adults let her and her brother down. Over time, she'll learn that you have resources and want to support her. But for now, her behaviors are a way of letting you know that she's had to take care of herself for some time. We call these behaviors *trauma symptoms*. They're going to show up from time to time because this little girl has been in protective mode for some time and it's been important for her survival. The longer she's with you and you're patient and reassuring, the more she will trust that you can meet her needs. But if you see her behavior as challenging, naughty, or frustrating, she'll likely stay in a protective mode. For her, these behaviors have meant survival."

Framing trauma that manifests as behaviors allows space and compassion for caregivers and acknowledgment for the child's pain.

Building Coping Skills

Coping skills include anything the patient or caregiver can do to help alleviate their feelings of stress. Our interventions in primary care may not ultimately be sufficient to help a patient or family heal, but they are a necessary part of our interim plan with the family until they can engage with a mental health professional. My primary goal in discussing coping strategies is to try to steer patients away from unhealthy or unhelpful coping methods and toward more helpful ones. It should be noted that while all coping skills are adaptive (and serve their purpose), some are helpful in providing positive outcomes, and some are not. During this conversation with patients and families, I often draw 3 buckets on the exam room paper to describe these categories of coping skills: helpful (ie, art, exercise, meditation), unhelpful (ie, drugs and alcohol, overeating), and neutral (mostly screen time, which probably doesn't help or hurt but delays coping with stress in the first place). This is an opportunity to learn about the coping strategies the child or parent currently uses; in turn, that creates the opportunity to suggest new tools they can keep in their toolbox—again, with the goal of replacing unhealthy or unhelpful coping methods with more constructive ones. (See **Box 10-2** for one helpful technique that caregivers can help children with.)

> ### Box 10-2.
> ### "Name It to Tame It"
>
> Dan Siegel talks about helping kids tell stories to calm big emotions, as it's a way to help kids engage their thinking brains to calm their feeling brains.[3] Kids who have experienced trauma will often have outbursts of big emotions where they are stuck on the scary or traumatic event. Parents and caregivers can help kids describe the experience, which is effectively creating a "trauma narrative" around the experience. This is meant not to take the place of a trauma-specific therapist to help the child heal from the event but rather to give caregivers a tool to use when their child is in a crisis.
>
> When a child is remembering a traumatic event, rather than dismiss the event as being "over" or "in the past," caregivers can help children process their memories by asking simple "And then what happened?" questions until the story comes to its end. The goal is to help kids remember the conclusion of the traumatic event—that although the event was scary or upsetting, there was an adult to help the child feel safe, or a particular resilience activity or intervention helped the child feel better. Caregivers can then remind children what to do if that situation recurs—that the child has their love and support, that they are there to help the child feel better, and that there are things the child can do to help process their fears.
>
> Again, if the thinking brain is engaged, the emotional part of the brain will start to be tamed and the child will have an opportunity to heal. Caregivers are meant to be facilitators in the conversation, guiding the story to the point where the child was safe, so the child can start to overcome their fears and bad memories by simply naming them.

If you or the patient is not sure where to start, go back to the pillars of stress health that we talked about in Chapter 8, Revamping Anticipatory Guidance: mindfulness, exercise, getting out in nature, sleep, nutrition, good mental health, and positive relationships. I used to tell everyone to do breathing exercises because they're so effective—there are a lot of studies that correlate the practice of deep breathing with a decrease in cortisol levels (it takes only 90 seconds of deep, belly breathing to reduce cortisol levels by 30 %)[4,5]—but the truth is, sometimes you just need to run around the block or go outside and do jumping jacks to metabolize a big emotion. See what resonates with the patient and their preferences. ACEs Aware has a great patient handout for identifying goals around self-care that may help you frame this conversation. A useful conversation prompt in this context is to ask the parent or patient "What helps you stay calm and in control when faced with something stressful?"

Most of the interventions we've discussed up to this point are intentionally designed to build resilience and enhance strengths within the caregiver-child relationship and should be used intentionally for children who have experienced trauma. Specific interventions that you may find helpful to enhance coping skills and resilience include the following:

Chapter 8, Revamping Anticipatory Guidance

- The Three R's (regulate, relate, reason)
- Time-ins and special time
- Looking Beyond the Behavior
- I Love You Rituals/I Love You No Matter What!
- Self-care routines

Chapter 9, Designing and Using Efficacious Interventions to Support Early Relational Health and Heal Trauma

- Yolky Feelings

Note From Amy

Sometimes, the most straightforward tool to offer a parent when they're overwhelmed is to give them permission to take a break, to walk away. When they recognize that they feel tense and want to lash out, it's important to encourage them to disengage from their child in any way possible. They can walk outside, go to their bedroom, or even shut themselves in a bathroom for a bit. Often, parents feel bad about leaving their child, but the alternative—to stay close but experience negative interactions and, even worse, anger and hostility—causes a lot more damage in the long run.

Reframing the child's or youth's behavior is another way to increase the family's safety. By reframing "difficult" or "acting-out" behavior as a way of communicating, caregivers can learn ways to address behavior that won't lead to physical or emotional punishment. This is a great example of when to use the Looking Beyond the Behavior intervention from Chapter 8, Revamping Anticipatory Guidance. Often, an effective intervention such as thinking about behavior in a different way may completely change an unsafe family interaction. As we've described, you've probably had cases in your own practice where parents describe a young toddler as "willful," "spoiled," "stubborn," or some other negative adjective that doesn't really match up with where the child is developmentally. I go back to the core axiom of collaborative problem-solving that says "kids do well when they can,"[6] because it's a reminder that if a kid isn't doing well, there's a reason for it. Something is getting in their way, typically a lagging developmental skill like being able to regulate emotions. Encouraging caregivers to become curious about a behavior (and not furious!), helping them understand development, and reminding them to approach their children with empathy may help avoid overly harsh punishments. It's one of the core parenting principles we espouse: love the child even if you don't love the behavior.

A good shared care plan will include patient and/or caregiver goals in addition to the instructions about what to do when you're in an exacerbation. When it comes to mindfulness, meditation, and other self-care techniques, practice makes perfect. If the patient or family isn't engaging in self-care skills and routines when they aren't in crisis, it's harder to tap into those skills when they are in crisis. Help the family set some SMART (**S**pecific, **M**easurable, **A**ttainable, **R**ealistic, and **T**imely or time-specific) goals about self-care routines that they can implement on a regular basis so they're more readily accessible to the patient when they need them. For example, a patient goal might say, "I will practice breathing exercises for 5 minutes a day for the next 2 weeks" or "I will reach out to someone in my support network and make plans to get together in the next week." Other potential goals can include contacting or accessing a community resource within a specified time frame or making a follow-up appointment with you or a mental health clinician.

Assessing social supports is an important component of this step in the safety plan, and it is essentially a list of whom the patient, caregiver, or family member can reach out to when they need help. When a person is in crisis, it's often hard to think about the people in their life who can help; the list makes it easier to remember. If a patient or parent is having a hard time identifying people they can reach out to, the Circles of Support intervention is helpful for fleshing this piece out (see Chapter 9, Designing and Using Efficacious Interventions to Support Early Relational Health and Health Trauma, for details on this intervention). As a sidenote, I also use the Circles of Support for parents with postpartum depression or teens who experience anxiety and depression; it's a good one to have in your toolbox.

Follow-up Tools to Assess Mental Health and Social-Emotional Development

Another component of safety is assessing the child's mental health. This may require additional screening tools that are specific to trauma and mental health; consider also that children who have experienced trauma may be experiencing suicidal ideation as a result of that trauma. Some specific tools include tools for general behavior and SE health that we discussed previously (see Chapter 6, Understanding Early Relational Health), as well as trauma-specific tools like the UCLA PTSD Reaction Index (PTSD-RI), the Trauma Symptom Checklist for Children (TSCC), or the Pediatric Trauma Stress Screening Tool (PTSST; available at https://intermountainhealthcare.org/ckr-ext/Dcmnt?ncid = 529795302). Specific mental health screening tools may also be appropriate, such as the Screen for Child Anxiety Related Disorders (SCARED) for anxiety, the Patient Health Questionnaire-2 (PHQ-2)/Patient Health Questionnaire-9 (PHQ-9) for depression, and the Ask Suicide Questions (ASQ; not to be confused with the developmental screening of the same abbreviation) or the Columbia-Suicide Severity Rating Scale (C-SSRS) to assess for suicidal ideation in older kids and teens. Remember that you must be ready to respond to any of these assessment tools with referral resources; it's another area where integrated behavioral health with the capacity for warm handoffs is particularly valuable.

Note From Amy

The other important factor to consider is systemic and historical traumas. We have to remember that not all families have had positive experiences in systems. The family you're working with may have experienced significant disservice from the medical field, mental health services, or systems such as child welfare. As well, children and families of color are overrepresented in our child welfare systems. Many such children and families are understandably skeptical of "help" that may mean they lose custody of their child.

Providing Referrals and Resources

Other resources to include in the shared care plan, depending on the needs identified by the family, include crisis lines, community-based organizations (CBOs) to help address any identified social drivers of health (SDOH) needs, mental health clinicians, parenting programs, and developmental supports. Common trauma-specific therapeutic modalities are listed in **Box 10-3**; if you're able, try to identify clinicians for these therapies in your community.

Beyond organizations and community-based supports, resources can also include handouts, websites, activity sheets, or books, depending on the patient's or caregiver's goals and priorities. Remember that when parents were asked about what resources they were most interested in receiving, education about trauma was near the top of the list. There's no need to reinvent these handouts; websites like PACEsConnection, ACEs Aware, the Centers for Disease Control and Prevention (CDC), and The National Child Traumatic Stress Network have great patient resources for education about trauma, ACE prevention, positive parenting, and parenting with ACEs (**Box 10-4**).

Summing It Up With a Written Shared Care Plan

Once safety planning is completed, it's helpful to summarize the information in a written document for the family; often, when a patient or parent is in crisis, it's hard to remember the steps

---

Box 10-3.
Trauma-Specific and Trauma-Informed Therapies

Attunement Therapies for Younger Children
- Child-Parent Psychotherapy (CPP)
- Parent-Child Interactive Therapy (PCIT)
- Circle of Security

Home Visitation Model to Promote Attachment
- Attachment and Biobehavioral Catch-up (ABC)

Therapies for Addressing Trauma
- Trauma-Focused Cognitive Behavioral Therapy (TF-CBT)
- Eye Movement Desensitization and Reprocessing (EMDR)

See The National Child Traumatic Stress Network website (www.nctsn.org) for more therapy types.

Box 10-4.
Websites With Patient Handouts

- PACEsConnection: www.pacesconnection.com/pages/handouts
- ACEs Aware: www.acesaware.org/resources/resources-by-type/patient-family-education-handouts-2
- Centers for Disease Control and Prevention: www.cdc.gov/violenceprevention/aces/index.html
- The National Child Traumatic Stress Network: www.nctsn.org/resources

---

they should take to care for themselves. The written plan will serve as a concrete reminder of what you discussed during your visit.

In the context of the medical home and caring for kids with special health care needs, the shared care plan is a written document that is created collaboratively with the primary care clinician, patient, behavioral health clinician, and other team members. This document is then given to the patient or family to help them in their ongoing care. In medical care coordination, it would include people who are involved in the patient's care, information to help the patient or family manage an exacerbation of their medical condition, and goals for their own self-care and health promotion. In the context of trauma, the shared care plan is essentially a document that covers the steps in safety planning that we've just discussed.

You'll find a template in Appendix K that will help get you started. Consider having the steps of the safety plan on one side of the page and the patient's completed Circles of Support on the reverse. The care plan should also be explicit about who takes responsibility for contacting resources and when to expect that to happen; it helps to ensure that no balls get dropped in the process, like if a family thinks that someone in your office is going to contact a community resource when you're anticipating that they will do it themselves.

Expanding the Care Team: Care Coordinators, Community Health Workers, and Peer Navigators

True care coordination involves helping patients and families navigate the health care system and all the other systems that intersect in a patient's life. Again, there are great resources for getting care coordination going within your practice, so we'll focus on the role of these team members in helping families that have experienced trauma. Needless to say, care coordination is a fair amount of work, so you'll need some staff to help.

Traditionally, care coordinators have been staff members dedicated to assisting patients who experience medical complexity, but it's not a stretch to extend those same principles and workflows to patients with trauma. In fact, the science of trauma and adversity would say that trauma leads to myriad medical conditions that add to a patient's complex needs, and medical complexity is conversely traumatizing to patients. Depending on the size of your practice, there may be one person who fits the care coordinator role into other responsibilities; larger practices will likely require a team. In my practice of almost 30 clinicians, we have a team of referral and care coordinators who have distinct roles in helping patients with community resources, mental health, or medical needs. Some days it's still not enough, but it would be a lot to try to handle without their help. Keep in mind that continuity of care is important for these families, so try to assign them to one clinician and one care coordinator; this way, families don't have to start over with their story every time they access care in the clinic.

Some practices are starting to include community health workers (CHWs) as unique team members who function as an adjunct to medical care coordinators, which is a promising practice for becoming a trauma-responsive office. The CDC defines a CHW as the following:

> [A] frontline public health worker who is a trusted member or has a particularly good understanding of the community served. A CHW serves as a liaison between health and social services and the community to facilitate access to services and to improve the quality and cultural competence of service delivery.[7]

As such, *community health worker* is a broad term that encompasses many types of health care professionals including promotoras, doulas, peer wellness navigators, and others. They generally work in concert with medical and mental health clinicians, which allows us to focus on more specialized tasks. Community health workers, being members of the community they serve, are often more trusted with sensitive information than those of us with a lot of letters behind our names. In Santa Barbara, CA, 77% of families with trauma histories accepted preventive services offered via wellness navigators.[8] Community health workers are often more in touch with the nuances of culturally specific care than we are, and they often readily know the resources available within their communities. The best CHWs have lived experience navigating the different systems of care and use that experience to coach families.

Alternatively called *wellness navigators, peer navigators,* or even *ACE navigators,* these individuals can help by meeting with families, eliciting their specific needs, connecting families with resources, and tracking referrals. Ideally, they would also help in some of the shared care planning process. They are often trained in enrolling patients and families in state and federal assistance programs to help with SDOH needs. To date, most of the CHWs are funded by public health or grant programs, but some Medicaid agencies are beginning to include CHWs in reimbursement policies.

Referral Tracking

In my opinion, referral tracking is one of the most labor-intensive parts of being a high-functioning medical home. At a minimum, it involves keeping track of all the referrals you make to outside clinicians and then figuring out a workflow to ensure that the patient made it to the appointment and that you got a note back from the specialist. That's the simple version of referral tracking, since you can passively wait to see if a note came back from the specialist, mark that referral as complete, and then follow up with families only where you don't see that information come into the chart. It's a little more complicated when you're dealing with trauma and referring to mental health clinicians and CBOs. A CBO isn't in any way required to tell you that they contacted a family, so you'll want to take a proactive approach to follow-up to ensure patients receive needed care.

In spite of being labor intensive, doing appropriate referral tracking has some real benefits. First and foremost, there is evidence that soft-touch referrals (giving patients a contact number or a handout) don't often result in patients resolving their social needs. There are a lot of reasons for this: the patient may experience shame or embarrassment in contacting the resource themselves, they may not understand the need for the referral or what the resource can offer, the resource may have eligibility requirements that we didn't take into consideration, the resource may have access or capacity problems, or the resource didn't fit with the patient or family priorities. Tracking referral completion can help you identify what barriers families experience while accessing CBOs, and it may influence what CBOs you refer to in the future depending on that organization's responsiveness and ability to meet family needs.

The general process is to document the patient information and the resource being referred to in some sort of tracking system like an electronic spreadsheet, give the family the information about the resource and what they need to do to access it, and then follow up with the family by phone to ensure that the referral was completed. If the family accessed the resource and got what they needed, you're done for now. Families often make their decisions about accessing a resource within a few days of the referral being placed, so it may be helpful to do the first follow-up call within that time frame to help reinforce the need for the referral, answer any questions, and assess whether the family needs any assistance with the process. If the family attempted to access the resource but experienced a barrier, you would either assist the family in contacting the referral resource or redirect them to an alternate resource. Even when a family has successfully contacted and engaged a community resource, it's important to still provide follow-up to the family to ensure that the service is still meeting the family's needs. This is particularly true for resources for social driver needs; food and housing insecurity may be fluid from month to month or even from day to day.

If you have referral coordinators, care coordinators, or CHWs on your team, this responsibility often falls to them. The way you track can be as simple as a spiral notebook: I've worked with practices that put a patient sticker on the notebook, write down the resource they referred to, and then check off when they reach the family and confirm that they accessed the resource. Simple electronic spreadsheets are another option; if those spreadsheets are on a shared drive, multiple team members can access them and contribute to the work. There's a sample spreadsheet that was created as part of the AAP Addressing Social Health and Early Childhood Wellness project, which can be accessed here: https://view.officeapps.live.com/op/view.aspx?src = https % 3A % 2F % 2Fdownloads.aap.org % 2FDOCHW % 2FASHEWKD4.5.1.xlsx&wdOrigin = BROWSELINK.

Conclusions

It's important to be prepared to support patients and families that have experienced trauma. Identifying patients and families that have experienced trauma is the first step in ensuring they receive appropriate care; however, their ongoing care requires specific medical home activities like tracking and care coordination. Families in crisis often have difficulties finding the resources and supports they need; one of the core responses of the pediatric medical home is to offer support during these times. As we mentioned at the beginning of this chapter, the same care coordination workflows used for medically complex kids (creating shared care plans, including safety planning, and helping ensure that patients connect to needed resources) should be used for patients and families that experience trauma. While labor intensive, these principles of care coordination greatly benefit families. You will need team members who are assigned the specific care coordination tasks; this may require tracking down funding for additional staff. Community health workers are a great option for helping patients achieve their goals, and they help clinicians and integrated behavioral health professionals focus on more specialized tasks related to patient care.

Questions to Consider

1. Do you have the appropriate staff to conduct care coordination functions? If not, whom do you need to hire to fill this role?

2. What funding do you need to support these roles?

3. What shared care plan template works best for your patient and practice needs? What common emergency or crisis lines are in your area that need to be included in the resource section of your shared care plan?

4. Do you have the contact information for your local child protective services agency? What are the specifics of the mandatory reporting laws in your state?

5. What is the best way to track referrals to CBOs for your practice, considering the staff and resources you have at your disposal?

References

1. Trzeciak S, Mazzarelli A. *Compassionomics: The Revolutionary Scientific Evidence That Caring Makes a Difference.* Studer Group; 2019

2. American Academy of Pediatrics. *Helping Foster and Adoptive Families Cope With Trauma.* American Academy of Pediatrics, Dave Thomas Foundation for Adoption; 2016. Accessed March 20, 2024. https://downloads.aap.org/AAP/PDF/hfca_foster_trauma_guide.pdf

3. Siegel DJ, Bryson TP. *The Whole-Brain Child: 12 Revolutionary Strategies to Nurture Your Child's Developing Mind, Survive Everyday Parenting Struggles, and Help Your Family Thrive.* Bantam Books; 2012

4. Perciavalle V, Blandini M, Fecarotta P, et al. The role of deep breathing on stress. *Neurol Sci.* 2017;38(3):451–458 PMID: 27995346 doi: 10.1007/s10072-016-2790-8

5. Ma X, Yue ZQ, Gong ZQ, et al. The effect of diaphragmatic breathing on attention, negative affect and stress in healthy adults. *Front Psychol.* 2017;8:874 PMID: 28626434 doi: 10.3389/fpsyg.2017.00874

6. Greene R. Collaborative & Proactive Solutions. Accessed March 20, 2024. https://www.cpsconnection.com/ross-greene

7. Centers for Disease Control and Prevention. Community health worker resources. Reviewed August 29, 2023. Accessed March 20, 2024. https://www.cdc.gov/chronicdisease/center/community-health-worker-resources.html

8. Barnett ML, Kia-Keating M, Ruth A, Garcia M. Promoting equity and resilience: wellness navigators' role in addressing adverse childhood experiences. *Clin Pract Pediatr Psychol.* 2020;8(2):176–188 PMID: 34194889 doi: 10.1037/cpp0000320

Chapter 11

Pulling It All Together

R.J. Gillespie, MD, MHPE, FAAP, and Amy King, PhD

> *Always work hard on something uncomfortably exciting.*
> **Larry Page**

R.J.: Early into my journey of implementing resilience interventions in my daily practice, I'm sitting across from the mother of a 9-month-old. I've been diligent about teaching the baseball analogy, being a baby observer, bids for attention, and time-ins at each of her previous well-child visits. Mom leans in and asks, "What are we going to learn about today?" The interventions are obviously landing well with this family, so she's eager to hear more. It's a reminder that we don't approach building early relational health (ERH) as a single effort in just one visit; rather, it's the 100 little doses we keep talking about. Giving caregivers a single, simple, developmentally appropriate tool to work on at each visit is key. And, in my experience, the parents and caregivers love it.

Amy: If caregivers and children are players on a team with pediatricians, then the pediatricians are the coaches. And these coaches experience increased competency when they have tools that nurture families and help them thrive. One physician told me that her patients put the intervention reminders on their fridge and look forward to the next "lesson" on ways to build resilience. Another has delighted in telling me stories about how talking with caregivers about relational health and connection has transformed his practice and relationship with his patients. In alignment with the guidance of the American Academy of Pediatrics (AAP), we want to build these buffering relationships early and often: 100 little doses, as R.J. points out. When pediatricians feel equipped to respond when adversity is present and to guide or coach parents on ways to respond to stressful events, adversity, or trauma, they're increasing the family's internal capacity to heal past hurts and create new patterns of relating with their child and family.

R.J.: Up to this point, we've shared a lot of interventions, tweaks to anticipatory guidance, surveillance questions, and critical screening and assessment tools that make up a family's relational health history (RHH). On the surface, it looks like a lot. In this chapter, we're going to pull it all together into a roadmap of how these interventions and assessment tools look over the first 6 years after birth. The RHH you're obtaining from a family is meant to be a longitudinal and flexible process over the child's life, rather than a comprehensive history taken or all your ERH promotion done at a single visit. Because you see families early and often, you have a unique opportunity to observe, encourage, and collect this information over time.

Within the AAP Bright Futures recommendations[1] are 5 priority themes to address at each of the well-child visits. The table of interventions and screening tools you're about to see is aligned with some of the priority themes at each visit; this is done not to dismiss the remaining themes but rather to highlight which of the themes are relevant to the ERH promotion work you're going to be doing in practice. The table will also help you in your quality improvement efforts that we'll describe in Chapter 15, Implementation Nuts and Bolts, as you'll be able to assess what you're already doing and see what you need to implement to make your RHH more complete. There are not always clear periodicity recommendations for some of the screening tools; we've marked these in the table, and they're meant to represent what has worked in my practice. Some of the interventions are also listed more than once—partly because it's OK to reinforce some of these key messages but also to indicate there's some flexibility in when you actually implement them based on how much time you have in a visit. There are some ages where a couple of interventions are listed; this again is to offer some flexibility in how you implement interventions, including how you align your interventions with what the parents or care-givers are most interested in hearing.

Amy: As R.J. points out, interventions are introduced early, at developmentally appropriate intervals, and then revisited often. We want to encourage families to go back to tools, rethink ways they're engaging with their children, and reinforce interactions that build relational health and improve social-emotional (SE) development over time. Special time (or time-ins, as R.J. mentions) represents a fabulous way for caregivers to interact with their children at any age, but how that looks differs over time. For instance, special time with a baby might be playing and splashing in the bath while narrating coos and giggles. Special time for a teen might be shooting hoops together or going for a drive. Both are critically important and build connection. So, we want to keep reminding and encouraging parents to revisit these interventions in little doses.

I notice that the more pediatricians use the interventions, the nimbler they become. For instance, we introduce a tool that explores parenting styles and discipline as early as 12 months. It's a strength-based way to reflect with caregivers about how they approach discipline, not only encouraging positive discipline but also modeling the continuum of styles from controlled to permissive and from distant to warm. One physician mentioned to me that she was struggling with a father and his son who was steadily gaining weight, with a body mass index in the highly obese range. She was worried about the eating patterns of this young boy and had tried many times to communicate about nutrition, activity levels, and healthy choices. Then, she reported to me, she had an aha moment. She pulled out the card that reviews parenting approaches and reflected with Dad about how he had been parented and how he thought he approached his son now. He shared with her that his parents had been quite militant in their approach, so he tended to be more permissive. Suddenly, his eyes lit up and he looked at her and said, "I'm doing it with food too, right?" Then they were able to partner on a more balanced way to approach food and activity; they not only provided lots of warmth and love, with no "bad" choices, but also set some boundaries and parameters on sugary, processed foods. The physician said she felt such greater competence and collaboration with this approach than she had with more traditional approaches to food and activity. And she was aligned with Dad to make different choices.

R.J.: Always put the family's agenda first, then include some key conversations to get deeper into the caregiver's concerns. That may mean that you don't get to every intervention at every visit if you run out of time (practice some self-compassion on this one), but I've found this approach to promoting ERH in well-child visits to be a lot more rewarding and satisfying than our traditional approach to well-child care. It's fun being able to provide something practical to caregivers, so I always prioritize these interventions in my visits. Plus, I've found that a lot of the interventions line up with things the family was curious about in the first place.

The Roadmap

R.J.: Here it is: **Table 11-1** shows the way I pull this all together in practice. I've included a chapter number for the interventions we've already discussed.

You may already have some interventions or scripts that work for you—so be sure to include ones that are already in your repertoire. The table also doesn't represent all the screening tools we use in practice (eg, dental risk assessments, tuberculosis and lead risk screenings) but rather represents the screenings and assessments that relate specifically to ERH. You'll want to keep those other tools in mind as you're choosing the schedule that works for your practice. We'll go more into the specifics of implementation in Chapter 15, Implementation Nuts and Bolts.

Table 11-1. The Roadmap

Age	Relational Health History Screening Tools or Assessments	Anticipatory Guidance Highlight/ Intervention	Bright Futures[1] Priority Alignment	Chapter to Find It in This Book
Newborn period	PMDs Food and diaper insecurity[a]	Circles of Support	Parent and family health and well-being SDOH	9
2 wk	PMDs Food and diaper insecurity[a]	Parent self-care/ baseball analogy	Parent and family health and well-being SDOH	8—Box 8-1
2 mo	PMDs Food and diaper insecurity[a]	Being a baby observer	Parent and family health and well-being Infant behavior and development SDOH	9
4 mo	PMDs Food and diaper insecurity[a] Caregiver trauma history[a]	Education about trauma and PCEs Bids for attention	Infant behavior and development (infant and parent communication) SDOH	8—Trauma Education section 6—Table 6-1
6 mo	PMDs Food and diaper insecurity[a] SE health[a]	Time-ins	Infant behavior and development (communication and early literacy) SDOH	8—Positive Parenting section
9 mo	Developmental screening	Time-ins Beginning discipline	Infant behavior and development Discipline	8—Positive Parenting section 5
12 mo	SDOH[b]	Beginning discipline Mealtime routines	SDOH Feeding (transition to family meals)	5 8—Nutrition section
15 mo	SE health[a]	Bedtime routines and reading Review of special time	Sleep routines Communication and social development	8—Sleep and Caregiver Self-Care section
18 mo	Developmental screening Autism screening	Positive parenting/ handling tantrums	Communication and social development Temperament, behavior, and discipline	8—Positive Parenting section
24 mo	SDOH[b] Autism screening SE health[a]	Looking Beyond the Behavior	Temperament and behavior SDOH	8—Positive Parenting section
30 mo	Developmental screening	Special time "Shark music"	Social development promotion Language promotion and communication	8—Positive Parenting section 12

Continued on the next page

Table 11-1 (*continued*)

Age	Relational Health History Screening Tools or Assessments	Anticipatory Guidance Highlight/ Intervention	Bright Futures[1] Priority Alignment	Chapter to Find It in This Book
3 y	SDOH[b]	Building family connections and routines	SDOH Playing with siblings and peers	8—Trauma Education section
4 y	SDOH[b] SE health[a]	I Love You Rituals/ I Love You No Matter What! "Highs and lows"/ "roses and thorns"	SDOH School readiness (ie, feelings, opportunities to socialize)	8—Healthy Relationships section 8—Nutrition section
5 and 6 y	SDOH[b]	Yolky Feelings Flipping Your Lid	SDOH Development and mental health (patience and control over anger)	9 8—Trauma Education section

Abbreviations: PMD, peripartum mood disorder; SDOH, social drivers of health; SE, social-emotional.

[a] No clear guidelines exist for periodicity of this tool/assessment; this is what has worked for us.

[b] No clear guidelines exist for periodicity of SDOH tools, with the exception of recommendations that The Hunger Vital Sign be used at every visit (https://frac.org/aaptoolkit).

After eliciting any caregiver questions and concerns, I recommend starting your ongoing RHH taking with some opening questions to probe for any changes that have happened since the last time you talked with the family. If you've identified specific family challenges in the past, ask for updates about those as well. Following are some sample questions:

- How are you doing emotionally?
- How's everyone in your family? Have there been any big changes in the family?
- How are you coping with the challenges of parenting?
- Tell me about some parenting successes you've had lately.
- What have you done for fun together as a family?

You will, of course, have families that are new to you and your practice at varying ages, so you won't always have the opportunity to do all the interventions in the table with every family. I use some of these opening questions to assess where they are in their parenting journey, identify what challenges they may be dealing with, and then pick an intervention that is appropriate for their needs. As Amy has mentioned, many of the interventions in the table are applicable to varying ages, but they look different depending on the developmental stage, so you can pull them out and modify them as often as applicable when the situation requires you to. Catch-up assessment and screening tools may be applicable to these new families as well, depending on family needs—so consider using SE screening tools and social drivers of health (SDOH) surveys at other visits than the ones we suggest, depending on your clinical judgment.

A Few General Principles of Screening and Assessment Tools

R.J.: In previous chapters, we've talked about screening and assessment tools that you'll need for the components of your RHH, such as peripartum mood disorders, SDOH, and SE health tools. We've also talked about assessing caregiver trauma, resilience, and PCEs through assessment surveys or surveillance questions. I'm going to back up a little bit and remind you of a few basic principles of screening and assessment tools to make the workflow go a little more smoothly. Remember that each of these tools is a part of a bigger picture when it comes to an overall RHH for the family, so consider how the information you obtain relates to other pieces of information you've collected in the past, rather than discrete data points.

First of all, screening and assessment tools should be applied universally, to all patients. You can't assume that you'll be able to tell which caregivers are experiencing depression, or which ones are struggling with social drivers, just by looking at them. As Amy points out in Chapter 3, Getting Your Organization Ready: Creating Compassionate Pediatric Practices, we want to assume that trauma is ubiquitous and that most people have experienced adversity, a social driver, and/or a struggle with anxiety and depression. Just screen everyone; you will keep your own biases in check by doing these tools universally, and you won't offend the patients who aren't having these problems—they "get it" even if things are going well for them. It's also easier to reassure the caregiver who is worried or concerned about the questions if you can state that they're something you ask of all your patients and that you aren't making assumptions about the caregiver who is sitting in front of you.

Second, be sure to include messaging about the tool itself. This includes scripts to give to the person handing out the tool (whether that's front desk or nursing staff), so they can not only explain the tool to the caregiver but also answer basic questions about it. I've found that cover letters—or even a brief sentence or two—for a lot of the tools are helpful for explaining the tool, why you're asking the questions, and what you intend to do with the information. You can include statements about confidentiality or that they can opt out of a tool if they choose, as needed. To note, Chapter 2, Addressing Barriers, points out ways to prepare your staff to answer questions about why we're screening for RHH. We encourage your clinic to ensure that everyone understands the importance of the tools you're using.

Finally, make sure you've matched all your screening and assessment tools to resources. We've said this before, but it bears repeating: you absolutely must be able to answer the question of what you're going to do with the information. This is a great place to lean on a care manager, behavioral health consultant, or social worker if you're part of a larger organization.

Conclusions

R.J.: We've covered a lot of ground in how to do RHHs and how you use resilience-based interventions to build ERH between caregivers and kids. Now you've seen how it all pulls together into a longitudinal curriculum of little doses that are spread out between all the well-child visits in the first 6 years after birth. Each of the interventions we've referenced is deliberately designed to align with the child's developmental trajectory, restore trajectories that may be off track because of adversity or trauma, and align with the Bright Futures recommended priority areas for each well-child visit. Implementing all the interventions is a major transformation to how you do well-child care; while it may be hard to imagine implementing them all, it may also be difficult to prioritize which to do first (I mean, they're all so good, right?). For now, keep it simple by picking 1 or 2 new interventions to try; we'll talk more about implementation in small steps in Chapter 15, Implementation Nuts and Bolts.

Questions to Consider

1. What tools are already in your toolbox for promoting ERH for your families? Do any of them need updating or replacing?

2. What screening and assessment tools are you already using that contribute to RHHs? What gaps are there?

3. If you were to pick 1 new intervention to implement, which would it be? Which one feels like a good fit for your practice style? Which visits could be enhanced by adding an intervention?

Reference

1. Hagan JF Jr, Shaw JS, Duncan PM, eds. *Bright Futures: Guidelines for Health Supervision of Infants, Children, and Adolescents.* 4th ed. American Academy of Pediatrics; 2017 doi: 10.1542/9781610020237

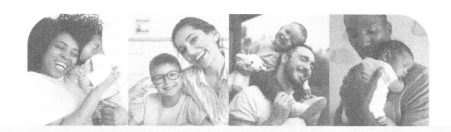

PART 4

Building Clinical Skills: Incorporating "The Most Important Medicine" Into Practice

In this section, we're going to tackle skill building for you and your colleagues. Since relational health histories (RHHs), and, particularly, addressing trauma in practice, are likely new to your skill set, some specific skill building support is warranted.

Some key points to consider: First, listening is therapeutic—it actually helps people heal. We've talked about this already, but it bears repeating. Second, being able to listen effectively is the key strategy for avoiding re-traumatization of patients or caregivers who have experienced trauma. Finally, bringing your whole self to this work will make you more effective as a clinician. To address these key points, Amy will talk about the art of listening and present the idea of "humanbeingness" in her chapters. This approach is perhaps contrary to how we've been trained in medicine—where we're expected to keep strict barriers between ourselves and our patients—but it's a transformative way to look at how we care for our families.

Again, the primary skill that is required of you to effectively address trauma in a clinical setting is your ability to listen. That comes from 2 interrelated concepts—not only how to enhance your listening skills but also how to compartmentalize challenging conversations to prevent burnout and overwhelm. That means taking care of yourself to be available to hear the difficult stories that may arise in your day-to-day work of addressing RHHs.

In case you're a novice to quality improvement (QI) in practice, we've included a chapter on implementation because a big component of what you're going to be doing is motivating change within your practice (see Chapter 15, Implementation Nuts and Bolts). For many clinicians, trauma doesn't feel like it's naturally in our wheelhouse, as we discussed earlier in Chapter 2, Addressing Barriers. Now that you're becoming a champion for trauma-responsive care in your office, you'll need some additional strategies and tools for motivating the rest of your colleagues as well as your practice's administrative team. We'll include QI basics to help you plan out changes in your practice when it comes to implementing the assessment tools and interventions that we've been exploring. We'll also address sustainability: once you've started this work, you'll need to engage in continuous QI to continue your trauma-responsive journey as the field evolves.

We've all been trained to disconnect ourselves from work or to behave in superhuman ways. We hope you find practical tools in these chapters so that you have to do neither.

Chapter 12

The Art of Listening

Amy King, PhD

Being heard is so close to being loved that for the average person,
they are almost indistinguishable.
David Augsburger

Pediatrician: I'm not a therapist.

Me: I know you're not a therapist; you don't have to be.

Pediatrician: But what if they *(the patient or patient's parent)* start talking about traumatic events? It's like opening a can of worms.

Me: They already tell you so many hard things and you already advise on difficult matters; we're just giving it a different frame now.

Pediatrician: What if I don't know the right thing to say?

Me: What if you don't have to say anything?

Pediatrician: [*blank stare*]

Me: What if you just ask questions, validate experiences, listen, and provide resources when asked?

Pediatrician: [*hesitantly*] I can do that. I already do that.

Sometime after this discussion, after putting this realization into practice and gaining some confidence, this same pediatrician told me, "Sometimes, after I ask my patients about ACEs, trauma, food insecurities, etc, they feel better *simply because I asked, then listened empathically.* And often when I ask if they want to talk more or need resources, they tell me that 'just knowing my doctor asked and cares' made them feel better."

In this chapter, we'll review fundamental concepts around listening. Being a compassionate, present listener is both a skill and an intervention itself. When done thoughtfully, it shifts the felt sense of safety between our patient and us. It creates a holding space that says, "Whatever you bring to this space is welcome." Once we review these fundamental concepts, we'll discuss 2 themes that often emerge and are related to how we listen: responding to positive findings on screenings and thoughtfully replying to disclosures of trauma. At the end, you'll have some tangible tools and reassurances that you can do this work and, likely, already embody so many of these necessary skills.

The Power of Listening

Stories create connection. Creating narrative and sharing history lay the foundations of healing. As health care professionals, we often look for cures, diagnoses, and treatment plans. It can be easy to forget that listening is a therapeutic treatment as well. Especially as we encourage and explore trauma-informed and trauma-responsive care in pediatric settings, listening proves to be an invaluable tool. We're putting our "intervention" symbol in the margin here to call it out, but really, this whole chapter constitutes an intervention.

Listening is a nonverbal skill. We do it with our whole body, and 90 % of all communication is nonverbal. So, *how* we listen proves to be critically important. I remember, back in my early days of graduate education, we endured an entire semester on nonverbal communication. For 3 hours a week over 12 weeks, faculty watched us through a one-way mirror as we interacted with clients, patients, students—whomever we could recruit to practice our listening skills. Then, as we engaged with our pseudo-patients, the phone next to us would ring and, on the other end, constructive feedback was provided about our listening skills:

Sit forward to look interested.

Don't cross your arms; your client might think you are angry.

Slow the cadence of your voice; that's more reassuring.

Don't look away.

Explain why you're writing things down.

And on and on…

In working with patients and families that have experienced trauma, these skills prove to be crucial for building alliance and trust and creating a space where people feel genuinely heard. The great news? These skills are teachable and learnable.

Think about how safety feels. Maybe you were chatting over coffee with your best friend or being embraced by a loved one. Maybe you asked for guidance from a trusted colleague or felt protected by a friend. Can you remember the last time you felt safe in the presence of another person? It's likely that this person created an environment that lent itself to physical and emotional safety. Together, you engaged in a dance where the environment felt safe, you leaned into the safety, the listener reciprocated, you shared more, you felt safe because of their response, and the dance continued. There are many ways we create safety in professional relationships, and listening provides a fundamental pathway toward safety.

Bessel Van der Kolk says that our bodies are continuously mapping what feels safe and what feels dangerous.[1] Stephen Porges explains that our bodies are shaped by past experiences and current cues from our environment, a process called *neuroception,* how we read the environment and determine if it is safe.[2] In Chapter 3, Getting Your Organization Ready: Creating Compassionate Pediatric Practices, we talk about becoming "maps of safety." Especially for individuals who've experienced complex trauma, paying attention to these cues and getting them right are survival mechanisms. Therefore, we must practice ways to listen artfully and become a map of safety for our patients and their families.

Components of Listening

Listen by Watching

As a clinician, you've honed an attunement skill of observing: watching for pathology, difference, and symptoms of physical ailments, disorders, and conditions. The same skill applies to trauma: we can learn to listen by watching for cues. For instance, even though you know that adverse experiences from childhood may increase the likelihood of certain diseases or poor health trajectories, it's only through a fine-tuned observational skill that you can parse out critical factors such as when, for how long, or how severe the adversities were that you noted.[3] And then, with increased awareness, you can ask questions that will inform you regarding who was there, what buffers were present, and so forth. You're watching and listening for both adversities and resilience builders. This process enables you to draw out specific information to circle back to that might promote wellness for the child and/or family or might inform what resources are needed to address stress within the family system.

Watching for our patients' internalized states is something that Hibbard and colleagues pointed out as critically important to identify emotional abuse.[4] These authors found that factors such as hostile parenting (eg, shouting at a child, spurning them, calling names) as well as abuse by omission and neglect were the number one predictor of emotional abuse. Emotional abuse correlates strongly with internalizing behaviors such as anxiety, harmful substance use, and attachment disorders.

Here's a practical example of how a clinician might observe and intervene regarding concerns about emotional abuse. Consider a parent responding to a child with language such as "He's such a jerk; I don't know what to do with him" or "Go ahead and open the drawer again and see what happens." Knowing that this type of emotional abuse from a caregiver to a child predicts long-term mental health difficulties, you may be more likely to find moments to intervene and educate caregivers about discipline styles. Or you might use the opportunity to ask more about the caregiver's family experience growing up and offer tools, support groups, or education. I might say something like this: "I notice that you seem frustrated with your toddler's behavior. I wonder if you respond with a bit more curiosity about the behavior, if they'll respond differently. You could say something like 'When you open drawers like that, you could get hurt. Can I help you get something?'" Or, to the parent using abusive language, I might offer, "I get that he seems like he's behaving like a jerk, and it's OK to feel overwhelmed with how to help. As a parent myself, I get to the end of my rope too. I've found that if I focus on behavior instead of referring to my child's character, we have more positive interactions and I feel less angry toward them. Let's try this: 'You're acting pretty feisty right now and I'm not sure how to help. What do you want Mommy to do?'" It's important that we empathize with parents while providing positive guidance and ideas. (See the acronym NOTES in Chapter 5, Guiding Principles of Resilience Education.)

Note From R.J.

This is so important—to learn how to read the exam room and respond appropriately. In his book *Your Brain at Work*,[5] David Rock describes this interpretation of body language as recognizing that a person is "leaning in" or "leaning back." If a person is leaning in, that means they feel safe and secure. You know what this comfortable, relaxed body language looks like. You also know the body language of leaning back—that is, what it looks like when a person feels under threat: arms crossed, no eye contact, short answers—all the things Amy's nonverbal communication class told her not to do. When you're assessing relational histories in practice, a patient or caregiver having completed (or even just read) the questions on an assessment tool about social drivers of health, depression, or trauma may already trigger that kind of reaction before you even walk into the room. It's one of the potential harms of caregiver trauma inquiries in the first place, particularly if the respondent doesn't know from the start that they can opt out.

The importance of that observation comes in how you approach the visit from then on. If a patient is leaning back, they aren't in receive mode—they won't be able to hear any of the advice or recommendations you're eager to give them. In those cases, it's more important to connect with the caregiver or patient first. Listen empathetically to their concerns. Reassure them about their privacy and confidentiality, what you're going to do with the information, and that they don't have to share anything they aren't comfortable with (which, ideally, should be part of your cover letter, or whatever scripting you use when introducing the questions in the first place, to give "choice and voice" about whether they're going to answer the questions at all). Let them know you're always willing to listen should they choose to talk in the future.

If the patient is leaning in, on the other hand, you're golden. They're ready to hear what you have to say.

Listen With Our Whole Bodies

What we do with our bodies when we are listening is just as important as the act itself. We know that individuals who have been maltreated have more heightened responses in the part of their brain that processes fear when they see angry faces. This means that as clinicians we should be aware of our body language and facial expressions because they may inadvertently communicate an environment that does not feel safe. Whole-body listening can be challenging. In a world of electronic health records, we are compelled to multitask. Often, multitasking is acceptable; but if you sense that someone is sharing a vulnerable story, they are implicitly asking you to reassure them they're safe. At times like these, listening with your whole body is important.

Ways to use our bodies and movements to create that felt sense of safety include the following:

- **Cast "warm eyes":** Soften your eyes toward the person who is speaking, looking down or slightly away at times to feel less intimidating; this creates empathy in your eyes.

- **Use a soft, calming voice:** Use a cadence that is slower than usual to let the speaker know that you are not scary; this speaks to their limbic system as it searches for cues of safety. Decrease your volume a bit, and make your pitch just a little higher.

- **Get down on the person's level:** Often we don't mean to, but we end up literally talking over people as professionals. Squat down by a child, pull up a chair or stool with a caregiver, sit next to or near a teenager, or simply lean forward.

- **Reassure safety:** This might seem implicit to you, but reassuring your patient that they are safe with you needs to be explicit. "I'm here," "You're safe," "You're not alone," and "It's not your fault" are all reassuring statements of safety that you can provide.

- **Give choices:** Often, a person who survived trauma is robbed of choice, which leads to feelings of helplessness. Provide choices to your patient whenever possible. It might be as simple as offering to give shots at the end or beginning of a visit or allowing choice around scheduling, screeners, or handouts.

- **Be predictable:** Do what you say you will. Follow through. These things create safety and show integrity. If you let a patient know you're going to call, follow up with laboratory results, see them in a week, or send materials to them, be sure to do so because you're building trust.

- **No fast movements:** People with histories of trauma have often experienced unwanted physical or sexual gestures. Let your patient know when you're going to touch them, how, and why. Move slowly and with permission. Explain every step.

- **Allow a safe person to be present:** Again, this may seem implicit, but offering to have another person in the room, whether it be a caregiver or trusted medical assistant, or inviting a spouse/partner or a behavioral health clinician to a future appointment can create an environment of trust because another safe person is present.

Listen With an Open Mind

In addition to being aware of what we're doing with our bodies, how we receive the information as well as what we do with it is equally important. Following are additional factors you might consider as a way to create safety with your patient or their family:

- **Set aside your own goals:** Whatever you might have in mind to cover today, if a caregiver arrives and begins talking about how their impending divorce is creating sleep disturbance and bed-wetting and children are witnessing hostile fights, it is important to delay your agenda and respond to the needs at hand. If you ignore the distress in the room and push forward with car seat safety, developmental milestones, or questions about kindergarten readiness, your patient and their caregiver will feel dismissed and you'll miss an opportunity to connect.

- **Don't personalize:** Often, people with histories of trauma can present in confusing or even frustrating ways. Caregivers may blame; teens may ignore medical advice or go completely against best practices; kids may shut down. In a trauma-responsive space, it's important that you know that how someone else is manifesting trauma has nothing to do with you. That's hard to remember, but if you can, it will help you depersonalize. You'll be able to stay in the moment with your patient or their caregiver and feel more helpful.

- **Respond to fears:** So much fear is expressed through anger. In previous chapters, you've seen that increasing staff awareness to this dynamic helps alleviate many mishaps. In an office visit, a teenager might brush you off, seem hostile or questioning, shut down, or withdraw. Often, the underlying issue is fear; and when we ask a simple question like "What's really going on?" it can get right to the heart of the matter.

- **Ask how you can help:** This is strongly related to our earlier discussion about providing choice. Often, people don't want us to tell them what to do; they want to be given choices and offered help. So many caregivers have told me that, often, they feel greatly cared for by being heard. Help or next steps may or may not be needed. Simply ask and allow your patient or their caregiver to be their own expert. Your patient notices if you listen for the purpose of caring versus listening as an agenda item. If they are comfortable charting their own course, often the physician can affirm and encourage this by asking, "How can I help with this?"

- **Acknowledge stress and pain:** We know that active listening has been shown to increase resilience during acute phases of stress. When a patient feels heard, they begin to heal. I still remember sitting with a young boy, forced to come to therapy because of his behavior in his home with foster parents. To me, it was clear that his behavior was a result of trauma and multiple miscommunications about unmet needs. When I offered to him how hard it must feel to talk with yet another new therapist, he relaxed a bit. And when I reassured him that we didn't have to talk about anything he didn't want to, he began to trust me a bit more. Finally, when I acknowledged how painful the loss of his parents was and that he never signed up for this circumstance, we began to build rapport. Acknowledgment of pain is often the first step toward a patient feeling validated and safe. It begins the healing process.

Listen Through Validation and Empathy

Patients are keenly aware of the difference between empathy and sympathy. To your patients, empathy exudes care, whereas sympathy indicates feeling sorry for them. Empathic listening means that you reflect the feelings of another person, show compassion, and validate their experience. Although your patient's, or their caregivers', experiences may be different from your own, it's important to validate their narrative as true and unique. You might say something like "Gosh, I remember those early days and how tough having a crying baby was. What has this been like for you?" or "That experience sounds really painful. Will you tell me more? What has helped you so far?" People's perception creates their reality, and validating their lived experience is crucial. Stay curious, ask questions, and acknowledge difficulties. When we validate experiences and provide empathy, we often bridge the gap between ourselves and the other person in the room.

Listen to Our Own Triggers

Trigger (or *activation*) is a therapeutic word conveying how our own history of trauma manifests when we hear stories of trauma from another individual. We could also refer to triggers as creating a state of activation in our nervous system when we're aroused or hypervigilant to cues. As we mentioned before, engaging in the work of trauma awareness, listening to stories, and eliciting stories from our patients and their families about complex trauma could certainly trigger us. Everyone has experienced adversity, so listening intently and purposefully to another person's story or disclosures—doing everything we've just described in this chapter—may inevitably cause discomfort and, sometimes, sharply painful reactions. The reactions (or activation) we experience may be a result of our own trauma we've experienced, past or unresolved, or the result of hearing suffering through the stories of others, what we refer to as *secondary trauma.*

When I work with pediatricians, I teach them to pay attention to their "shark music": if they were approaching a neutral stimulus, such as a body of water, but what they heard was ominous music indicating that a deadly shark was about to appear, the music would be a cue because it warns the person that something frightening is about to happen; in other words, it's a trigger.

If you're approaching a body of water and you hear shark music, you're not diving in, right? Your whole body tells you, "Don't go in there!" "It's not safe!" and "You'll get eaten alive!" Every part of your body tenses and signals danger. The same is true when our own trauma becomes activated. If I'm working with a patient's caregiver who has experienced domestic violence and I'm attempting to listen to her story, provide resources for the family, educate about how witnessing domestic violence can cause harm to children, and describe ways to break cycles of intergenerational trauma, I need to be aware of my own triggers. If my body and brain are activated and all I can see and hear is my mom crying when I was little or fearing my father, I'll feel overwhelmed, less helpful, and drained from the experience. By the way, it's a great time to offer Circles of Support for clinicians (see Chapter 9, Designing and Using Efficacious Interventions to Support Early Relational Health and Heal Trauma). We, too, need people we can process our experiences with, people whom we trust and whom we know will hold our stories in confidence.

The first step is recognizing when we're in an activated state. The second step is addressing our triggers so we can hear the shark music and not be activated but rather remain present with the patient or caregiver. Being aware of our own shark music helps us provide exceptional patient care because we're aware of what activates us and we have greater insight into some of the triggers our patients may experience. See Chapter 3, Getting Your Organization Ready: Creating Compassionate Pediatric Practices, and Chapter 13, Self-Care and Sharing Our Humanity, for more on this.

Defining shark music is helpful for parents too. From Circle of Security, shark music to parents is how their body elicits and experiences stress or activation from a cue.[6] Once parents can identify their shark music, they can decide to respond to the cue differently and create a more positive interaction with their child. Following is a story I often share with parents:

> "It's about 7 in the morning and I'm in a frenzy to get ready for work. I can hear my kids downstairs begin to fuss and fight about breakfast, sharing the bathroom and getting ready for school. My cortisol level begins to rise. I can hear my shark music, and this is what it tells me: I *know* things are going to go horribly wrong. I'm already running late for work; my kids are misbehaving and we're all going to have a terrible morning. Because my shark music is guiding my next response, I respond out of fear, frustration, and survival (similarly to how you would if you thought a shark was nearby). I go downstairs, yell at my children, threaten consequences if we don't leave on time, and send them both to their rooms. They're tearful and ashamed. And, just as I expected, our morning is off to a horrible start. However, once I begin to recognize my shark music, in my case, children yelling or a parent running late, I can decide how I want to respond differently and how I want the outcome to feel. In the same scenario, I recognize that I'm hearing shark music, but instead of responding to my children with anger, this is what I try: I go downstairs and say, 'Hey, you two, it's getting pretty loud down here and we have to leave for school

soon. How can I help?' Or I might try, 'Remember last night when we made a plan for the bathroom so we could be on time? Can we try that?' Or 'I'm really confused why you're using mean language with each other. It's really unkind. Let's try this a different way.' Having more positive, proactive responses with my kids allows me to enter the day with a greater sense of peace and a lot less shame. Shark music thwarted!"

Notice Whom We're Not Hearing

Part of being a trauma-aware professional means recognizing that many patients we see have histories of intergenerational trauma and historical trauma. We may have lived experiences that allow us to relate to these patients or we may not. It's important that we take inventory and increase awareness of people with histories of trauma, especially marginalized voices, which we may not recognize unless we make concerted efforts to do so. Following are some examples:

- A caregiver refuses to allow a vaccine for his child because of his distrust of the medical system based on a history of racial inequities within our health care system.
- Resources and handouts at a clinic are provided only in English, and patients are expected to navigate a health care system that is unfamiliar to them. Or a clinician uses a child as a translator for their caregivers.
- A teenager refuses to disclose important medical information about sexual behavior because she fears judgment about her sexual orientation.
- A single mother experiences criticism for her "lack of compliance" to treat her daughter's asthma with appropriate care and feels shamed. She's reported to child protective services for neglect.

Let's reframe one of these experiences into a more positive response. If you're sensing that a teenager is not disclosing important medical information about sexual behaviors, you might offer what you believe about sexual development, sexual health, partners, and relationships:

> "I've found that some of my patients are hesitant to talk with me about sex or partners because a lot of adults tend to judge them. I won't do that. Your sexual health is part of your overall physical health. And your sexual orientation is part of figuring out who you are. In my office, I believe that people should be able to love and have sexual, consenting relationships with whomever they choose. Please know that what we talk about is just between us. I won't disclose information about your partners or your sexuality without your permission. But I do want to help and be a supportive adult in your life when it comes to being physically, and sexually, healthy."

Applying the Art of Listening

To bring this matter full circle, listening offers a bridge of caring to our patients. Listening is made up of how we watch, what we do, how we respond, creating a space of empathy, recognizing our triggers, and making a commitment to listening to voices that may have been marginalized. Listening is an art, but it is an applied art. We practice it every day in our work and life.

> What I've realized in my work is that I simply need to ask a question, pass the tissues, and be quiet. Just listen. Listening is so powerful. —Dr Eric Wiser

Now that we've laid the foundation around listening from a trauma-informed perspective, let's use our skills to respond compassionately to 2 commonly experienced themes: how to define a positive screening finding from a trauma assessment and how to thoughtfully reply to disclosures of trauma.

Defining and Responding to Relational Health Histories or Disclosures of Trauma

A word of caution: When it comes to utilizing questionnaires about trauma in practice, there's a tendency to want to base your response workflow on how many adversities an individual endorses on the screening tool or on a set score based on that number of traumas. This comes from the tendency in the research to classify risk from the number of experienced ACEs: the more ACEs an individual has, the higher their risk for any number of health outcomes. Although this is true at a population level, it can be problematic at an individual level, and this is one of the reasons that ACE screening itself is controversial and not particularly helpful. In the paper *Beyond the ACE Score,* The National Child Traumatic Stress Network provides a beautiful overlay of additional adversities that families face as well as factors to consider when thinking about screening scores,[3] such as frequency of adversity; severity; access to other caring, supportive adults; and the length of time the trauma occurred. In R.J.'s practice, even though clinicians are asking about parental ACEs, we want to remind folks that asking about parental adversities is only *part* of a relational health history; it begins to validate experiences and open up further conversations about trauma and ways to intervene with support. We talked about these pitfalls of using ACE surveys in depth in Chapter 1, The ACE Debate and Ethical Considerations.

Since screening scores for trauma don't measure the frequency or severity of each trauma, a score of 1 could indicate a divorce—even an amicable one—or it can represent years of repeated sexual abuse. Are those 2 traumas equal? A person may have experienced severe bullying or houselessness but had strong, stable adult figures who helped them find meaning in and protection from those adversities. More advised is to screen for symptoms with measures and ask about strengths and supports.

The best way to decide how to respond to a "positive" score on your assessment tool is to ask the patient. They're an expert on how the adversity affected them and how it continues to do so. If you start with the assumption that any endorsed trauma is potentially significant to the patient, then your natural next response is to figure out what importance the patient places on that trauma. That means you should have a follow-up conversation about *any* disclosure, rather than rely on a potentially misleading score for your assessment tool. The conversation can proceed like this:

1. Thank the patient for sharing the disclosure with you. After all, you've clearly created a map of safety and a space that feels reassuring and empathic for your patient's disclosure.

2. Ask a follow-up question. It's best to follow up with an open-ended question to gauge their feelings about how the trauma impacted them. Felitti used the question "How did that affect you later in life?"[7] In R.J.'s assessment of parental ACEs, he starts with the question "Do any of these experiences still bother you now?" I ask, "Which of these would be helpful to talk about some more?" That way, we respond to any disclosure that patients share.

3. Remind the patient they're not alone. Reassure your patient that you're part of their health care team and want to help.

4. Ask them if they'd like to talk more or need additional resources. You'd be surprised at how often we, and other clinicians who ask questions about trauma, are told, "I don't want to talk more right now, but I'm glad someone else knows what I've been through. And I'm glad you're asking." It's often that straightforward. Being asked is a first step in healing. In Chapter 10, Supporting Families That Have Experienced Trauma, we covered targeted therapies for times when a different approach is needed. But for now, trust that listening is the best first step.

5. Create a safety plan if needed (see Chapter 10), assessing how the trauma currently impacts your patient.

It should go without saying that when a patient discloses a trauma, you should put aside your laptop or paper chart and listen attentively.

Note From R.J.

I've found that disclosures come in all shapes and sizes, so to speak. As Amy said, let the patient tell you how big their trauma was, rather than make assumptions.

One recent parent disclosure revealed that a mom not only had experienced all 10 of the classic ACEs and all 4 of our "expanded ACEs" but also was currently experiencing food, housing, and diaper insecurity. As she told me more about her story, it emerged that her preteen was born after she herself had been raped when she was only 12 years old, and she had been experiencing intermittent homelessness since that age.

If you haven't stopped to take a breath after reading that, please do so.

Clearly, it's a *lot* to untangle and is, to date, one of the biggest disclosures I've ever had, so I had the choice of dumping a bunch of resources on her or letting her prioritize what she needed and in what order. This is why we talk about the art of listening in the first place: the obvious, correct answer to this life test is to let Mom do the prioritizing.

Gentle readers, I know some of you are concerned for this mom, and others of you are concerned that you're going to face a disclosure like this and have the visit consume too much of your precious time, so I'll treat it as a teachable moment and walk through how I approached it. First of all, I asked the preteen to go out to the waiting room and check out the fish tanks to help Mom feel more comfortable with the rest of the conversation (this happened before she discussed the rape and houselessness history). I shut down my laptop and sat down, keeping my voice low and calm and maintaining eye contact with Mom. Remember the HELLPPP mnemonic from earlier in the book (see Chapter 2, Addressing Barriers)? I'll highlight the pieces I used in the dialogue. Feel free to pick apart my response to see how you would (and can) do better.

Me: Thank you so much for sharing this with me. You've truly endured quite a lot (EMPATHY). Have you ever talked with anyone about all of this?

Mom: No, I've never had the chance.

Me: Again, thank you for sharing this. I'm going to do what I can to help you (PARTNERSHIP), and I think we can provide you with some resources that would help (HOPE). What do you think would be most helpful to start with?

Mom: I'd like to have a counselor or someone I can talk to.

Me: I can help you find that. Would it be OK for me to pass your information to our mental health care coordinator? She knows all the counselors in the area and might be able to help find a match for you (PERMISSION).

Mom: Yes, I'd like that.

Me: You also said you're having some trouble with food and diapers. I can get you connected with some resources to help with that if you want. Would that be OK too (PERMISSION)?

Mom: Yes.

Me: OK. So, for now, I'm going to have our mental health care coordinator get some resources; she should call you in the next few days with some places you can go. I'll get your information to some food and diaper banks, so you should hear from them in the next few days as well (PLAN). Is there anything else you feel like you need right now?

Mom: Not that I can think of.

Me: We'll get those things started. If you can think of anything else you need along the way, let me know. I'm always here to help.

Now it's up to me to ensure that I—and my staff—follow through on my promises, so I set a reminder for myself to follow up in a few days to see if Mom got the resources she needed and to see if there was anything else she thought would be helpful.

Questions to Consider

1. Are you surprised that we use listening as a therapeutic tool? Are there ways we could hone our listening skills more by using one of the strategies listed in this chapter?

2. Are you aware of your own triggers that might come up (ie, your shark music) as you work with patients who have trauma histories?

3. What voices should we pay greater attention to in our practices?

4. How might you respond differently to disclosures of trauma using the information and guidance provided in this chapter?

References

1. Van der Kolk B. *The Body Keeps Score: Brain, Mind, and Body in the Healing of Trauma.* Penguin Random House; 2015
2. Porges SW. The polyvagal perspective. *Biol Psychol.* 2007;74(2):116–143 PMID: 17049418 doi: 10.1016/j.biopsycho.2006.06.009
3. Amaya-Jackson L, Absher LE, Gerrity ET, Layne CM, Halladay Goldman J. *Beyond the ACE Score: Perspectives From The NCTSN on Child Trauma and Adversity Screening and Impact.* National Center for Child Traumatic Stress; 2021
4. Hibbard R, Barlow J, Macmillan H, et al; American Academy of Pediatrics Child Abuse and Neglect; American Academy of Child and Adolescent Psychiatry. Psychological maltreatment. *Pediatrics.* 2012;130(2):372–378 PMID: 22848125 doi: 10.1542/peds.2012-1552
5. Rock D. *Your Brain at Work: Strategies for Overcoming Distraction, Regaining Focus, and Working Smarter All Day Long.* Harper Business; 2009
6. Zanetti CA, Powell B, Cooper G, Hoffman K. The Circle of Security intervention: using the therapeutic relationship to ameliorate attachment security in disorganized dyads. In: Solomon J, George C, eds. *Disorganized Attachment and Caregiving.* The Guilford Press; 2011:318–342
7. Felitti VJ, Anda RF, Nordenberg D, et al. Relationship of childhood abuse and household dysfunction to many of the leading causes of death in adults. The Adverse Childhood Experiences (ACE) study. *Am J Prev Med.* 1998;14(4):245–258 PMID: 9635069 doi: 10.1016/S0749-3797(98)00017-8

Chapter 13

Self-Care and Sharing Our Humanity

Amy King, PhD

My brokenness is a better bridge for people than my pretend
wholeness ever was.

Sheila Walsh

At the beginning of every training I do, I provide the following brief disclaimer:

> Anytime we deal with trauma, discuss its origin, or learn new ways to deliver trauma-informed care, there are inherent risks. Participants may feel triggered by the work or need space to process their own trauma, unresolved or current. Dr Amy is available for support and resources and can direct you toward specific assistance, should you need help. Please know that any person can choose to participate as much or as little as feels comfortable.

Heads nod, acknowledging the disclaimer. And yet, it feels impossible to prepare people for triggers that may arise. I feel protective of our collective process, I recognize the need for the important work we are embarking on, and I wish to create a space for us to deeply process what adversities we face and find compassion for those who face them as well. This work of providing trauma-informed care (TIC) is so completely transformational that I can feel it in my soul. Often, physicians approach me during and after trainings to express a variety of manifested feelings.

> I lost my husband and my children lost their father last year. It's affecting every aspect of my practice.

> My mom was beaten in front of me when I was little; now I see why every time I have a hunch about domestic violence, I feel sick.

> I was so harsh with a mom this morning who seemed angry and dismissive to her children. Now I get it.

> If I had known this earlier this morning, I would have changed the way I interacted with 3 different patients. It could have gone so differently.

As we've mentioned before, part of the readiness for practices is shoring up skills and tools for yourselves and your staff. But the first person to show compassion to is you.

Caring for Yourself

As medical experts and part of a larger health care system, we're not trained to engage in self-reflection on such adversities or in forms of self-care. We're trained to compartmentalize: there is heroism in long hours, delayed breaks, sleeplessness, and denial of food or of time with loved ones. We operate in a performative society that emphasizes outcomes and results above collective care. Martyrdom is celebrated. Medicine is seen as distinct from mental health, and taking time to look after ourselves may feel too vulnerable or may feel like a luxury we can't justify indulging in.

The emphasis on TIC and relational health shifts this dynamic to encourage us to reflect on past adversities and ways to mitigate relational trauma through protective relationships. Yet, the internal work of doing this is tough. It is hard work! And it's activating. If you've experienced your own trauma, which we all have in some capacity, then doing this work around becoming trauma informed, building awareness of childhood adversities, attuning to parental stress, and preparing your workforce to become more compassionate, engaged, and understanding is going to be very difficult if you haven't engaged in some self-reflection about your own adversities and begun to address the need to take care of your own whole self.

Before we can ask others (ie, our colleagues, our medical assistants [MAs], our staff) to do this important and hard work, we have to muck through it ourselves. So, where do we begin? I always encourage physicians to take inventory of their own childhood adversities. I don't ask them to "disclose" to me or anyone else what they've endured; rather, I ask it for their own self-reflection. If you acknowledge (even if you haven't shared) what you've been through— what trauma, complexities, challenging experiences, or stressors you've experienced—you'll have a greater sense of what may become activated in the work you do. What matters most is, how have you dealt with these adversities? Who was there for you? Have you processed and grieved and come to terms with any of them? What we know for sure as mental health experts is that if we have not attempted to resolve our own past trauma, it will get activated in the important work we do as we ask others to navigate theirs.

The other point of encouragement lies in knowing the importance of wellness—internally, relationally, and organizationally.

So, what are the barriers to these kinds of wellness? Often, there are messages that self-care and personal wellness are selfish or self-absorbed. Cultural messages tell us that we need to take care of *all* our other obligations, and then, if there is time left over, we can take care of ourselves in some capacity. We're encouraged to put the needs of others before our own and then pick up little scraps of time for "self-indulgences." But self-care is not selfish; it's absolutely necessary. In this chapter, we'll focus on care for physicians. In our chapter on getting your organization ready (Chapter 3), we focused on ways to address more systemic change too.

We often end up as healers and helpers because we want to give of ourselves to others. We feel compelled to help others, heal others, find cures, sit with pain, create change, and give of ourselves. But often that comes with a message of "to no end." One aspect that becomes clear over time, however, is that if we practice total selflessness, the end result is burnout.

The Baseball Analogy for Self-Care

I encourage physicians to think of their own wellness like a baseball field. Similar to Circles of Support, layers of self-care begin close and move outward—or, in this analogy, around the bases. On first base lies whatever you enjoy doing that fills up your cup. It need not be traditional forms of self-care such as eating better or sleeping more; nor should it be elaborate ways to escape from our lives (eg, "I'll go to this amazing yoga retreat for 3 weeks and then I'll feel better"). Rather, self-care should be consistent, sustainable steps toward giving yourself energy in whatever capacity that can occur: movement, music, laughter, breathing, spending time with others, reserving time to yourself, or setting appropriate boundaries are all forms of caring for yourself.

On second base, you will find relationships with others who can also reciprocate care for you. This means making time for your partner, your friends, clubs and organizations, playing cards with buddies, or hiking with a friend. Second base is for mutual relationships with shared interests.

Next, as you round to third base, you'll see relationships in your life that require caregiving— your children or other dependents. Notice that nowhere on the infield is your job or other obligations? Those are in the outfield, after all the bases have been covered.

I joke with physicians that watching others engage in this process is like watching Little League. We step up to the plate, hit the ball, and run…who knows where? Like some Little Leaguers, we may run to the outfield, run to third, stand still, and do nothing, or chase after our own ball. My encouragement: play like a Major Leaguer. Start on first base. Everything and everyone else on the field is depending on you to hit first base in order for the run to be counted.

Note From R.J.

I once read a book by Wayne Muller called *Sabbath*,[1] which talks about the need for all things to cycle through periods of productivity and periods of rest—that you can have a productive spring only if you've "lain fallow" for the winter. I love that analogy because it reminds me of the natural flow of our professional lives. Constant productivity leaves us feeling empty inside, and being busy day after day takes its toll. You've noticed it too—how the first patient visit of the day usually feels easy and light compared to the last. It's usually not the patient who changes as the day goes on; it's us, carrying more and more in our minds as we progress through our days. If we're going to do this meaningful work, we have to spend time filling our own cups once in a while.

That said, I think there's a misperception that a Sabbath has to be a big event, partly because *Sabbath* and *sabbatical* have the same root, *sabbaton*, which is Greek for "rest." When you think of rest, do you think about bigger things like a day off or a vacation or a sabbatical? Or are you focusing on the small things you can do throughout your day? It needs to be both, in my opinion, but this is Amy's point here—that there are consistent steps we can take to give ourselves energy. A few of my own workday practices are the following:

- I meditate daily at work with whatever time I have leftover in my lunch hour after charting and finishing phone calls. I don't treat this as an optional luxury; it's literally every workday. Sometimes it's 5 minutes; sometimes (although rarely) it's 20 minutes.

- I use common touch points in a visit to clear my head. For example, before knocking on an exam room door, I take 2 deep breaths to clear my head and let go of the last interaction I had with a patient. Same thing when I'm washing my hands.

- On particularly challenging days, my "work spouse" and I will message each other with "3 good things" as a way of improving our mindsets and practicing gratitude in a real-world, practical way.

- On the inside of my office door are 3 poems that I find inspiring, that I read through once or twice a week.

In 2014, I was lucky enough to have an actual sabbatical—an extra 4 weeks I could take to rebuild my reserves and spend time with my partner and in-laws. I wanted to spend some time reflecting on the direction my career had taken and be sure that the remainder of my career was as fulfilling as possible. So, I took the time to go a step further and wrote a personal values and mission statement, modeled after Stephen R. Covey's *The 7 Habits of Highly Effective People*. It's written down in my yearly planner (I'm old fashioned and keep my to-do lists in a paper calendar book instead of online; there's nothing more gratifying to me than ticking boxes of things I've gotten done), and I review my values and mission statement as one of my monthly to-do tasks. It helps keep me grounded to know that the work I do is a reflection of who I am as a person. I have since learned to never say yes to a new project, committee, or other responsibility without first sitting on it for 24 hours—partly to keep boundaries for myself but also to ensure that the request aligns with my values and mission statement.

Ultimately, the sum of the big and the little Sabbaths is what helps us keep going, so think about ways to build self-care into your daily flow.

Another way to engage in self-care is the radical act of self-compassion in being fully human.

Being Fully Human

I'm sitting in the office as a young graduate student, when my new therapist, Eric, enters. He walks in, threadbare tee and khakis, barefoot, longish hair, and an easy smile. He greets me with warm, brown eyes and asks me to talk about why I'm interested in working with children, especially children and families that've experienced complex trauma. My first thought: This guy? This hippie-looking guy is going to psychoanalyze me and let my dean know that I've been declared "ready" to be a psychologist? Second thought: Defend. You'll know only what I share. Third thought: This could be tough work; he seems pretty seasoned…and kind.

In many doctoral programs throughout the United States, therapy is a required component of graduate work. And many of us continue to work with our own therapists throughout our lives, having it destigmatized early on. Part of this journey of self-awareness and self-care will hopefully lead to self-compassion and help us navigate what is sure to be triggering work. It's a slog at times to do this work and continue to show up for others. It can feel scary and overwhelming at first. And often, when I talk with physicians, that fear bubbles up to the surface for them as well—especially given that self-disclosure and introspection are not necessarily core parts of medical school training.

Fast-forward a few years. I'm working with a young boy who is suffering significant emotional abuse and, I suspect, physical abuse at home. There are also signs of neglect as witnessed in his lack of readiness at school, his acting-out behaviors, the dark circles under his eyes, and lunches that aren't nourishing. He hasn't reported physical abuse to me, as we're still establishing trust. As I report to my clinical supervisor about this slow but steady progress, he indicates, "Sometimes you have to lose a battle to win the war." I'm confused about the war analogy, but what he's suggesting is that the progress with the boy is too slow and I need to move on to help other students at my placement. Another time, this same supervisor indicated to me that he witnessed a little girl hug me after a session (in actuality, she threw herself into my arms after processing horrific sadness) and reminded me to be sure to establish clearer boundaries. On yet another occasion, this supervisor scoffed when I declared that, rather than do a quantitative dissertation, I wanted to listen to stories of families with complex medical needs and draw qualitative findings on what made them resilient, despite adversity. Sigh.

Thankfully, a female professor who would become my mentor rescued me: She scooted me into her office one day, witnessing my tears after a long day at a psychiatric hospital. She closed the door behind me and said, "As a woman in academia, you'll be judged for having emotions. Seen as weak. You'll be your clients' mothers, sisters, aunts, and friends; they'll project their losses onto you. You'll be told what's professional and what's not, based mostly on standards from white men. Stand in your feelings. Embrace them. Don't avoid them. *Crying is not a sign of weakness. It's an indication that you're human. Fully human.*"

Thank you, Dr Scott. She introduced me to who would become my dissertation chair, and, together, we set a path for understanding resilience in children and families that has now become my passion.

Anyway, fast-forward again to about 10 years ago. I'm sitting in a different psychologist's office, sweaty having just come from the gym. I apologize for my unkemptness and sit on the floor to avoid getting his couch grimy. He asks me why I apologize for coming in sweaty. I tell him, "Well, it's just not how I usually present myself." He responds with wisdom and insight, "I'm curious about those parts too." And he asks me how I would feel if everyone walked around with little sticky notes on them, letting us know what was actually going on inside of them or what they might be struggling with, hiding, embarrassed of, or the like. Things like these:

- I'm still grieving the loss of my mother.
- I'm afraid you won't like me.
- I'm getting over a cold.
- People at work harass me.
- I can't get pregnant.
- My spouse drinks too much.

Although this idea would have terrified me as a young graduate student, at this point in my life, it excited me. Sticky notes on all of us? Yes, please! It would feel so validating and create so much less aloneness in the world. That way, when we have a regrettable interaction with the barista at the coffee shop, rather than assume she's a horrible person, we would see—she's barely making rent. This is the underpinning of our chapter on becoming a trauma-aware and trauma-responsive environment, to flip the script from "What's wrong with you?" to "What happened and how can I help?"

But it begins at an individual level. That's why I am sharing these uncomfortable stories about a younger version of myself. We're all scared at first. We're all taught what it means to be a professional. Stoic. Controlled. Authoritative. We have answers, insights, and a plan. People look to us for solutions. Patients trust us with their health—mental and physical well-being. And the unspoken curriculum of medical school (or, in my case, graduate school) is to close off parts of ourselves in order to be that professional. Unfortunately, that leads to a great deal of burnout. Continuously compartmentalizing our humanity means that we're turning away from parts of ourselves that are most relatable to others and missing an opportunity to connect.

Thankfully, my path was righted by Dr Scott; and many times, throughout my tenure, I've had to reground myself. That being human and whole is more important than being a professional. That aligning with someone is more important than knowing more than them. That being present with a person's problem is more important than solving it. That *power with* is more important than *power over*.

Think of someone who has inspired you. Someone whom you would trust to care for your mother. Your child. Your loved one. My guess is that your trust is based not on the degree hanging on the wall but on *the way they make you feel*. That's their "humanbeingness." What we're urging here is that part of the preparation for this work is being in touch with your *whole* self—your humanbeingness—and then deciding what you feel comfortable bringing into the exam room. It will be different for all of us.

It's hard to operationalize this concept, which is why we rely on stories. But here is my best attempt.

Genuine Effort

People are doing the best they can with the information and circumstances they are in. If they're not doing well or behaving well, it's likely they are lacking one or both of 2 things: information and support. Information might be medical, physiological, behavioral, or insight about patterns of behavior. Support might be resources (financial or otherwise), transportation, coaching/suggestions, encouragement, or referrals. Regardless, if we shift from thinking about humans as being "noncompliant," "difficult," or "acting out" and begin to think with curiosity—"What's behind this behavior?" "What else might be going on?" and "If I believe he's trying his best, then what's the barrier?"—we'll discover more compassion and understanding of *why* someone is engaging in a certain behavior. We may realize they truly are doing their very best with what they have.

Humanizing Experiences

When we humanize and normalize another person's experience, it helps them feel less alone. In Kristin Neff's work,[2] the term *common humanity* is at its core. Common humanity acknowledges that all humans suffer. The very definition of being *human* means that one is mortal, vulnerable, and imperfect. Therefore, when we recognize that suffering and feelings of inadequacy are part of the shared human experience—something we all go through rather than something that happens to "me"—it creates less aloneness. You will not be able to relate to every experience another person has. So, search for the common humanity, as Neff points out.

A parent feels overwhelming grief. The loss is unexpected. You may have never had the same loss, but you have lost. Sit there. Offer that to your patient. Your resident feels inadequate. Offer times you've felt the same way. Your colleague is going through a divorce. Reassure them that many people have gone through the same experience and that they're not alone. If the heavier stuff feels hard, start with more lighthearted content: "Gosh, before I became a parent myself, I gave lots of advice about croup. Now, I just want to say, 'I'm sorry you're going through that. My husband and I sat up so many nights with our baby. What have you tried so far?'" Being a parent: common humanity. Experiencing loss: common humanity. Negotiating complicated medical decisions: common humanity. Joy of milestones: common humanity.

Beyond Validation

Implicit in this work is moving beyond validation and toward compassion and empathy: "I see you." People need their pain to be seen. Their experiences. Their anger. Although it can feel hard, even scary, most people calm and regulate themselves almost immediately when they feel seen and heard. Often, when parents are feeling inadequate or even triggered by their child's behavior, I encourage them to do one of 2 things: Get small, on the child's level; reassure them of their safety; and don't leave them. Join them. The child will begin to calm down and regulate. Or, match the child's arousal level but not their dysregulation: "I know! Can you believe how crummy teachers can be! I can't wait to hear more!" Same outcome—the child will feel seen and begin to downregulate. By the way, this is also true for parents feeling angry or overwhelmed. Check out Chapter 12, The Art of Listening, for more insights on how we can empathize and listen from multiple vantage points.

Lay Down Goals

This is likely the hardest for all of us. We go into the office or exam room with a lot to check off on our lists and a short amount of time. But if there's tension between what you feel you *have* to cover and what the patient and family *want* to cover, you'll spend a lot of energy and end up with a great deal of unmet needs. Let me offer you a script from a family practice physician I know and respect.

> "Good morning. I'm sure we have a lot to cover in about 10 minutes today, so what's your priority? What are 2 or 3 things you want to be sure to talk about? If we need to schedule another appointment, we can, but let's be sure to cover what's most important to you today."

This physician shared with me that so many other things can be handled in the laboratory, on a portal, with the MA, or at a later visit; but when coached about the importance of prioritizing, the patient and family feel that their time is valued and the physician has been clear about the unfortunate boundary of time. Notice the duality here: our time is important *and* so are your goals.

Holding Spaces

A held space may be an environment you create that feels safe, both physically and emotionally; or you can hold space for someone, meaning you are fully present with them and allow them to be vulnerable. You may not realize it, but you're creating a holding space in your exam room. A holding space is physical space where a relationship manifests and safety is felt (or not). And holding space for someone means being physically, emotionally, and mentally present for someone. People hold space for us multiple times throughout a day if we're fortunate. In the exam room, you have an incredible opportunity to let someone know that "I see you. I'm here. I can be present for you."

From The Trauma Healing Project, based out of Eugene, OR, and their Survivor Voices survey,[3] we know that people feel "mostly healed" simply by being heard. In R.J.'s clinic, they found that it did not add significant time to ask patients about their adversity. But it went a long way in healing.

That's a sacred holding space.

Let me give you an example of how this has played out in my practice. I grew up with a father who was an alcoholic. I've also experienced a divorce, both as a child and as an adult. I don't share that with all my patients, but I tend to know, in my gut, when it's appropriate to share. My golden rule: When it's about them and not about me. So, when a young teen asks me with trepidation, "What's a normal amount of alcohol my mom should drink?" I encourage them to trust themselves if it feels like too much. And later, when they share more (weeks or months or years later) and they share hurt and disappointment, I may offer, "It's hard growing up in a home with an alcoholic. It can feel confusing and sad. Let me know if you need any pointers." Or if parents are struggling to navigate divorce and want to know if their kids will be OK, I reassure them that it's possible. When a mom looks down, ashamed and worried she's ruining her children's lives, I can calmly say, "I've been there. It gets better." I can't relate to everything and I don't disclose most things. But I do share some of what makes me fully human because it creates a safe holding space.

Conclusions

We're encouraging ways to allow yourself to be fully human in your work. Being trauma aware and trauma responsive means being self-reflective. It means acknowledging how hard our work is at times, recognizing triggers and seeing pain in others. When possible, offer humanizing experiences to your patients to create trust in your relationship. This is what will ultimately allow your patients to share experiences that are greatly impacting their lives and, therefore, their health. When they feel comfortable with sharing experiences in their lives with you, you'll get to the heart of the matter—and, therefore, underlying health problems, barriers, and manifested symptoms—much sooner than if you remain the consummate professional.

Questions to Consider

1. What messages do we give ourselves about self-care and personal wellness? Are those messages helpful? How might we reframe some of our unhelpful attitudes toward self-care?
2. Have you taken a fundamental inventory of your history of trauma?
3. What gets in the way of wellness for you? How might you address those barriers?
4. Before now, had you thought about patient encounters as an opportunity to hold space?
5. When is it comfortable to self-disclose, or offer common humanity, to a patient? What type of information do you feel comfortable with sharing?

References

1. Muller W. *Sabbath: Finding Rest, Renewal, and Delight in Our Busy Lives.* Random House; 2000
2. Neff KD. Self-compassion: theory, method, research, and intervention. *Annu Rev Psychol.* 2023;74:193–218
3. Barrett P, Zhang Y, Davies F, Barrett L. *Clever Classrooms: Summary Report of the HEAD Project.* University of Salford Manchester; 2015. Accessed March 20, 2024. https://healingattention.org/wp-content/uploads/Clever-Classrooms-A-Summary-Report-of-the-HEAD-Project.pdf

Chapter 14

Addressing Physician Overwhelm

Amy King, PhD

The expectation that we can be immersed in suffering and loss daily and not be touched by it is as unrealistic as walking through water without getting wet.

Rachel Remen, MD, Internal Medicine Physician

As I sit on a panel of experts for the Lane County, OR, quarterly meeting for physicians, many appear bleary eyed. They're hungry for validation and resources as we discuss "How to Handle Medical Misinformation" during the height of the Omicron surge in the COVID-19 pandemic. I sit on this panel with our health authority experts and 4 other physicians. As a psychologist, I'm there to provide insight into why patients question authority and to encourage self-care and talk about boundaries for physicians.

As we write this book, the World Health Organization continues to mark this time in our history as a global pandemic. We're not out of the woods. The world, seemingly, has gone back to normal; but the crushing effects on our health care systems, especially physicians, proves to be monumental. Experiencing moral injury, vaccine hesitancy, and large expanses of the public questioning medical authority, physicians are weary. They're more exhausted than ever before. They're overwhelmed.

Physicians were experiencing high rates of burnout even before the pandemic. There was enough overwhelm to go around without a global pandemic and patients questioning scientific authority. The pandemic only heightened already existing rates of burnout and deepened feelings of moral distress. Yet, to be a physician who's not only trauma aware but trauma responsive entails recognizing stress, overwhelm, and symptoms of burnout. First and always, physicians must address their own physical and emotional health to provide compassionate care to others.

In this chapter, I use the term *physician overwhelm* for the sake of convenience; but, of course, professionals of all kinds throughout the health care system are experiencing high levels of overwhelm. This chapter's guidance is meant to be of help to all of us.

Sources of Physician Overwhelm

Why does our work feel so much heavier now? Overwhelm is an extreme level of stress and emotional or cognitive intensity to the point of feeling unable to function.[1] It's as though the world is spinning faster than we can comprehend. While there are many contributing factors to overwhelm, let us point out a few that are especially burdensome. Later, we'll break down both individual and organizational responses to overwhelm.

Lack of Resources

There has been a national problem in primary care that has been growing over the past decades. The COVID-19 pandemic compounded these deficits. What was already a problem due to the pressure of increased productivity, administrative burdens, regulations, and expectations without supports (eg, staffing shortages, electronic health record demands, and lower salaries than other physicians) only worsened with a pandemic. Many child-serving professionals felt and continue to feel undervalued and overburdened. The pandemic and the anti-science movements were layered onto an already existing crisis in pediatrics. Now, we're seeing a compounding effect due to these poor resources and unmet needs for patients like never before. Continued lack of resources during the pandemic and the de-prioritizing of patients with non–COVID-19 needs created a heavy burden for physicians and engendered feelings like "We did our best with the staff and resources available, but it wasn't enough."[2] Unmet mental health needs, postponed medical treatments, and delayed preventive care have left physicians with a feeling that, despite their best efforts, patients are more complex than ever and the outlook for resources is bleak.

Challenges to Decision-Making

Another contributing factor is how folks are making decisions. Treatment delays, medical misinformation, ethical choices about appropriate support, physical isolation of patients during the pandemic, and denial of social-emotional support for caregiving are a few examples of how complicated care has been for several years. This also means that it feels nearly impossible for physicians to navigate decision-making without feeling questioned or ethically challenged. A prime example of distress around decision-making has been vaccine hesitancy. Although physicians, especially pediatricians, are accustomed to answering questions about vaccines, this time in our history has been unprecedented. In a politically charged environment, physicians are navigating patient education while combatting "Dr Google." Over time, it can feel hopeless.

Moral Distress/Moral Injury

Physicians are accustomed to difficulty, long hours, heavy responsibility, and high stress. Death and dying, life-altering decisions, families with limited resources, and uncertainty have been part of the territory for as long as there have been healers. But simply acknowledging this does not resolve the conflicts created by responsibility without autonomy.[3] In other words, physicians feel immensely responsible for the care and outcome of their patients without the autonomy to make decisions they feel are in their patients' best interests. Enter moral distress.

Moral distress is the gap between what a professional feels they should do for their patient and what a system, an organization, a payer, or circumstances allow. The resulting feelings are guilt, shame, anger, and disgust. Common factors that compound feelings of moral distress include the following:

- Knowing what resources may benefit your patient or family but being unable to provide them because of limitations such as lack of access, lack of payers, or lack of suitable providers
- Impossible (life-or-death) decisions combined with pressure
- Balancing the physical and mental health needs of the patient with your own
- External stressors such as the political climate, significant losses for groups of people who've experienced systemic injustice and inequity (eg, job, food, or housing insecurities), and natural disasters

Compounding Stressors

Compounding stressors, or additive stressors that create a cumulative weight, increase psychological harm to physicians. Here are some examples.

CONCURRENT CATASTROPHES

A pandemic or natural disaster has international and national effects. What compounds the losses of those catastrophic disasters is other concurrent local, national, and international stressors such as natural disasters, political conflict, and war. For instance, political upheaval or the threat of war in other countries compounds loss and worry during an already stressful event.

Local weather events, fires, or community traumas heighten an already significant obstacle. Local, national, and international stressors create additional turmoil for a physician who may be already barely hanging on.

PERSONAL STRESSORS

Unfortunately, life does not stop even when more public tragedies are occurring. Divorce, job loss, illness, and personal strife are stressors that have a cumulative effect on physicians. Many physicians suffered their own personal losses or illnesses due to the pandemic. Often, physicians feel they are expected to overly compartmentalize their personal life from their professional life. So, in addition to the personal stress, an immense feeling of isolation can co-occur.

PATIENT LOSS AND/OR SIGNIFICANT LOSS OF LIFE

Patient death, the significant loss of lives, or knowing that you have the expertise to recognize what children need but cannot help them because of lack of services, lack of specialty care, lack of mental health services, or the like all significantly impact physician wellness. During the height of patient deaths in the Omicron surge, one physician disclosed to me that if he had to stop and "debrief" every death he'd experienced in a given day or week, he would have to stop providing patient care. And yet, the impact of loss is monumental. The grief, overwhelm, and distress to physicians who, often, are not offered a space to process such feelings represents a significant addition to compounding stressors. Another physician told me that, after losing 5 patients in 1 month, she questioned whether or not she could come to work and provide patient care without "falling apart" at her clinic.

INCREASED MENTAL HEALTH NEEDS

While physicians' mental health needs may be unmet, their concern for the unmet mental health needs of patients is noteworthy. Often, physicians cannot rely on outpatient mental health needs being met, because therapists who specialize in complex behavior or complex trauma are nearly impossible to find; or they're faced with a lack of outpatient therapists, in general, and long wait times. They feel compelled to address serious mental health needs during short visits, which leads to a great deal of personal angst. As a physician, you recognize that you're not trained to address complex mental health needs, but you also recognize that doing nothing feels horrible and wrong as well.

UNALIGNED DECISIONS

As mentioned before regarding moral distress, when health care professionals cannot meet patient needs because of strained resources or resistance to medical recommendations, a great deal of distress is experienced.

Burnout

Burnout is a combination of 3 factors: emotional exhaustion, depersonalization, and decreased sense of personal accomplishment. To note, *burnout is a result of unmet needs due to overwhelm.* It is an unfortunate result of not addressing overwhelm soon enough. Maslach and Leiter have done extensive work in this area and further define the 3 dimensions of burnout[4]:

- Emotional exhaustion
  - Wearing out
  - Loss of energy
  - Depletion
  - Debilitation
  - Fatigue

- Depersonalization
  - Cynicism
  - Negative or inappropriate attitudes toward clients/patients
  - Irritability
  - Loss of idealism
  - Withdrawal
- Decreased sense of personal accomplishment
  - Inefficiency
  - Reduced productivity
  - Reduced capability
  - Low morale
  - Inability to cope

Physician burnout is at an all-time high. Sheather and Fidler point out that "simply working harder cannot resolve the conflicts caused by responsibility without autonomy."[3] The COVID-19 pandemic has only heightened the feeling that physicians have to make impossible decisions and work under extreme pressures. In addition, burnout is compounded by a mixed message to be both boundaryless and completely boundaryed at the same time.

On the one hand, the messaging to medical professionals is one of boundaryless sacrifice and selflessness. Most physicians go into health care to make a difference, help others, and change lives. Medical schools have taught physicians to be self-sacrificing—to ignore their needs for sleep, food, breaks, and personal time. Because of this training, physicians are at high risk for burnout.

At the same time, physicians are expected to be completely boundaryed with their emotions: the consummate expert and professional. Physicians are not trained to self-disclose, share their humanity, or appear anything less than heroic and stoic. This environment creates an insurmountable pressure to be performative, unfazed, and self-assured at all times. Many physicians I talk with disclose to me that they don't seek out mental health and addiction services, request time off, or discuss family stressors with anyone for fear of losing their license, being reported or demoted, or losing their ability to provide for their family.

Remedies

I wish R.J. and I could wave a magic wand and create systemic change to health care systems and organizations that are perpetuating messages that lack self-care and dismiss the idea that physicians need to be professionals *and* humans—meaning, physicians cannot be unemotional robots without needs; they need to be recognized as fully human. In this book, we want to encourage some proactive measures that go a bit beyond traditional self-care and may offer you actionable steps to combat overwhelm and prevent burnout. We're offering organizational shifts as well because the hard work of combatting overwhelm cannot be the work of individuals alone. But let's start with you. **Box 14-1** lists 5 supports for individuals and 5 supports for organizations. My guess is that every person and organization will have their own inventory of strengths (what we're already doing well) and needs (where we could use more help or support).

For Individuals

DIFFERENTIATE BETWEEN STRESS AND OVERWHELM

One of the best-received workshops I've provided is on helping health care organizations and clinicians differentiate between stress and overwhelm. Physicians, clinic managers, and new employees often approach me after the workshop and say, "I had no idea. I've actually been

---

Box 14-1.
10 Considerations to Address Physician Overwhelm

Support for Individuals
- Differentiate between stress and overwhelm.
- Embrace uncertainty.
- Create boundaries.
- Find community and connection.
- Be your whole self.

Support for Organizations
- Ask for help from outside consultants who specialize in wellness.
- Encourage staff to ask for help and support.
- Encourage discussions about how to address stress.
- Encourage discussions about how to address overwhelm.
- Address administrative burdens.

---

overwhelmed this entire time but acting as if it was just stress. I was beating myself up because none of the tools I was trying were working. Now I get it: I'm overwhelmed."

Stress is manageable. To be clear, the stress we're talking about in this chapter is tolerable stress. That's different from the complex stress we're referring to when we are discussing complex trauma. We feel stressed when we evaluate environmental demand as beyond our ability to cope successfully for a period of time.[1] This includes elements of unpredictability, uncontrollability, and feeling kind of overloaded. But stress is manageable. And it's manageable because we have relational supports to ameliorate the stress. Think about stress like a Monday morning at your clinic: calls are coming in, huddles are happening, messages are picked up from weekend hospital stays, colleagues are exchanging post-call information, and patients are anxious to be seen for visits. You'll get through it. It will feel hairy, but manageable with some strategies and supports. That's stress.

Overwhelm is different. As noted earlier, overwhelm is the feeling that our lives are somehow unfolding faster than our human nervous system and psyche are able to manage.[5] Overwhelm is a Monday morning when all the previous statements are true and then you find out that one of your patients died by suicide over the weekend. The world stops. You wonder what you missed. There's no "going on" with your day; you must stop and absorb what's happening. It can also be overwhelming that you're expected to see 20 + patients, work through lunch, or see kids with inadequate staff. All of it is overwhelming.

It's essential to differentiate between the two. Often, in medical systems, we continue to insist we're "OK" when we're really overwhelmed. In fact, we've been trained to do so—to ignore our physical triggers or emotional cues—and keep on working. But there's only one cure to overwhelm: we must give ourselves time to absorb the impact of trauma that's occurred, feel the feelings, and take care of our bodies. The result of ignoring this many times over is burnout, leaving the profession, turning to substances, or, even worse, physician suicide. Physician suicide rates,[6-8] at a conservative estimate, are between 300 and 400 deaths per year. And suicide rates are higher among female physicians. I've been fortunate to run a physician support group this past year, specifically aimed at decreasing physician suicide. Please take advantage of all the available resources (**Box 14-2**). You are not alone.

Box 14-2.
Physician Resources

- Physicians Anonymous: Visit www.physiciansanonymous.org.
- The Physician Support Line is a free and confidential service open Monday through Friday from 8:00 am to midnight (ET): Call 1-888-409-0141 or visit www.physiciansupportline.com.
- 988 Suicide & Crisis Lifeline: Dial 988 anytime.

EMBRACE UNCERTAINTY

This might seem like another radical type of self-care, but embracing uncertainty can be quite powerful. First, acknowledge what you know and what you're good at. Second, acknowledge what you don't know. Then, decide how you'll proceed. For instance, I was working with a pediatrician recently who was unable to identify a nasty infection that a teenaged boy had on his hand. He shrugged his shoulders and said, "I just don't know what this is." He referred the boy to a dermatologist and infectious disease expert. He said, "I'm not sure, but we'll find out together." It allowed this physician to be both human and collaborative. Or, in another example, when you start your day but know that it might go sideways, you can create a plan. So, when your patient reports that they're without shelter, and the visit goes longer than anticipated, you have a plan to help yourself (asking for help, taking a deep breath, or asking for more resources for the family). When you embrace uncertainty, you relieve the pressure of perfection.

Once you've done this, redefine what you do know. It's empowering to take inventory of your expertise. You can reground yourself in "knowing" versus "not knowing" and reassure yourself that you can both embody answers and seek them out.

CREATE BOUNDARIES

As I mentioned earlier, physicians are taught to be boundaryless, and this can be tremendously taxing. To start bringing some boundaries into the picture, create some short- and long-term measurable goals for yourself. Short-term goals might be things like leaving the office by 6:00 pm, delegating responsibilities to a care manager, or hiring some help at home to offset your work pressure. Long-term goals might be addressing workplace violations, creating affinity groups with other physicians (eg, Black physicians, LGBTQ+ physicians, single-caregiver physicians), asking to change your patient workflow, or creating a specialty within your practice that you feel passionate about.

Boundaries feel so hard because you're unlearning something that's been ingrained in you for so long. It will take time and practice to prioritize boundaries, but you can definitely create boundaries without sacrificing patient care. In fact, learning to create boundaries can help you feel more purposeful in patient care.

PRACTICAL EXAMPLES

1. At R.J.'s clinic, they had an intentional discussion about how much information exchange and suggestions should be put into the patient portals. It was taking minutes to hours to respond to patient needs in the portal. So, their team chatted about the patient portal and began to be specific about when, if, and how much they should respond. Concurrently, they created a system to explain to patients when the needs they had went beyond the portal experience and needed to be a separate appointment.

2. Another physician uses the first few seconds of a visit to prioritize an agenda with her patient. She says, "We only have about 15 minutes together today. I wish that wasn't the case, but it's what we have. What 1 or 2 issues do we need to tackle?" When the patient begins down the list of 15 items, she gently says, "We won't get to all those today. What are your top 2 issues? Can I help you prioritize?" And then she encourages her patient to make a follow-up appointment for other issues as well as differentiate what she might delegate to a community health worker, behavioral health consultant, or health coach.

3. After many months of overwhelm, a family practice physician asked her practice manager to do 3 things: (1) no double-booking; (2) protect her lunch hour with fewer meetings; and (3) give the front desk permission to triage patients whose presentations seem more complex by having them see the behavioral health clinician before she comes into the room. When I asked her if these changes were hard, she answered, "Of course. They felt impossible at first. But the choice was either workflow change or I was going to quit. I was sacrificing my mental health and the quality of patient care to see more people in less time."

4. Grannies and nannies! I'll never forget talking with Dr Nadine Burke Harris after we presented on a panel together. When we were commiserating about being busy, working moms, we both agreed that, when possible, physicians should hire and enlist help. She said that if she didn't have "grannies and nannies," she wouldn't be able to do her job. I've spoken with many physicians who've hired nannies, scribes, personal trainers, and personal assistants to free up their time and create more balance in their lives.

5. I've included a letter in Appendix T at the end of the book. The letter outlines what feels OK and what does not feel acceptable given a situation. It helps break down what's negotiable for you and what is not. And then it helps you craft a specific request to ameliorate the boundary that has been crossed. It's a good first step at creating workplace boundaries.

FIND COMMUNITY AND CONNECTION

Having meaningful social interactions is probably the greatest factor to mitigate burnout. Maybe it's your spouse. Maybe it's your "work spouse." Perhaps it's volunteering, dates, book clubs, cycling, or doing something creative with your mind or hands. Social interaction and connection create resilience and meaning in our lives. We've discussed the baseball analogy for caregivers in previous chapters (see Chapters 8, Revamping Anticipatory Guidance, and 13, Self-Care and Sharing Our Humanity). This applies to you too! You have to hit second base to take care of others. We want you to say yes to date nights, time with your dog, hiking with friends, and laughing with your family. But we also need to embed care into our work routines every day, not simply save it for later "when we have time" because that time may or may not come. Look around the baseball field: there are so many other competing demands!

In speaking with a physician at a busy diabetes clinic, he said that he makes sure his charts are done before he leaves the office. "Work hard, play hard" was his motto. While it's a grind to get charts completed before he leaves, it means he can be fully present when he goes home. And then when he's home, he's constantly reflecting on all the parts of himself that need tending to; he bikes, hikes, does yoga, spends time with his kids, and volunteers. While he admitted he's not always been good at this, he said that when he listens to his body, he becomes aware of where gaps are that need to be paid attention to.

Other physicians have shared how they embed self-care into their work. For instance, I work with a pediatrician who does mindful breathing in between exam rooms: "It might look silly, but I try to walk and breathe slowly in between patients. I know my body needs a break, and if I breathe, I go into the next exam room with more calm and presence." Another physician has shared that he started a meditation group for peers during the lunch hour. He was afraid no one would join him, only to have to find a bigger room because so many colleagues showed up when it was offered.

Being connected and in community will heal your soul. Sharing your stories and being vulnerable are a great first step in how important this is. It is the healing balm to burnout. R.J. has a great story about why this is important.

Note From R.J.

Last spring and summer, I felt like I was hitting a particularly difficult patch. The pandemic plus the adolescent mental health crisis meant that literally everyone in my practice was experiencing some sort of trauma. Lost jobs, food insecurity, and losing family members were daily stories. I had some days when 5 or 6 of the 20+ patients on my schedule were teens whom I was newly diagnosing with anxiety or depression, and the wait list for mental health clinicians was somewhere within the 8- to 10-month range, even for those patients who were experiencing suicidal ideation. Instead of getting the help of a mental health professional, my patients got me. I crammed in watching 18 lectures on cognitive behavioral therapy so I could at least get my patients started, but I was listening to other people's pain, day in and day out. I found myself praying to see a simple ear infection so I could be in and out of the room without taking on any more stories.

One Saturday, my partner dragged me out to Silver Falls to go on a 9-mile hike. Even though I've lived in Oregon for over 50 years, I'd never been; but the idea of getting up early on a Saturday morning and driving an hour to the middle of the woods seemed completely unappealing compared to burying my head under my blankets for the rest of the day.

An hour into the hike, I muttered under my breath, "Getting out in nature is one of the 7 pillars of stress health."

From a few feet ahead, my partner replied, "I know."

(Wait, you were listening to me all these years? When did that start?)

Naturally, I felt better after that day. How could I not? Several of the waterfalls in Silver Falls State Park are carved out of the rock cliffs in a way that you can actually hike behind them and stare through the cascading water into the dappled sunlight filtering through the forest. It's magical. Plus, I reconnected with my partner, who was feeling powerless in watching me struggle and who wanted to help in whatever way possible. Human connections are healing, plain and simple.

Heading back to work after that weekend, I knew that something had to give. In spite of how I was feeling at work, I had been following my training and keeping my personal stress to myself. I had kept up the professional boundaries that we all strive so hard to meticulously maintain.

However, there's some power in letting those boundaries down. It doesn't harm our patients if they see us as human; in fact, they can often learn from our experiences (in mental health, it's called *parallel process* when you use your own experiences for the benefit of the patient). So, that Monday morning I talked about my weekend with some of my staff and with my patients. I called out how burned out I had been feeling and how doing that small bit of self-care helped me heal a small part of my soul. I talked about what I hoped to do next to get out of my rut a little bit and continue to work on taking care of myself.

Did it help my patients and families at all? How could it not? I connected with them on a real level. I gave them examples and ideas from my own experience about what might help them feel better, because it helped me feel better. And it also helped me feel better when I put words to my own emotional state, using my thinking brain to start to organize and make sense out of the tangled ball of spaghetti that my emotional brain was cooking up. It felt better to let myself be human (letting go of the physician mode of needing to be superhuman); and when we're connecting with our patients, they end up feeling a little bit better too.

That said, I'm not naive enough to believe that a walk in the woods will completely cure something as complex as burnout. It takes the sum of all my coping strategies to manage it—daily meditation, exercise, vacations both big and small, spending time connecting with friends, and so on—but bottling up the feelings isn't an option. Keeping strict boundaries with our patients, where we don't admit to our own humanity and discuss the complexity of our own lives, often compounds the problem and isn't realistic. It's not about whether we have it tougher than our patients, or unloading all our problems on them, but rather about how we reveal enough about ourselves to help them identify how to collaboratively problem-solve and manage their stressors.

BE YOUR WHOLE SELF

I do a fun activity called "Mad Libs for Humanity" when I work with physicians. One thing I ask them to identify is something that makes them "pretty much a rock star" that's also a nonphysician trait or interest. It's amazing what I find out about them in groups.

- "I'm an incredible gardener."
- "I love writing."
- "I work incredibly well with pastels."
- "I can build homes."
- "I sing at my synagogue."
- "I've traveled to 34 countries."

And on and on… And yet, I almost *never* know this until I ask. One aspect of radical self-care is being your *whole self*. I'd like to encourage you to think about investing serious time into the activities, people, and experiences that fill up your cup. And then tell other people what makes you human.

The other activity I do with physicians is to explore what makes them "messy" humans. Often they laugh at this activity and then sheepishly squirm, waiting for colleagues to answer first. Finally, someone will bravely speak up and share something like this:

- "I'm probably drinking too much."
- "I overeat."
- "I avoid chart notes for too long."
- "I'm considering a divorce."
- "I hate administration."
- And always: "I think I'm the only one who feels this way…"

Remember: your humanity will help others heal. Your patients and your colleagues do not expect perfection. In fact, they're hoping you're just like them so they'll feel less alone. Don't miss an opportunity to connect with yourself, your colleagues, or a patient by being too guarded. For more ideas on ways to show compassion and connect, see Chapter 13, Self-Care and Sharing Our Humanity.

For Organizations

We want to underscore the importance of organizational shift. Too often, wellness programs focus solely on professional wellness and neglect significant changes that must be made at an organizational level. Such a focus also has the effect of placing the responsibility for overwhelm and burnout on the people who are experiencing it, which can communicate the message that these things represent personal failings.

ASK FOR HELP AS AN ORGANIZATION AND ENCOURAGE STAFF TO ASK FOR SUPPORT

In 2021, in response to the COVID-19 pandemic and the resulting overwhelm that so many of our health care professionals were experiencing, I partnered with another consulting firm to create a program called THRIVE, a year-long learning collaborative for primary care teams. We surveyed over 300 staff at the beginning of the year and then created a curriculum to focus on workforce wellness over the ensuing 11 months. The survey was adapted from the work of Daniel Shapiro at Penn State, who mapped health care professional and organizational wellness onto Maslow's Hierarchy of Needs.[9] Each month, we focused on either a team or a topic. For instance, from our survey, we discovered that more than a third of all staff were experiencing anxiety and/or depression "often" or "always"; if we included the response of "sometimes," the number went up to 86%. So, for one month, we focused solely on mental health. For other months, we ran affinity groups for medical assistants, practice leaders, or nonclinical staff. These groups allowed folks to brainstorm and provide resources to each other while gaining validation from their peers that they were not alone in the difficulties they faced.

The results were promising and important. Although clinics varied in areas of improvement depending on their individual base scores, all clinics saw improvements overall. Most significantly, changes were seen in cultures of respect and appreciation. In other words, having a space to get needs met, engage in conversations, and receive support, as well as increasing the intentionality of appreciation, changed the workplace culture in several practices. Having outside consultation allowed information to be shared anonymously and support to be provided externally, 2 key indicators of success.

THRIVE is just one example of how outside consultation may benefit your team. There are fabulous organizations, psychologists, and coaches who can provide curriculum, training, and materials regarding workforce wellness. It's also important to encourage staff to be aware of and make use of internal support systems. Examples include employee assistance program resources, affinity groups in hospitals and clinics, wellness programs and luncheons, free continuing education, and peer coaching. Often, what I find is a lack of awareness that programs exist more than a lack of desire to participate.

ENCOURAGE DISCUSSIONS ABOUT HOW TO ADDRESS STRESS AND OVERWHELM

On an organizational level, it's important to have discussions about how secondary stress, stress that is manageable (see the Differentiate Between Stress and Overwhelm section earlier in this chapter), and overwhelm are different and, crucially, what to do to address each.

Over the years, I've seen physicians dramatically impacted by this differentiation in terms. For the first time, they're able to verbalize what's happening internally. They recognize what they've been trained to ignore: that voice inside that says, "I need a break." One head of human resources told me that, after a training where we differentiated the 2 terms, she had a physician bravely approach her and discuss what it might mean to take a sabbatical.

Encourage discussions about stress versus overwhelm in your office. It's part of being trauma informed—to resist re-traumatizing folks and create systems that are responsive. For a more extensive explanation of how your organization can become trauma informed, please see our previous chapter on creating compassionate pediatric practices (Chapter 3). Simple things like email reminders, flyers, and check-ins can encourage folks to reflect and seek out help.

Conclusions

Addressing physician overwhelm requires both individual and organizational commitment. In many ways, it means relearning ways to take care of ourselves and ask for help—or unlearning behaviors and messaging that require self-sacrifice and detachment from our basic human needs. Our encouragement is that health care organizations and professionals begin to ask questions and collect data regarding overwhelm and burnout in their organization. Then, take steps to ameliorate through actions laid out in this chapter. We cannot lose more colleagues to the unwritten messages of martyrdom and perfection.

Questions to Consider

1. Of the 10 considerations for individual and organizational wellness, how do you assess wellness within your clinic or factors that might be addressed to mitigate overwhelm?

2. What do you see as the most significant barriers to your wellness? To your colleagues' wellness?

3. Is there one component in this chapter that feels actionable? One factor you might consider or felt was especially impactful?

4. Do you know folks you can turn to for support or guidance? Groups or programs?

References

1. Brown B. *Atlas of the Heart: Mapping Meaningful Connection and the Language of Human Experience.* Random House; 2021
2. Greenberg N, Docherty M, Gnanapragasam S, Wessely S. Managing mental health challenges faced by healthcare workers during COVID-19 pandemic. *BMJ.* 2020;368:m1211 doi: 10.1136/bmj.m1211
3. Sheather J, Fidler H. COVID-19 has amplified moral distress in medicine. *BMJ.* 2021;372:n28 doi: 10.1136/bmj.n28
4. Maslach C, Leiter MP. Burnout. In: *Stress: Concepts, Cognition, Emotion, and Behavior.* Academic Press; 2016:351–357. Handbook of Stress; vol 1
5. Kabat-Zinn J. Overwhelmed. *Mindfulness.* 2019;10(6):1188–1189 doi: 10.1007/s12671-019-01150-6
6. Ye GY, Davidson JE, Kim K, Zisook S. Physician death by suicide in the United States: 2012–2016. *J Psychiatr Res.* 2021;134:158–165 PMID: 33385634 doi: 10.1016/j.jpsychires.2020.12.064
7. Irigoyen-Otiñano M, Castro-Herranz S, Romero-Agüit S, et al. Suicide among physicians: major risk for women physicians. *Psychiatry Res.* 2022;310:114441 PMID: 35183987 doi: 10.1016/j.psychres.2022.114441
8. Shanafelt TD, Dyrbye LN, West CP, et al. Suicidal ideation and attitudes regarding help seeking in US physicians relative to the US working population. *Mayo Clin Proc.* 2021;96(8):2067–2080 PMID: 34301399 doi: 10.1016/j.mayocp.2021.01.033
9. Shapiro DE, Duquette C, Abbott LM, Babineau T, Pearl A, Haidet P. Beyond burnout: a physician wellness hierarchy designed to prioritize interventions at the systems level. *Am J Med.* 2019;132(5):556–563 PMID: 30553832 doi: 10.1016/j.amjmed.2018.11.028

Chapter 15

Implementation Nuts and Bolts

R.J. Gillespie, MD, MHPE, FAAP

The journey of a thousand miles begins with a single step.
Chinese proverb

We've covered a lot of ground to get you ready for this point, so now we're going to get into the nuts and bolts of implementing the screening and assessment tools that make up the components of relational health histories (RHHs), as well as implementing the resilience-based interventions. This section is heavy on quality improvement (QI) skills. Hopefully, you've done some QI projects before and the work is not entirely new ground; so, we're going to focus on the nuances of implementation of more delicate assessment tools than some of the screening tools you already use.

My first QI job was teaching clinicians across the state of Oregon about developmental screening tools with the Oregon Pediatric Society (OPS). We had a perfect storm of clinician interest, improved payment for screening tools from policymakers, and recently formed relationships between clinicians and the community-based organizations (CBOs) that helped manage kids' needs once they'd been identified. It didn't hurt that the president of the OPS was a developmental and behavioral pediatrician, in addition to being an amazing mentor and teacher.

As I traveled around the state training practices on this new workflow, I ran into all types of people—those eager to adopt developmental screening and those completely resistant—but a lot of the people I met were somewhere in the middle: well intentioned, interested in doing better for their patients, but in need of some guidance and support in creating a practice change. Someone to "bring the bagels" to a practice meeting and walk them through the details of implementation.

In following up with some of these clinicians, I learned that one of the big barriers they experienced was getting patients connected to services. They had no problem getting the tools distributed and completed. But things fell apart after that, because the clinicians would collect the completed tools and review them at the end of the day while they were doing their charting. This meant they didn't have a conversation about the tools at the point of service and were stuck trying to contact families afterward to complete their referrals.

When it comes to trauma, social drivers of health (SDOH), or mental health assessments (including peripartum mood disorders [PMDs]), you simply can't do this.

As we talk through implementation, let's commit to reviewing every tool that we implement during the visit with the family. The message of silence, which we've talked about before, implies that the history you've just obtained isn't important or that the person completing the tool is not safe disclosing their history. This is perhaps the most important nuance of implementing assessments about trauma (although I believe it applies to PMDs and SDOH as well), so keep this in mind as you make decisions about how and in what circumstances you conduct your pilot implementation.

As a starting point, let's go back to the table from Chapter 11, Pulling It All Together, which gives you a roadmap of what it looks like to conduct an RHH as well as what resilience-based interventions align with Bright Futures priority areas and the developmental status of the child's age. This time, in **Table 15-1**, look at the assessment and screening tools on the left, and the interventions on the right, and assess where you and your practice are starting from.

If you aren't doing any screening or assessment tools in your practice, you'll need to prioritize where to start. I would suggest PMDs and social-emotional (SE) health first, then SDOH, and then parental trauma assessments. As mentioned in the Introduction, when implementing a new screening or assessment tool, I tend to break the process into
4 fundamental questions:

- Why am I looking?
- What am I looking for?
- How will I find it?
- What will I do when I find it?

Once you've answered these 4 questions—or, in the case of the *why* question, figured out how you're going to articulate your answer—you're ready to go. So, let's walk through them one at a time.

Why Am I Looking?

By now, you've already learned a lot about the barriers to early relational health that we see in practice, so you have a reasonable handle on why you want to address these. Otherwise, you probably wouldn't have picked up this book in the first place. That said, if you're a champion of this concept, you're likely going to have to motivate other people in your practice to get on board, which means you need to be able to put your why into words—clear, succinct, motivating words. I've found that this is particularly true about why we would want to assess caregiver trauma and SDOH in practice (it seems easier for most clinicians to understand the why behind PMD screening), so a lot of this discussion will be anchored to the process for explaining why trauma assessments are something we should implement in primary care. Think about who in your practice needs to be involved in your pilot implementation and who needs to be informed. There are at least 4 groups of people you'll likely need to convince: clinicians, administration/clinic leadership, staff, and caregivers and families (**Table 15-2**). I'm going to talk through the nuances of explaining your why to each of these groups.

Clinicians

You know how busy you and your colleagues are, so if you're going to convince them to adopt this change, you're going to have to talk fast. This comes down to creating an elevator pitch—a quick, 30-second or less description of your project that you could say in the time it takes an elevator to go from one floor to the next. One of my mentors described a simple process for creating this elevator pitch: the Story of Me, the Story of Us, the Story of Now. This communication tool is known as the public narrative,[1] and it's used to motivate change in all kinds of settings.

The Story of Me is pretty simple: it's describing a story from your own clinical experience that illustrates the need for change. People can usually identify a similar example in their own practice, which is why this story is such a motivating place to start. The Story of Us is how the story of that one patient that sticks out in your memory broadens into what you and your fellow clinicians see on a day-to-day basis and illustrates the depth of the problem and how it affects us in practice. The Story of Now is a brief synopsis of what we can do about it and how that would improve the wellness of our patients, our practice efficiency, or other important outcomes.

Table 15-1. The Roadmap Assessment

Age	Relational Health History Screening Tools or Assessments	Am I Already Doing These Tools/ Assessments?	Anticipatory Guidance Highlight/Intervention	Am I Already Doing an Intervention?
Newborn period	PMDs Food and diaper insecurity[a]		Circles of Support	
2 wk	PMDs Food and diaper insecurity[a]		Parent self-care/baseball analogy	
2 mo	PMDs Food and diaper insecurity[a]		Being a baby observer	
4 mo	PMDs Food and diaper insecurity[a] Parental/caregiver trauma history[a]		Education about trauma and PCEs Bids for attention	
6 mo	PMDs Food and diaper insecurity[a] SE health[a]		Time-ins/special time	
9 mo	Developmental screening		Time-ins/special time Beginning discipline	
12 mo	SDOH[b]		Beginning discipline Mealtime routines	
15 mo	SE health[a]		Bedtime routines and reading Special time (play based)	
18 mo	Developmental screening Autism screening		Positive parenting/handling tantrums	
24 mo	SDOH[b] Autism screening SE health[a]		Looking Beyond the Behavior	
30 mo	Developmental screening		Special time "Shark music"	
3 y	SDOH[b]		Building family connections and routines	
4 y	SDOH[b] SE health[a]		I Love You Rituals/I Love You No Matter What! "Highs and lows"/"roses and thorns"	
5 and 6 y	SDOH[b]		Yolky Feelings Flipping Your Lid	

Abbreviations: PMD, peripartum mood disorder; SDOH, social drivers of health; SE, social-emotional.

[a] No clear guidelines exist for periodicity of this tool/assessment; this is what has worked for us.

[b] No clear guidelines exist for periodicity of SDOH tools, with the exception of recommendations that The Hunger Vital Sign be used at every visit (https://frac.org/aaptoolkit).

Table 15-2. Messaging Considerations

Group	What to Consider in Your Messaging
Clinicians	Time Support for skill building
Administration/clinic leadership	Alignment with mission/patient care Operational impact Financial bottom line
Staff—both clinical and nonclinical	Relevance to their role Time
Caregivers and families	Relevance to health/wellness Getting input on the process

Here's an actual example from my clinical practice, focused on food insecurity screening, which our practice decided to implement a few years ago. As with any effective public narrative, it's based on a true story that you've heard referenced already.

> "Last week, I had a patient in for a well-child visit who experiences profound developmental delay, cerebral palsy, and chronic, uncontrolled seizures. I noticed they weren't making most of the appointments with the specialists, so when I asked if there was anything they needed, the caregiver said, 'I know that all those appointments are important, but right now, we're struggling to put food on the table, so I just can't make it in for all those doctor visits.' (the Story of Me)

> "It turns out that as many as 1 in 7 kids is living in a food-insecure household; that means we're seeing at least 3 or 4 kids a day who don't have enough food to eat. (the Story of Us)

> "There's this simple 2-question survey that helps identify families that experience food insecurity called The Hunger Vital Sign, and it's pretty easy to use. If they say yes to either of the questions, we can do a referral to community action or to the local food bank." (the Story of Now)

Granted, the QI process behind implementing a screening tool is a little more complicated than the story makes it sound. But the point is that this simple communication tool helps improve motivation for change. It quickly helps people see the why behind the change and gives a simple answer to what their clinical response includes. Imagine how much more achievable it seems to implement food insecurity screening with this narrative than if you'd approached a clinician and said simply, "We need to screen our kids for food insecurity." When this need is stated in such broad terms, it's easy for clinicians to get lost in the details of how complicated screening sounds, so it's easy for a colleague to simply say no.

Remember from Chapter 2, Addressing Barriers, that the main reason clinicians say no to a change is that they lack either skill or will to implement the change. An effective public narrative will address those particular root causes of resistance by including how you will support your colleagues during the implementation of change, as well as by providing a rough overview of the resources that will be used if needed. It may be as simple as "I've done this, it worked out well, and I'll teach you how to do it"; it's important to reassure your colleagues that they won't be left on their own to implement a new workflow like this.

In Appendix J, you'll find a worksheet for creating your own public narrative. Keep it brief, so you can remember it on the fly with your colleagues, but make sure it's honest and specific. More often than not, the response from your partners will be "Tell me more!"

Administration/Clinic Leadership

When it comes to explaining to leadership your reasons for implementing RHHs, the approach may vary depending on the structure of your practice. In some cases, there may be overlap between leadership and practicing clinicians; for example, I work in a physician-owned practice, so I have to convince the same people as leaders and as practice colleagues. If you work in a larger system, you may be in a position of having to convince administrators who do not have direct or specific clinical experience. Using the public narrative approach is still appropriate for this group, but the key message may be slightly different, particularly for leadership members who don't have direct clinical experience. The difference between convincing leadership and convincing practicing physicians is that you have to consider the operational bottom line when crafting your arguments with leadership; alternatively, one potentially powerful approach is to align your explanation to your system's mission, vision, or values.

Let's use my own clinic's mission statement as an example:

> The board-certified pediatricians of The Children's Clinic are committed to providing the highest quality care to our patients from birth to young adulthood. Our goal is to provide this care with compassion, integrity and continuity. We are devoted to these goals while developing a trusting and lifelong relationship with our families for generations.[2]

There are a couple of key pieces of our mission statement that can come into play in this conversation. The quality angle is one potential approach—that by implementing RHHs and the associated assessment tools, we are improving the quality of care that we provide to families. Another approach would be to pull out the concept of compassion—that having a better understanding of our families and their trauma histories would increase the compassion and empathy we have for them or that creating a trauma-informed or trauma-responsive culture within the practice would increase that compassion. Finally, in this case we could touch on how RHHs help build trusting relationships with families by better identifying and responding to their needs.

As I mentioned, administrators are often concerned about the bottom line, so addressing how you intend to minimize schedule disruptions, increase efficiencies, or improve patient satisfaction by being a trauma-responsive organization may work to garner support for your proposal. The communication with leadership also should include what resources will be needed to start and maintain implementation. For example, do you need funding for purchasing screening tools? Do you need stipends, space, or dedicated time for team meetings? Do you need dedicated administrative support, such as time from care coordinators, leadership, or administrative staff? Be prepared to talk about what implementation will cost.

It can be a tricky conversation—most administrators are highly focused on the bottom line (as they should be)—but addressing trauma may help alleviate some of their pain points. For example, given that there's a correlation between parent ACEs and utilization patterns,[3] you can address how you hope that addressing trauma will improve no-show rates in the clinic. Since no-show rates affect other quality metrics, like developmental screening and immunization rates, if your practice is part of a pay-for-performance program, you'll see financial benefits from focusing on getting your patients through the door in the first place. There's also a shift toward effective utilization by addressing trauma in practice—fewer emergency department visits, for example[4]—so if your practice is being held to ambulatory-sensitive emergency department utilization or a total cost of care metric (like we are), addressing trauma will give your practice a chance to do better care coordination for families that might be at risk and, ultimately, lower costs. If staff and physicians have a better understanding of trauma, and if they have skills to more compassionately interact with patients and families, you may be able to improve burnout rates, which improves the clinic's bottom line as well. Let's face it, turnover is expensive with training costs, fees for job postings, and so forth—so giving staff tools and skills to be trauma responsive and to feel more supported in their work as well as addressing root causes of burnout in your institution will save administrative costs down the road. We'll talk more about tool selection in a minute, but cost is (and should be) one of the criteria you think about in your decision-making process for what tool you're going to implement. In my practice, we started with tools that were freely available in the public domain; in fact, most practices that aren't grant funded as a research project take this approach to avoid burdensome costs.

Staff—Both Clinical and Nonclinical

The next group of people you will need to communicate your why to is your staff—both clinical and nonclinical. They're also busy folks, so be sure to anchor your reasoning to how addressing trauma in practice will help them get a handle on their day-to-day work. In my experience, the people in my office who have the most firsthand exposure to how trauma manifests in practice are the front desk staff and the advice nurses. Going back to the FRAYED mnemonic (see Box 7-2 from Chapter 7, Supporting Caregivers to Strengthen Safe, Stable, Nurturing Relationships), front desk staff often see parents with emotional dysregulation and are often yelled at by angry parents when things aren't going smoothly. Similarly, advice nurses often hear the frets and fears as well as the yelling when they help families on the phone. Teaching clinical and nonclinical staff that these are symptoms of trauma or stress and then teaching them the classic mental frameshift from "What's wrong with you?" (our natural, pre–trauma-informed reaction) to "What happened to you?" as part of their trauma-informed training will help them compartmentalize how they react to these challenging behaviors instead of seeing them as personal attacks. It increases compassion and empathy for the families as well, which ultimately defuses tense situations and provides better care. We discussed this in detail in Chapter 3, Getting Your Organization Ready: Creating Compassionate Pediatric Practices.

Note From Amy

My experience in working with staff at health care organizations is that these folks are the most impacted by families' traumas and the most moved by learning what trauma is and how it presents. Often, they start trainings with skepticism asking questions such as "How does this apply to my job?" With specific examples about how trauma shows up in their work, they're motivated to understand more and help patients and colleagues at their practice.

I fondly remember a billing/coding expert from a large federally qualified health center whom I consulted with about how trauma presents in patients and in her colleagues. We discussed how angry people are often hurt people with defenses up because of past experiences. And we problem-solved one particular case about a family that didn't understand an explanation of benefits. There were language barriers, service barriers, and multiple misunderstood charges amid a lengthy, jargony billing statement. We used that family's experience as an example of how folks might have experienced a lot of systemic injustices, felt judged because English was their second language, or were met with impatience as they attempted to navigate a confusing health care system. She was tearful and sincere as we used this family's experience as a case study for understanding trauma in health care systems, saying to me, "Now I get it. I can help families feel like they have an advocate and someone who wants to understand their circumstances." I truly believe that once staff understand trauma, they see the world through a different lens.

Remember that all your staff, colleagues, and leadership may also have experienced trauma themselves. When communicating about why you're going to embark on this process, include messages about how you intend to keep staff safe throughout the process.

Caregivers and Families

The last but most important group to whom you will have to explain your why is caregivers and families. We use a cover letter on our assessment tools that helps explain why we're asking the questions and what we intend to do with the information (it's included in Appendix F). Remember that caregivers are generally willing to talk about trauma with their pediatricians, but they also need explicit, transparent communication about the purpose of the questions before you can expect them to trust you and respond comfortably and honestly. As mentioned previously, the goal isn't to obtain the disclosure of trauma; the goal is to create a culture change in practice that normalizes conversations about trauma. That means that the way you explain trauma is probably more important than the tools you use or the answers you get on those tools. Spend some time thinking about how you want to communicate this information to your families. Other methods for communication include informational posts on social media, exam room posters, flyers taped to the clipboards that caregivers use to fill out office paperwork, and information on your clinic's website.

Of course, to hone your messaging to caregivers and families to be as effective as possible, you may want to seriously consider inviting them into the process. The QI committee in my clinic has always included a parent advisor. In fact, one of our early learning collaborative experiences centered on implementing trauma-informed care principles into practice—and our parent advisor traveled to all the learning sessions and helped develop our assessment workflows side by side with me and the nursing staff. When we started doing caregiver ACE assessments in our office, she reviewed our cover letter and gave feedback. It's pretty eye opening to learn how our words, written or spoken, are received by caregivers, so get their feedback on revising any information you present to families.

We'll talk more about family engagement in Chapter 16, Sustaining Trauma-Responsive Practices, but for now, just know that the feedback you get from families is invaluable in creating meaningful change. Parents ultimately have the same goals we do: to have their children experience the best care possible. We may feel uncomfortable asking parents for their advice because telling a family that we need to improve our clinic feels like an admission of weakness, but believe me, they don't see it that way. In fact, guidance on trauma-responsive environments points out that utilizing "voice," especially those of our patients with lived experiences, proves to be invaluable and often prevents us from re-traumatizing patients who have experienced adversity.[5] Asking for their advice and direct input on making the clinic better is a real game changer.

What Am I Looking For?

This comes down to which tools you're going to implement for each of the components of the RHH, but you'll need to think about which interventions you want to implement as well. Start with the priorities of PMDs and SE health, then SDOH, and then caregiver trauma history. As we've mentioned before, the caregiver trauma history may be a survey or it may be a series of guided questions to walk through the caregiver's experiences. Use **Table 15-1** to guide your decision-making, and choose relevant tools from Tables 6-1 and 7-1 in the previous chapters. As far as the interventions go, consider doing some of these resilience-based interventions, including a discussion about PCEs, before talking about trauma in caregivers. In the HOPE model developed out of Boston,[6] clinicians use this sequence with parents and caregivers, typically beginning with resilience before addressing trauma and adversity. Basic QI principles suggest doing "small tests of change"—starting with a small, manageable process change— rather than trying to "boil the ocean" by doing too much at once. As you become more adept at using the assessment tools or delivering a specific intervention, you can then build on what you've done and potentially add tools or another intervention as you see fit, to make your approach more comprehensive. But to begin with, choose just one tool, one intervention, and one visit.

How Will I Find It?

You may already be familiar with the idea of a Plan-Do-Study-Act (PDSA) cycle[7] (**Figure 15-1**), but if you aren't, I'll walk you through it. There's a blank planning form in Appendix S that you can use to document your implementation process.

At this point in your practice, you've probably implemented other screening tools; it may be helpful to look at previous workflows to see what worked and what needs to be adjusted when it comes to this implementation. A basic workflow for screening or assessment tools would typically look like **Figure 15-2**.

FIGURE 15-1.

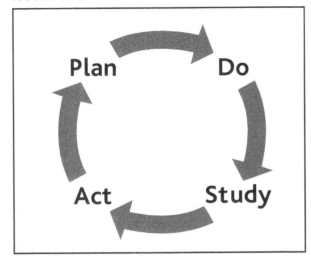

The Plan-Do-Study-Act cycle.

FIGURE 15-2.

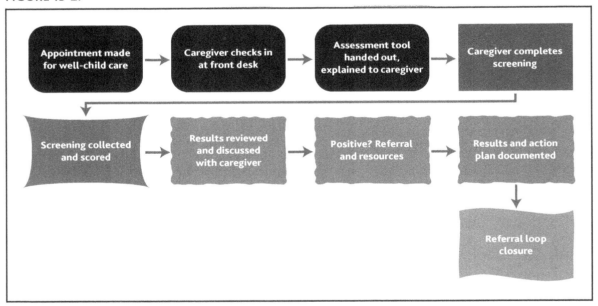

Basic screening workflow. Shapes indicate which team members will be responsible for which steps. Rounded box = front desk staff; squared box = caregiver; ragged box = health care professional; stretched box and wavy box = variable members of the office team.

In this simple workflow, the different shapes represent different team members who are involved in the screening workflow and, therefore, the different groups within your office that you need to engage to make the project successful. As noted in the figure, the stretched and wavy boxes may represent different people in the office, depending on your resources and how your office flow works. For example, screening tools may be collected by a medical assistant or a clinician, depending on your office flow. Referral loop closure may be done by a care coordinator if you have that role in your office or by someone else if you don't. This workflow analysis is fleshed out further in the workflow breakdown document in Appendix D. Use this appendix to analyze the nuances of your practice, then move into your first PDSA cycle.

Plan

Keep in mind that as a trauma-responsive practice implementing a complete RHH over the course of a child's life, you will need to implement multiple assessment tools, and some of the tools will need to be repeated over time. However, in the spirit of QI, remember the concept of small tests of change: choose one tool to start with. If you're feeling low confidence in addressing these subjects in practice—particularly trauma—starting with a tool may feel more comfortable, as it gives you a jumping-off point for the conversation. With experience, you may realize that a series of questions may lend itself better than another survey or assessment tool.

That said, a subtle but important decision point with regard to caregiver trauma histories is whether you're going to use a written tool or conduct a specific interview during the visit. When talking about more sensitive issues like trauma, written tools may be preferred over a set of verbal interview questions, as it's easier to ensure privacy and it gives the person completing the tool a chance to mull over the questions and decide if they feel safe answering in the first place. In studies of screening for intimate partner violence, written tools were generally more comfortable for patients to complete compared to interview questions.[8,9] Nonetheless, there are visits where surveillance questions are easier to implement because they don't interrupt the flow of a clinical visit; for example, if I'm in a visit with a person who has a mental health or behavioral concern, it's pretty easy to ask, "Did anything scary or upsetting happen before these symptoms began?" instead of pulling out a specific trauma assessment tool. In practice, using an assessment tool versus surveillance or history questions is not an either-or situation; they are both useful for different reasons, and they are both a part of my usual practice.

To be successful, the tools you select should be relatively quick to complete—the longer the tool, the less likely that it will be finished by the time you walk into the room. Other considerations for tool selection include cost, available languages, the types or categories of adversity or SDOH being assessed, and whether there has been any study of validity or reliability for the tool itself.[10]

The same PDSA cycle can be used when thinking about implementing resilience interventions, as listed out in the table at the beginning of the chapter (see **Table 15-1**). The same QI principles of small tests of change apply: start with 1 or 2 interventions that you want to implement, see how that goes, and then expand from there. Think about getting some simple feedback from caregivers as you implement the interventions; it can be as simple as "Is this helpful information? Is there any part of this that I could explain better? Do you think this will be a useful intervention to implement at home?"

When choosing your pilot group, you'll want to start with a small group of interested clinicians rather than roll the tool out to the whole group at the beginning. When my practice started to assess caregiver ACEs, we started with a small group of motivated, interested clinicians, which played a crucial role in making the pilot implementation successful. We were all willing to deal with the uncertainty of how the process was going to work and willing to get our hands dirty while we learned how to do the survey effectively. It would not have worked to implement the tool with the entire practice at the same time: we were spread over several sites, and most of the other clinicians weren't yet familiar with trauma or ACEs, so they weren't necessarily motivated to implement a tool yet.

Once you've picked your tool, the visit, and the pilot group, create a SMART (**S**pecific, **M**easurable, **A**ttainable, **R**ealistic, and **T**imely or time-specific) goal statement to focus your work.

✔ Each of the clinicians in the pilot group will survey 5 caregivers for ACEs at their child's 4-month visit in the next month.

It's a short statement, it describes exactly what we're going to do and when we're going to do it, and it's achievable. Another example of a SMART goal for implementing a resilience-based intervention might be the following:

✔ I will discuss "yolky feelings" with caregivers during every 5-year-old well-child visit for the next week.

During the pilot implementation, the physicians were looking for a few data points to evaluate. Our primary question was "Is screening for parental ACEs feasible in the course of a visit?" Having this question in mind helped us frame what data we needed to evaluate to know if the pilot implementation was successful. My colleagues were specifically looking for whether or not the tool could be completed by the caregivers efficiently, if the conversations during the visit were manageable, and how the caregivers responded or reacted to the tool itself. We also wanted to know how the physicians felt during the visit: Was the information obtained by the assessment tool useful? Could the physician navigate the conversation? Did the physician need to do any referrals and, if so, to what resource? During the pilot implementation, participating physicians kept notes on each of these pieces of information.

Furthermore, feedback from parents and caregivers is important, so make a point of asking them what they thought about the tool you've selected, how you explained the tool to them, and what concerns they had in completing the tool. Typically, our pilot group would be up front with the families during the visit by stating that we were piloting a new workflow and a new assessment tool, so their feedback would help us improve the process for everyone.

Do

The Do part of the PDSA cycle is self-explanatory, right? Just go for it.

Study

At the end of the pilot implementation, the Study phase of the improvement cycle is when you gather the data from what you've done and evaluate if any changes need to be made. This includes feedback gathered from families during the pilot stage.

If the pilot implementation was successful, you can plan to expand either scale or scope in your next PDSA cycle by screening more patients or involving more clinicians or by adding another resilience intervention for a different age-group. You might also consider small changes to the existing process (eg, trying a new script with families, testing a set of conversation prompts to navigate the conversation, or trying out a new resource for families).

If the pilot implementation was unsuccessful, try to determine why, and make changes to address the reason for the failure. And don't worry about failing; to paraphrase from one of the characters in the movie *Meet the Robinsons,* "From failure you learn; from success, not so much."

Act

The Act part of the PDSA cycle is when you use what you've learned from the Study stage and come up with a new SMART goal, plan a new improvement cycle, and then implement the changes you've made. In this way, PDSA cycles build on each other until you're ready for clinic-wide implementation. When you get to this point, you'll need to look at how screening tools are typically completed in your office through a workflow breakdown: examine the specific steps in a screening workflow that take place from the time a patient checks in at the office until the screening or assessment tool is completed, in the hands of the clinician, and documented in the chart. There are a series of questions in Appendix D to work through on your own, which will help you analyze your own clinic's processes to ensure that the tool is well embedded within your workflow.

Part of what we're doing when we pilot with a small group of clinicians is ironing out the wrinkles of implementation before rolling it out clinic-wide. Every practice has someone who is resistant to doing the proposed change. If you roll it out to a large group and something goes wrong, you've just validated what the resistant clinician thought all along and your implementation will stop right then and there; you'll have a really difficult time getting the resistant folks back on board. The pilot group typically can figure out the sticking points and resolve them before involving your "naysayers," making the change as easy and as clear as possible. That said, if you have a physician who remains skeptical or doesn't want to implement trauma assessments in practice, it's actually OK if they stay on the sidelines (as we've mentioned before). Because these are sensitive issues to talk about in the clinical visit, I'd rather have a resistant practitioner stay out of the game than approach the assessments half-heartedly. The patients will notice and might be harmed by this.

When you get to the point of clinic-wide implementation, you're going to want to think about building a multidisciplinary QI team to help with maintenance if you don't have one already. We'll talk more about that in Chapter 16, Sustaining Trauma-Responsive Practices, but ultimately, you're going to want to think about who is able to troubleshoot new problems and make changes as needed. Since we started our trauma assessments in practice, we've made 4 major revisions to the trauma questions, revised our cover letter (included in Appendix F), used 3 different resilience tools, added a list of resources that parents can tear off and take home, and so on. There are always ways to improve, particularly as the science around trauma evolves, so having a multidisciplinary team that oversees the initiative is vital.

What Will I Do When I Find It?

There are 2 ways to answer this question, as we've mentioned before. The first is the personal question about keeping yourself engaged, regulated, and calm (we talked about this more in Chapter 13, Self-Care and Sharing Our Humanity). The second is the clinical response, which comes down to implementing a basic 4-step safety plan that we talked about in detail in Chapter 10, Supporting Families That Have Experienced Trauma:

1. Assessment of child/family safety
2. Assets, resources, and resiliencies in the family—including coping and self-management strategies and an assessment of support networks
3. Follow-up tools for assessing mental health or SE development in patients as needed; in other words, assessing for symptoms caused by the traumatic event
4. Connecting with appropriate resources

Having a set of conversation prompts at your fingertips is the easiest way to navigate the subsequent conversation. Anchor your questions to the components of the safety plan to efficiently get through the rest of the visit. Before you begin with your questions, be sure to thank the patient or caregiver for disclosing a trauma to you. It means they trust you, but it is also a big step for someone to disclose to anyone, so acknowledge that.

Note From Amy

Here's a short script. "I see that you've endorsed some items on this questionnaire that are pretty personal. That's vulnerable and brave of you. Thank you so much for trusting me with this information" and, if needed, "Can we talk about this a bit more?" Providing affirmation and choice is a key element of trauma-responsive care; it shows compassion and awareness of sharing vulnerable information.

When thinking about which families need a safety plan, any disclosure of trauma deserves further follow-up, and any disclosure of trauma should be followed by an assessment of safety and symptoms or consequences of trauma. That doesn't mean you have to implement a written plan for everyone; I tend to use written safety plans in situations where the child has experienced trauma (we discussed this process in Chapter 10, Supporting Families That Have Experienced Trauma) and tend to use my clinical judgment for parent and caregiver trauma, although there are a few nuances to these conversations that are worth mentioning. There are 2 types of caregiver disclosures that you may face: the distal traumas that happened in childhood and more proximal traumas like domestic violence, SDOH, or episodic traumas like death of a family member or community violence. The basic sequence of the conversation follows the rhythm of the safety plan: assess safety, ask about strengths, and determine the need for further resources for the caregiver or child.

The first step in the safety planning process for more proximal traumas is to assess if there are any immediate threats to the child or family, including abuse, domestic violence, or acute social drivers that need to be addressed. I think about safety in terms of both physical and emotional safety. Remember your role in mandatory reporting if there is an immediate threat to the safety of your patient or family. Sometimes, assessing immediate safety is as simple as asking the patient or family, "Are you safe?" When assessing caregiver ACEs or histories of adversity that are more distal, I typically start by asking, "Do any of these experiences still bother you now?" which gets at the emotional safety concern. I then ask the caregivers what they need, rather than just hand them resources that I think would be helpful. The answers to these questions help determine what resources I'm going to need to connect with the family.

The best way to figure out resiliencies in the caregiver is, once again, to ask them. I like the question from Bethell and colleagues' work: How do you "[stay] calm and in control when faced with a challenge"?[11] It helps you get a sense of what coping strategies the caregiver is already using and helps you figure out where you might be able to offer some tips on effective coping strategies. As I've mentioned, I have a list of Ken Ginsburg's 7 Cs on my exam room wall that I refer to during these conversations; when families know the components of resilience, they often can start to identify where they need to shore up their own systems.[12] In my experience, most of the resilience tips relate to either Connection or Coping, so those are the ones I touch on the most; again, bonus points if you can get caregivers to do coping strategies together with their kids, as this means they're tapping into connection and building safe, stable, nurturing relationships (SSNRs). Another strategy is to discuss PCEs during the clinical visit and assess how families feel they are doing in making those experiences happen for their kids and whether they need support for it. You've been learning strategies throughout this book, so teach some of these skills during your visit. Some of the relevant resilience interventions to reinforce for more recent traumas include Circles of Support and parent self-care (the baseball analogy).

When a disclosure is a more distal event, such as when parents disclose trauma histories, I get at the resilience question by asking, "Of those experiences that no longer bother you, how did you get to the point that they don't bother you anymore?" It's another way of assessing resilience skills; I can further probe into their answers to figure out if those resilience factors still exist for the individual. For example, if it was connection with another adult in the family, is that person still around to turn to when the parent needs help? If it was therapy, do they still have access to mental health resources if they need them?

For younger kids, think about an assessment of SE health, as we mentioned in Chapter 6, Understanding Early Relational Health. The SE screeners will detect problems in the SSNRs between children and caregivers, so they are an appropriate screening tool to use to assess the sequelae of trauma in children younger than 5 years. Our practice does universal SE screening at 6, 15, 24, and 48 months, so it's again a dual application situation where a positive finding on screening during our routine assessments makes us probe for trauma or problems with SSNRs, and a caregiver trauma history makes us think of looking at SE health.

All the RHH assessment tools will need to be documented in your chart in some way. Be sure you have the ability to do this, either by adding forms into your electronic health record or by creating quick texts to streamline documentation. Typically, the documentation of any screening tool that you use needs to include the tool used, the score, your interpretation, and that you discussed the results with the family or patient. Some of the mental health and SE screening tools may be billable; these are the required charting elements to validly bill the tools.

The last component of the safety plan is to connect the family with resources. There is a temptation to think that if you detect trauma, the main resource is a mental health referral, but that really depends on what you find in the rest of your safety plan. To be sure, mental health resources are important, but if you're finding caregiver trauma, SDOH, or other factors, you'll also want to think about resources for parent coaching and positive parenting skill building, peer support groups, mentorship programs for older kids, domestic violence services, and social service resources. We've said this before, but it bears frequent repeating: you'll want to be sure you've done some degree of community asset mapping before starting your assessments to ensure you have adequate referral resources (both mental health professionals and CBOs) for any trauma or SDOH disclosures. A list of parent supports and trauma-specific therapies that have good evidence are listed in Box 6-2 from Chapter 6, Understanding Early Relational Health, and Box 10-3 from Chapter 10, Supporting Families That Have Experienced Trauma; see if any of them exist in your area.

Mental health resources include a myriad of evidence-based therapies for patients or parents, but also consider resources for PMDs, dyad therapies that involve caregivers and their children, and other support groups if you have them available. These therapies are reviewed in detail in the chapter on integrated care in Forkey, Griffin, and Szilagyi's *Childhood Trauma and Resilience: A Practical Guide.*[13]

All in, that's a lot of resources, so you're going to need some help. Hopefully, you have care coordination services in your practice to help you maintain some of the resource lists, but try to figure out who in your community is already keeping lists like this so you don't have to do it on your own. Many communities are building out systems like Help Me Grow (HMG; www.helpmegrow.org), Unite Us (https://uniteus.com), Aunt Bertha (https://helpfinder. auntbertha.com), 211Info, or United Way to help serve as a clearinghouse for resources for families. Rather than duplicate efforts by maintaining your own resource lists, build a relationship with the organizations that already do this work and figure out a referral system that works for you. Many of the practices in my area have been working on a referral system for HMG, where we send a referral to HMG and then it contacts the family, provides resources and supports, and, finally, closes the referral loop by sending us a summary of what it did for the family. Remember that Medicaid often offers care coordination services for patients with complex needs; our care coordinator knows the team within Medicaid, and they work collaboratively to help solve some of these referral issues for families.

Conclusions

There's a lot to think through as you're preparing to implement an assessment tool, isn't there? Breaking down the implementation process into 4 key questions—Why am I looking? What am I looking for? How will I find it? and What will I do when I find it?—helps organize your project into a logical process. Chances are, you've done some QI projects before, so this work isn't completely unfamiliar ground, but remember to break down your implementation into small steps of change. Build a team, talk it out, and make careful plans for a PDSA cycle and an initial pilot implementation before you begin. Use the resources in the appendixes, particularly Appendix D and Appendix J, to help facilitate the planning process.

You can do this!

Questions to Consider

1. Who in the practice will be impacted by implementing the tools needed to gather RHHs, and who needs to be involved? What communication needs to happen with each of these groups before implementation can take place?

2. What team needs to be assembled to help organize an implementation process?

3. What decisions need to be made to help decide on an initial PDSA cycle for implementing an assessment tool? What tool will you use and at which visits?

4. What decisions need to be made to help decide on an initial PDSA cycle for implementing a new resilience intervention? Which one will you implement first?

5. What conversation prompts make the most sense to you for navigating the conversations after a disclosure of trauma? Are they simple enough for you to remember during a visit, or do you need some type of reminder for the questions?

6. Are you familiar with the follow-up mental health assessment tools for when an RHH results in a trauma disclosure for patients? Are there any you need to locate? Do you know how to score them and document them in your chart?

7. Are there resource clearinghouses in your region that can help you organize referral resources for mental health, caregiver supports, and social service supports?

References

1. Narrative Arts. What is public narrative and how can we use it? Accessed March 20, 2024. https://narrativearts.org/article/public-narrative

2. The Children's Clinic. Accessed March 20, 2024. https://www.childrens-clinic.com

3. Eismann EA, Folger AT, Stephenson NB, et al. Parental adverse childhood experiences and pediatric healthcare use by 2 years of age. *J Pediatr*. 2019;211:146–151 PMID: 31079855 doi: 10.1016/j.jpeds.2019.04.025

4. Felitti V, Anda R. The relationship of adverse childhood experiences to adult medical disease, psychiatric disorders, and sexual behavior: implications for healthcare. In: Lanius RA, Vermetten E, Pain C, eds. *The Impact of Early Life Trauma on Health and Disease: The Hidden Epidemic*. Cambridge University Press; 2010:77–87

5. Substance Abuse and Mental Health Services Administration. *SAMHSA's Concept of Trauma and Guidance for a Trauma-Informed Approach*. HHS publication (SMA) 14-4884. Substance Abuse and Mental Health Services Administration; 2014

6. Sege RD, Harper Browne C. Responding to ACEs with HOPE: Health Outcomes From Positive Experiences. *Acad Pediatr*. 2017;17(7)(suppl):S79–S85 PMID: 28865664 doi: 10.1016/j.acap.2017.03.007

7. Langley GJ, Moen RD, Nolan KM, Nolan TW, Norman CL, Provost LP. *The Improvement Guide: A Practical Approach to Enhancing Organizational Performance*. 2nd ed. Jossey-Bass Publishers; 2009

8. Chisholm CA, Bullock L, Ferguson JEJ II. Intimate partner violence and pregnancy: epidemiology and impact. *Am J Obstet Gynecol*. 2017;217(2):141–144 PMID: 28551446 doi: 10.1016/j.ajog.2017.05.042

9. O'Doherty L, Hegarty K, Ramsay J, Davidson LL, Feder G, Taft A. Screening women for intimate partner violence in healthcare settings. *Cochrane Libr*. 2015;2015(7):CD007007 PMID: 26200817 doi: 10.1002/14651858.CD007007.pub3

10. Oh DL, Jerman P, Purewal Boparai SK, et al. Review of tools for measuring exposure to adversity in children and adolescents. *J Pediatr Health Care*. 2018;32(6):564–583 PMID: 30369409 doi: 10.1016/j.pedhc.2018.04.021

11. Bethell CD, Gombojav N, Whitaker RC. Family resilience and connection promote flourishing among US children, even amid adversity. *Health Aff (Millwood)*. 2019;38(5):729–737 PMID: 31059374 doi: 10.1377/hlthaff.2018.05425

12. Ginsburg KR, Jablow MM. *Building Resilience in Children and Teens: Giving Kids Roots and Wings*. 4th ed. American Academy of Pediatrics; 2020

13. Forkey HC, Griffin JL, Szilagyi M. Integrated care. In: *Childhood Trauma and Resilience: A Practical Guide*. American Academy of Pediatrics; 2021:159–167

Chapter 16

Sustaining Trauma-Responsive Practices

R.J. Gillespie, MD, MHPE, FAAP

I have no special talent. I am just passionately curious.
Albert Einstein

I'm sitting around a conference table with half a dozen of my colleagues at my clinic site, and we're spending our lunch hour exchanging scripts for how we introduce our caregiver trauma assessment tool to our families.

I say: "I talk about how most of what we learn about being parents comes from how our parents modeled it to us. If that was a good experience, we want to think about how we capture those positive aspects and make sure that happens for our kids. If it wasn't a good experience, we want to think about how we might do things differently. Looking at the past helps us be more mindful about how we parent."

Another colleague shares: "I talk about 'shark music'—how everyone has triggers that remind them of something stressful or dangerous. When we know what tends to make us anxious, we can prepare for it and hopefully respond differently."

And another: "I usually talk about the effects of ACEs on health and how one way to try to keep toxic stress from happening is by building strong relationships with our kids."

Some people are nodding and reflecting; others are scribbling notes and asking for us to repeat our scripts. We move on to talking about what has been helpful—and what's been challenging—about our workflow. What cases were difficult, and how would other colleagues handle them? What resources are we using, and how have families reacted to them? It's called *reflective practice* (more on this in a minute), and we're using the process to grow and improve. It's a major part of our sustainability plan for ensuring that our practice keeps trauma-responsive care front and center in our daily work.

Whenever you implement a new workflow in practice, it helps to think about sustainability from the outset. In Chapter 3, Getting Your Organization Ready: Creating Compassionate Pediatric Practices, and Chapter 15, Implementation Nuts and Bolts, we talked about how to engage leadership, staff, other clinicians, and patients before implementation. Getting that buy-in changes the culture of the practice and is foundational to sustainability in the long run.

That said, things will change in your screening and assessment protocol over time, as you learn new information and get feedback from clinicians or patients and as you evaluate the efficacy and practicality of the tools you've chosen or developed. In my practice's workflow for assessing caregiver trauma, we've been through numerous revisions of our tool—we're currently on our fifth version—and have responded to my colleagues' educational and skill-building needs, expanded our screening for social drivers and social-emotional (SE) health, and made many other changes to enhance our ability to be trauma responsive. These changes reflected how our practice approached maintenance and sustainability, including how we adapted to new information as it emerged in the literature. To effectively adapt and sustain your assessment protocols, there needs to be a structure within your practice to bring these changes to life.

Sustainability is enhanced when you become a part of a network of care; think about the saying often cited as an African proverb "Alone we go faster; together we go further." When we work in isolation, there are limits to what we can do, but following a collective impact framework means that our individual efforts—when aligned with the efforts of community-based organizations (CBOs), education systems, and mental health clinicians—add up to a lot more than the sum of their parts. Models for trauma-informed networks of care based on collective impact ideologies are emerging all over the country, including sanctuary models,[1] Blue Zone Communities,[2] and others; the idea is that your work will be more sustainable if it's buffered and supported by the efforts of others.

There are 3 general areas to consider when it comes to sustainability: monitoring and improving the clinical systems that support assessments for trauma or relational health history (RHH) taking; continuing to improve your knowledge and skills in trauma-responsive care; and maintaining and improving your clinical response to trauma, including your referral and resource network. Some of these areas are an organizational-level responsibility; some, clinician-level; and some, joint responsibility—so you'll need to continue to engage your administration to get all the support you need, particularly when it comes to financing educational or training opportunities, participating in community-wide networks of care, and supporting quality improvement (QI) infrastructure within your practice. We'll dive into each of these areas of sustainability in order, with tips about how to make each area practical and efficient. This work is best enacted when you have a champion or champions within your practice to lead the process, as well as a QI team that can support systemic change and address challenges as they arise.

A key component of sustainability is self-care and self-compassion, as we discussed in Chapter 13, Self-Care and Sharing Our Humanity. This can be hard work, as you've probably figured out. Remember the principles of self-care that we outlined earlier as you think about sustainability for the future: you can't continue to do this work without taking care of yourself, your staff, and your colleagues first.

Monitoring Your Clinical Systems

The Institute for Healthcare Improvement (IHI) identifies 6 key domains in sustainability of QI processes, all of which imply a specific structure within your practice to address these domains.[3] Specifically, there should be a multidisciplinary team within your practice that can proactively address changes, respond to problems, and ensure consistent workflows within the practice. It perhaps goes without saying that your sustainability efforts depend on having clinic champions who lead this team. The 6 IHI domains in sustainability are Integration, Accountability, Problem Solving, Visual Management, Escalation, and Standardization.

Integration

Integration refers to understanding the reason for the change and linking that change to a higher purpose. As mentioned earlier, a big part of this is understanding how assessments for trauma and social drivers of health (SDOH) link into your clinic's mission or vision for how it delivers care to patients and families. This means that trauma assessments should be integrated into your clinic's culture—with *culture* being loosely defined as "the way we do things around here." The challenge lies in keeping that connection to your clinic's vision front and center for existing clinicians and staff after implementation and in introducing the project purpose to new staff as part of their onboarding and orientation. One way to keep the project front and center is to schedule regular report-outs to leadership or to your provider group, such as a quarterly update on progress toward specific goals.

Clinical workflows are also generally more sustainable if they are anchored to patient and family needs and preferences, so obtaining ongoing feedback from families should be part of your sustainability strategy. This helps with the overall idea of integration: if a project is reflective of what patients and families expect from their care, it becomes a stable part of clinic culture. Take this testimonial from one of my parents, for example. She was interviewed about her experience being asked about ACEs as part of an RHH at her son's 4-month appointment—and the conversation that followed—as part of an article on PACEsConnection (not a formal mechanism for getting feedback, but still…). She said:

> "Just knowing that he was taking the time to listen to me, and validating that I was doing everything right, and that I was doing a great job, meant a lot to me....I have no idea how I got through it, but I did. Having the support of my pediatrician who genuinely cared about me definitely helped. By the six-month appointment, things were much better."[4]

Knowing that this is how parents and caregivers feel about the conversations in assessing their RHH helps anchor me in remembering why I do this work. This is the real power of patient and family feedback: that feedback gets woven into your core reasons for doing this work and stays with you as you move forward.

There are different ways to get family feedback, each serving its own purpose within your QI structure. There are some great resources for how to engage families in QI projects, including a toolkit from the National Institute for Children's Health Quality for implementing family advisory councils, but here are some high-level ideas for implementation.[5,6]

SURVEYS

Surveys are a great way to get broad feedback from patients or families on a wide variety of subjects. The strength in this approach is that you can get anonymous feedback from families, which might be more honest and direct than asking patients face-to-face about their experiences. The drawback is that the feedback may be selective, coming from those families that are willing and able to answer survey questions, which could be based on literacy, language that the survey is offered in, interest in the subject of the survey, and general time considerations. If surveys are open-ended, it may also be difficult to interpret the answers from a patient perspective.

PARENT ADVISORS

These are parents or caregivers from your practice who are brought on as established members of your QI committees. It's preferable to have parents or caregivers with lived experience, if possible (ie, people who have experienced trauma, peripartum mood disorders [PMDs], or SDOH), and are willing to not only share their experiences with your practice but also advise how they would experience the process of assessment and share their opinions on how to conduct the assessments meaningfully and sensitively in practice. Parent advisors usually work side by side with other members of your QI team and help inform all aspects of the clinic's workflow. That said, it's a big burden to expect just one caregiver to represent the opinions of all the families in your practice, so consider having multiple parent advisors if you're able to. Invest the time in onboarding them to your committee—when you're deep in QI and quality measurement, you end up using a ridiculous number of acronyms that can make meetings seem like you're living in the Tower of Babel. Help your parent advisor catch up to all the jargon and terminology they're likely to find. Also, if you have the resources, pay your parent advisor at least the same hourly rate that you would pay a staff member who attends the meetings; your parent advisor's time is just as valuable as everyone else's, and they often have to figure out child care arrangements to be able to fully engage and participate.

FOCUS GROUPS

Focus groups are a way to get a little broader representation of the experiences of families within your practice. Focus groups are groups of caregivers or patients who are brought together to give more detailed or in-depth feedback about aspects of your clinic's workflows around trauma assessments. Usually, this type of group is a limited commitment on the part of caregivers—typically a handful of meetings that are targeted to a specific subject that you're trying to obtain feedback about. Again, it's preferable to have people with lived experience who can use their wisdom to give feedback on your clinic's workflow. A focus group may also be helpful in fleshing out the information obtained from patient surveys if you are having a difficult time interpreting why caregivers responded the way they did.

FAMILY ADVISORY BOARDS

These are groups of parents or guardians that are an official committee within the structure of your clinic, as opposed to focus groups that may be a one-off. When implemented in practice, your family advisory board can be consulted on any number of clinic-based operations. In my experience, these are highly engaged people who really care about how your practice runs and are invested in helping ensure that your clinic delivers the best possible care. Their participation may be enhanced if you recruit a nonphysician staff member to help coordinate the committee; it's safer for parents and caregivers to express open and honest opinions if they aren't simultaneously worried about maintaining a positive relationship with their child's individual clinician.

Accountability

The IHI describes accountability in the QI context as "keeping an eye on the work being done."[3] Quality improvement projects are more sustainable if they have regular oversight and management by a team, preferably an ongoing, multidisciplinary team of staff and physicians who can reflect on the way screening or other processes are operationalized in the office. This team is also responsible for implementing changes based on new information in the literature and feedback from families, staff, or clinicians. In our practice, the QI Committee oversees these types of changes, including all our medical home efforts; our committee includes nursing, physician, and administrative staff, as well as parent advisors.

Once RHH assessments are well established, this team can also monitor SMART (**S**pecific, **M**easurable, **A**ttainable, **R**ealistic, and **T**imely or time-specific) goals related to the project and collect information related to assessment rates, referral loop closure, patient satisfaction, and other data points relevant to those goals. As with any continuous QI project, once goals from one Plan-Do-Study-Act (PDSA) cycle are completed, the team can link them to a new set of goals and a new PDSA cycle to strengthen or expand the assessment process. Once the assessment process is streamlined, the same QI processes of creating SMART aim statements and PDSA cycles can be applied to implementing resilience interventions and improving tracking and referral systems and other elements of the overall clinical response to trauma disclosures.

Problem Solving

Problem-solving in the context of sustainability refers to addressing any changes in practice, such as new electronic health records (EHRs), additions or changes to assessment tools, new front desk workflows, and so forth. It also refers to responding to changes in the literature that may influence how you conduct assessments in practice. As mentioned earlier, we've been through numerous revisions in our assessment tool over the years, and thanks to our multidisciplinary team, we're able to implement these changes efficiently. Many of the changes have been a result of looking at our own clinic data and doing "sense making" of that data—that is, trying to interpret what story the data are trying to tell us.

For example, when we first started assessing ACEs in caregivers, we were asking about each of the ACEs individually, so we looked at what ACEs they most commonly reported. Not surprisingly, experiencing divorce or separation was the most reported ACE. Looking in more detail, however, we realized that caregivers were more likely to disclose a parent having been incarcerated than to endorse a history of sexual abuse. In terms of mere prevalence of those 2 ACEs, that didn't make sense: sexual abuse is known to be a lot more common, after all. So, what's the story that the data are telling us? We considered if it was a reflection of the demographics of our population or if there was something missing in how we demonstrated the compassion and safety needed to create a safe space for sensitive disclosures. We also considered that perhaps caregivers didn't want to disclose that level of detail about sensitive information to their child's pediatrician, so we started with that assumption.

Our team decided that in the context of asking caregivers to disclose ACEs, it's better to ask an aggregated number; that is, rather than tell the details of which ACEs they experienced, the caregiver could simply read the statements and disclose a total number instead. If caregivers felt comfortable discussing it further with their child's pediatrician, they could, but the structure of the tool didn't force any specific disclosures.

After that change, caregivers were much more likely to reveal more ACEs, indicating that revealing a number was probably preferable to discussing more specific details. Given that we wanted to de-emphasize the importance of the ACE score, we then went on to embed the 3 follow-up questions from Chapter 2, Addressing Barriers, into our EHR as a form of decision support to remind pediatricians to expand the conversation and not simply stop once they've counted a score:

1. Do any of these experiences still bother you now?
2. Of those experiences that no longer bother you, how did you get to the point that they don't bother you anymore?
3. How do you think these experiences affect your parenting now?

In addition, we added an open-ended question to our tool to consider other types of adversity. These refinements helped move us away from labeling a patient as an ACE score and toward understanding whether or not the RHH of the caregiver might be impacting the child-caregiver dyad.

Visual Management

Visual management refers to how data are presented to staff and clinicians; as previously mentioned, this is a key component of sustainability. As part of the sustainability of your assessment process, there should be a plan for how to continue to review data. Your team can help you decide what pieces of data will be most helpful for maintaining gains made during the project; depending on where you are in your assessment journey, this can be as simple as a screening rate, or it may be something more complicated, like how many patients or families are connected to services. In our practice, we looked at some key outcomes that we were interested in—we discovered a correlation between caregiver ACEs and risk for developmental delay in the child—and presented that data to our physicians. Those data were extraordinarily motivating to my practice colleagues. When you're looking at data from the literature, it's easy to think of them as abstract or less relevant to your patient population; but when you're looking at data related to the patients you see in your own office, it's far more powerful as a motivating force because the data are personal.

The point here is that presenting data back to staff and clinicians helps provide motivation for continued work in your assessment workflow, but it also helps highlight opportunities for improvement. Data can be presented not only formally in meetings but also informally with posters or other visual media in the break rooms that include messages about data being collected, changes to your assessment protocols, goals of any SMART aim statements that your team is working on, results of patient feedback around assessment processes, and so forth. If your practice has a clinic newsletter, include some information about what you're doing to become more and more trauma responsive. Consider also presenting data to families and patients; it may help them understand why the workflows exist in the first place.

Escalation

Escalation refers to addressing specific problems as they occur during patient encounters, such as patient concerns or complaints about the assessment process. In the years we've been doing assessments of caregiver ACEs in my practice, I've had very few complaints from caregivers that have landed on my desk, but they do happen. One particular parent complaint stands out in my mind, because when I explored the context of what happened in her encounter, I learned a lot about how to improve the process. We were relatively early in our screening process, and when this mom was handed the assessment tool, the cover letter wasn't attached. When the mom expressed to her child's physician that she wasn't comfortable filling in the questions, the physician responded, "OK, I'll pass that on," and then referred the mom to me for feedback about our screening protocol.

There were, of course, some missed opportunities in that interaction. When I talked with her, I learned this mom had experienced several ACEs, which is what had led to her initial discomfort with the tool. Since the cover letter was missing, she didn't get any context about why the assessment was being done in the first place, nor did she get the information about what we were intending to do with her responses. It turns out that the front desk had been running out of tools, so they'd made some quick photocopies of the tool to hand out to caregivers who were coming in that day, and to save time, they copied only the questions themselves. Issue number one: staff training on how to explain the tool to caregivers and on the importance of the *entire* tool. Issue number two: maintaining office supplies and making sure someone is keeping track of what the front desk staff need to do their job.

Issue number three: the physician's response. Mom's discomfort could have been addressed differently in a couple of different ways; at a minimum, the physician could have reassured her that the tool was voluntary and she didn't have to fill it out if she wasn't comfortable. They could have taken the time to explain the purpose of the tool, how the information would be treated confidentially, and what we intended to do with the information. More importantly, the physician could have recognized that this mom's distress was because the tool had been activating to her given her own experiences; the physician could have empathetically explored that with the mom, if she was willing to disclose more details.

To be clear, I didn't blame my colleague for the interaction. Generally speaking, when errors happen in any area of medicine, it's far more meaningful and effective to explore the system that led to the error and turn it into a teachable moment, rather than point a finger at an individual. In this case, part of what was missing for the physician was some scripting for how to address the encounter, which signaled that more training was needed before we proceeded much further with our screening process. When the problem was brought back to the QI Committee, we were able to address it quickly and efficiently: administrative staff from the committee was able to address the workflow issues that the front desk experienced, and clinicians on the team were able to reflect on the clinician and staff needs for further training and support. We scheduled some lunch and learn sessions with our colleagues to discuss what scripts others use in their interactions with families—in other words, reflective practice—which helped the physician strengthen skills for future encounters.

As for the mom who raised the complaint, the conversation was helpful in a lot of ways. She was grateful to be heard and that her complaints were being taken seriously to help improve the practice workflows. When I explained the purposes of our assessment tool and how we intended to use it to help identify parents and caregivers who might need more support in their parenting skills, she offered to look at our cover letter (which had been missing in her encounter) to provide feedback and to decide if it would have been adequate for addressing her concerns. For my part, I learned a lot about how the workflow operated for other people in the practice and was able to identify needs on the part of the staff and my colleagues.

Standardization

Quality improvement projects are more sustainable if it's easy for clinicians and teams to "do the right thing" and ensure that assessment tools or screeners are done on time, every time. This comes down to decision support for staff and clinicians and to integration of the assessment workflow into staff training.

Decision supports are the prompts in documentation reminding a clinician that a screening is due at a particular visit. For example, if you're using an EHR and the 9-month visit template doesn't have a place to document the results of a developmental screening tool, it's easier to forget that the tool was supposed to have been done. On the other hand, if the visit template has a clear place to document results, the tools are more likely to be completed because the staff and clinician look for the completed tool and can encourage the caregiver to finish it if necessary. Taking it a step further, you can program in quick texts with follow-up questions or conversation prompts to help clinicians navigate the conversation. When we assess parental ACEs at the 4-month visit, underneath the spot where results are documented are the 3 follow-up questions that we recommend for the ensuing conversation, so it's a lot easier for clinicians to remember how to proceed.

As you experience staff turnover, principles of trauma-informed care (TIC) will need to be a part of your onboarding and training process. Similarly, new staff will need to be oriented to their role in the assessment process and be given scripts for how to introduce the assessment to parents and respond to their questions.

Continuing Development of Trauma-Informed Skills and Knowledge

Reflective Practice

As you learn from your clinical experiences in addressing trauma in practice, it's helpful to process that learning, either alone or with other partners. This is the idea of reflective practice: creating space to reflect on patient encounters that went well or those that were a little more challenging.[7] This process helps you gain insight into professional practice by thinking analytically about what factors may have led to either positive or negative outcomes and how you can learn and improve your practice from those factors.

Journaling is a flexible way to explore reflective practice on your own, although some people prefer a more structured template. The important thing is to focus on what was learned, not just create an account of the event. A simple template from the literature would be the following[7]:

1. Describe the situation.
2. Reflect on your emotional state at the time.
3. Make sense of the situation or why it happened the way it did.
4. Consider if anything could have been done differently.
5. Think about what changes you can make in practice.
6. Consider what will happen when you put this change into practice.

I find the reflective practice process to be most meaningful when it's done with a colleague or a group. This is the whole idea behind the "morning report" or "morbidity and mortality rounds" that are done in training—to figure out how to learn from challenging cases and put changes into practice. I think that often the residency training focus is to look at negative outcomes or things that didn't go well, but remember that reflective practice can also be used to explore positive outcomes to try to ensure that they're repeated in the future.

Consider establishing a regular process for reflective practice in your own professional life. It will not only give you insights into the way you do trauma-informed patient encounters but also highlight future educational needs, allow you to compare experiences with peers and learn how they manage challenging encounters, and allow you to celebrate things that went well. This is an area where you might want to consider consultation with outside professionals: psychology colleagues can help facilitate the reflective practice process, either external mental health practitioners or your internal behavioral health clinicians if you have them.

Another clinic structure that helps staff is the creation of affinity groups, where staff in similar roles can periodically get together and talk through how trauma has shown up or does show up in their day-to-day work. After all, reflective practice doesn't apply just to clinicians. Staff will also benefit from having the opportunity to problem-solve challenging interactions and share their collective experiences.

Note From Amy

There's so much growth that occurs from reflective consultation, with an expert, about trauma-informed practices. Finding an expert who intersects medicine, mental health, and trauma awareness creates a space for physicians to talk about tough cases, their own triggers, and ideas about how to approach patients and families that are experiencing trauma. First, it allows you an outside guide with perspective on mental health and trauma-informed practices. Second, it allows you to step away from being the expert and gain insight for your practice and patients. Third, it allows you to be in community with peers, which leads to less isolation.

This space is one where R.J. and I share our experiences, and it's where community, competency, confidence, and connection all grow. I've had the privilege of going into his clinic and consulting with clinicians about TIC and how patients present. Even more important is the ever-present question "Now what do I do about it?" It's inspiring and joyful to see physicians responding to the needs of patients in a compassionate way (As we keep saying, you're already doing it!) and, when they feel stuck, to see how responsive they are to gaining support and insight into their patients and their behaviors. Often, because time is set aside to brainstorm tough cases and consult, there are lots of insights and aha moments that are shared. There's something magical that happens when they sit and discuss how to go about supporting patients and building resilience in their clinic. I see their overwhelm decrease, their purpose surge, and their sense of connection rise.

Ongoing Education and Keeping Up With the Literature

Since the publication of the original ACEs study in 1997, the literature in this area has exploded. It can be a bit challenging to keep up with all the new information and changes. A quick search in PubMed revealed over 800 new articles about ACEs in the first half of 2022 alone.

If you are regularly doing reflective practice with your colleagues, educational needs will often be highlighted by this process. In our practice, we decided that we needed to do further structured training in positive parenting and SE health and eventually become certified as a No Hit Zone, which included education on how to talk with parents about alternatives to spanking as part of the curriculum. This reflective practice also helps you narrow what parts of the literature you're paying particular attention to.

Personally, I find it helpful to subscribe to a few key newsletters that summarize new information for me, and then I can dig deeper into articles or information that is relevant to my professional interests. Some journals, like the *Journal of Child and Adolescent Trauma*, will email you the table of contents when new issues are released, so you can scan the titles for relevant articles. The Center on the Developing Child at Harvard (https://developingchild.harvard.edu), The National Child Traumatic Stress Network (www.nctsn.org), and PACEsConnection (www.pacesconnection.com) have regular emails and updates that you can subscribe to. Some states have local organizations that keep track of training opportunities and literature updates, like Trauma Informed Oregon (https://traumainformedoregon.org) or the ACEs Aware initiative in California (www.acesaware.org); these organizations also provide electronic mailing lists and email updates. It's impossible to list all the amazing resources out there, but some of our favorite resources are in **Table 16-1**.

Obviously, conferences are a great way to keep up with changes in the field as well. The American Academy of Pediatrics (AAP) has an intermittent conference series called Trauma-Informed Pediatric Provider; the Academy on Violence and Abuse and the Chadwick conferences are other opportunities to keep up with colleagues in the field.

Practicing Resilience Interventions and Ongoing Consultation

It can feel a little awkward when you first get started on some of the resilience interventions, particularly as you decide how to work them into your clinic visit and practice the scripting for those interventions. This is another area where reflective practice, particularly in small groups with your partners, may be helpful. Through the reflective practice process, you'll be able to share scripts and problem-solve for how to best integrate interventions into the way you do your day-to-day visits. It may also be helpful to engage psychology colleagues to help you maintain these new practices.

Over the years, in my practice, we've engaged colleagues to help us develop and implement many of the resilience interventions that we've covered in this book (Thanks, Amy!), learning more about SE and early relational health (ERH); they've also helped with positive parenting tips and techniques to use in practice. We hired outside trainers to help with our basic TIC training at a practice level, joined learning collaboratives to learn more about TIC and resilience and get help with screening for SDOH and SE health, and so on. All these processes were ways that we engaged in ongoing consultation to stay up to date, expand our skills, and refresh ourselves on the basic concepts of trauma-informed and trauma-responsive care.

It can be challenging, as the practice champion for TIC at a practice level, to be the main person charged with keeping TIC fresh in the minds of the clinicians and promoting TIC as a practice priority. Bringing in outside expertise helps bring new voices and perspectives to the conversation. Through your reflective practice process, you'll identify needs for the clinicians in your

Table 16-1. Resources for Further Education on ACEs

Resource	Description	URL
American Academy of Pediatrics Preventing ACEs toolkit	Practice resources, infographics, videos, and articles about trauma and resilience	www.aap.org/en/news-room/campaigns-and-toolkits/preventing-adverse-childhood-experiences
Early relational health messaging guide from the Center for the Study of Social Policy	Lots of briefs and resources	https://cssp.org/resource/early-relational-health-messaging-guide
ACEs Aware initiative	Training guides, webinars, and other resources	www.acesaware.org
Johns Hopkins Pediatric Integrated Care Collaborative	Toolkit describing trauma-informed practices, resilience, and implementation in practice	https://picc.jhu.edu/the-toolkit.html
Zero to Three	Resources for providers and patients in promoting developmental health in early childhood	www.zerotothree.org
Center on the Developing Child at Harvard	Latest research, policy briefs, and other resources related to early childhood development and the effects of toxic stress on children	https://developingchild.harvard.edu
The National Child Traumatic Stress Network	Tracks and consolidates research on trauma and adversity in children; of particular interest is their paper *Beyond the ACE Score*.	www.nctsn.org

office; from that, you can create an academic calendar of continuing medical education or training events for related subjects that will strengthen your current efforts and hopefully take things to the next level.

Sustaining a Meaningful Response to Trauma

Maintaining Resource and Referral Networks

In the best-case scenario, you are using a community-based referral platform rather than trying to keep a list of resources on your own. Like we've mentioned, many states are building and enhancing Unite Us (https://uniteus.com), Aunt Bertha (https://helpfinder.auntbertha.com), or other platforms to help connect families with CBOs. Other organizations that keep catalogs of resources include 211Info and United Way. If you're able to connect with one of those types of organizations, let them do the legwork for you. It really does take a village to address trauma effectively.

If you are in a smaller community, or don't have these types of referral platforms available, that means you'll have to assign someone in the practice to take responsibility for maintaining your list of resources. This should be a living document that reflects changes in all the CBOs' current contact information, capacity, and eligibility requirements. Some organizations are well funded and have a strong foothold in the community, so not much changes; but other, smaller organizations that rely on grant funding for their sustainability may have regular changes to their ability to survive. Keep a spreadsheet or a contact list and create a work plan for how often you'll keep in touch with resources. The resources you're compiling should match the things you're assessing in practice (eg, resources for trauma will be different from resources for social drivers or PMDs). If you're doing referral tracking (see Chapter 10, Supporting Families That Have Experienced Trauma), you may get feedback from families about the effectiveness or availability of the resource; you can incorporate that information into your resource lists.

Mental health resource lists also require a lot of legwork. You should know the different types of mental health therapies available, including individual therapies, dyad therapies, and group therapies. Their access may wax and wane as well, so keeping up to date is vital for helping patients access services. We have a mental health care coordinator as part of our care coordinator team; her primary responsibility is keeping track of mental health clinicians so she can match up patient insurance with the type of therapist that is needed and the expected wait time for an appointment with that therapist.

Integrated Behavioral Health

The gold standard in integrated behavioral health (IBH) is to have mental health practitioners in your office who do a blend of warm handoffs while the patient is in the office for a visit, as well as separate appointments for short-term, problem-oriented patient care. This model of integration means that mental health practitioners are working side by side with physicians and nurse practitioners, and they are available for real-time support and conversations as problems are identified during office visits; this is in contrast with colocated models where a mental health practitioner shares space with your colleagues but keeps their own busy schedule, so the practitioner doesn't have the capacity for warm handoffs or immediate support as problems are identified in the course of routine clinical care. It probably goes without saying that there are currently challenges in finding/funding IBH professionals, given workforce shortages, practice capacity, and a host of other barriers—but like I said, it's the gold standard.

The advantage of a truly integrated model is the connection you have with your behavioral health practitioners and that you can engage those practitioners to become part of your response to trauma disclosures in practice. As you've noticed, sometimes trauma is present but there isn't an immediate consequence to that trauma; IBH can help with caregiver support as part of mental health preventive care. For example, in our practice of assessing caregiver trauma, if caregivers disclose trauma and are interested in support for positive parenting, IBH practitioners can spend a little more time with the family, do some short-term work on promoting SE health, and then assess which families might benefit from more long-term Parent-Child Interaction Therapy or other parenting programs. Ideally, IBH practitioners would be able to conduct group visits or support groups as well; remember that one of the resources caregivers are most interested in is support groups.[8]

I think there's a misperception of the role of mental health practitioners as simply responding when there's an identified mental illness or behavioral problem. Although that's an important part of mental health for older kids, there's a role for mental health promotion and prevention by mental health clinicians that is integrated into pediatric primary care. Having IBH gives you the opportunity to think creatively about how you can promote ERH, strengthen parenting skills, and respond to minor child behavior difficulties or parenting challenges early—before they become bigger problems.

Advocacy

The reality is that you may not have everything you need to respond adequately to trauma in practice; none of us have enough time or money to build the comprehensive care systems that we wish for. It would also be great if every community was flush with home visitation programs, caregiver supports, funding for IBH, care coordinators or peer navigators, appropriate CBOs for social needs, community-based referral platforms, trauma-informed mental health practitioners, and everything else you need to provide a good response for your patients and families. It would be amazing as well if we all could find, hire, and bill for IBH practitioners in our offices. Garner and Saul identified a lot of advocacy ideas in their book[9]; the list is extensive and reflects the need for greater partnership between health care and other public sectors to effectively address trauma at a societal level.

You're only one person, and you have a lot on your plate. If you don't have the bandwidth to advocate on your own, you should at least know where to send your best advocacy ideas. In many state AAP chapters, there is a legislative committee that takes ideas and carries them to the appropriate audiences at the state legislative level, so shoot them an email to tell them about what you're experiencing on the ground and what resources would be helpful—whether that's a concrete practice support or an underfunded community resource. State medical associations also often have legislative groups that can advocate on your behalf; in my state, the Oregon Medical Association often solicits ideas from members to carry forward. Most AAP chapters also have a pediatric council, which is a committee that is tasked with addressing payment or reimbursement challenges. Of course, advocating directly to Medicaid, your state's health authority, or state and federal legislators is also an option if you have the time and energy.

Conclusions

Implementing RHH assessment tools and resilience interventions in practice is the first step to becoming trauma responsive. Attention must be paid to how your efforts are sustained over time. This means maintaining your focus on trauma, responding to changes in the literature, and identifying educational needs for the clinicians and staff in your office. This maintenance is best done by a committee or group of champions who can carry this work forward.

This sustainability work helps keep your workflow from becoming stale by continually updating and improving what you do. For example, I found that changing from resilience surveys to asking about PCEs gave amazing life to our screening process and revitalized our interest in doing this work. This example of a major shift in our RHH process was possible only because of our ongoing efforts to learn and improve.

Questions to Consider

1. What are you doing to take care of yourself and your colleagues as you address trauma in your practice?

2. How can you implement reflective practice into your professional routine? What model for reflective practice—individual, with a colleague, or with a group—fits best into your practice life?

3. What electronic mailing lists, email subscriptions, conferences, or other educational opportunities are available to you to continue your journey toward trauma-responsive care? Where have you gone for education in the past?

4. What structures do you need to put in place to ensure sustainability in your practice? Do you have an existing team that can help manage ongoing QI?

5. How have you integrated TIC into your clinic's culture? What do you still need to do to keep TIC front and center within your practice?

6. What colleagues in the community can you enlist for ongoing consultation? What skills will your practice and colleagues need to enhance to take their TIC skills to the next level?

7. Do you have appropriate staff to maintain referral and resource networks? What plan can you develop to ensure that your information about CBOs and mental health practitioners is current and relevant?

8. What needs have you identified for advocacy? Payment, access to resources, better IBH? Where can you pass on your ideas?

References

1. The Sanctuary Institute. Sanctuary model. Accessed March 20, 2024. https://www.thesanctuaryinstitute.org/about-us/the-sanctuary-model

2. Blue Zones Project. Accessed March 20, 2024. https://info.bluezonesproject.com/home

3. Scoville R. 6 essential practices for sustainable improvement. Institute for Healthcare Improvement. October 26, 2017. Accessed March 20, 2024. https://www.ihi.org/insights/6-essential-practices-sustainable-improvement

4. Stevens J. To prevent childhood trauma, pediatricians screen children and their parents…and sometimes, just parents… for ACEs. PACEsConnection. July 30, 2014. Accessed March 20, 2024. https://www.pacesconnection.com/blog/to-prevent-childhood-trauma-pediatricians-screen-children-and-their-parents-and-sometimes-just-parents-for-aces

5. National Resource Center for Patient/Family-Centered Medical Home. Accessed March 20, 2024. https://www.aap.org/en/practice-management/medical-home

6. National Institute for Children's Health Quality. *Creating a Patient and Family Advisory Council: A Toolkit for Pediatric Practices.* 2012. Accessed March 20, 2024. https://www.nichq.org/resource/creating-patient-and-family-advisory-council-toolkit-pediatric-practices

7. Koshy K, Limb C, Gundogan B, Whitehurst K, Jafree DJ. Reflective practice in health care and how to reflect effectively. *Int J Surg Oncol (NY).* 2017;2(6):e20 PMID: 29177215 doi: 10.1097/IJ9.0000000000000020

8. Gillespie RJ, Folger AT. Feasibility of assessing parental ACEs in pediatric primary care: implications for practice-based implementation. *J Child Adolesc Trauma.* 2017;10(3):249–256 doi: 10.1007/s40653-017-0138-z

9. Garner AS, Saul RA. Implications for pediatric advocacy and public policy. In: *Thinking Developmentally: Nurturing Wellness in Childhood to Promote Lifelong Health.* American Academy of Pediatrics; 2018:133–142

On Being a Snowflake

Courage doesn't always roar. Sometimes courage is the quiet voice at the end of the day saying, "I will try again tomorrow."
Mary Anne Radmacher

By now, you may be feeling a little overwhelmed. This work is a lot to take in, and the idea of building relational health and changing outcomes for patients and families that have experienced trauma may feel a bit like moving a mountain.

But there is a force in nature that can move a mountain—a glacier (which is about as upstream as you can get!). Glaciers are formed by snowpack, and snowpack is formed very simply by individual snowflakes, falling softly one at a time, in just the right place.

Maybe the snowflake is the one simple step you make in your practice toward becoming more trauma responsive. Maybe the snowflake is you, knowing you're joined by others who are engaged in this work, both inside and outside the health care system. Maybe the snowflake is the one family that you helped today with your compassionate, diligent attention to the forces that shape their lives. However you look at it, know that you're not expected to be the entire glacier; just be a snowflake. We know how that sounds. A lot of unkind things have been said about snowflakes lately. But collectively, snowflakes are powerful. Snowflakes are heroic. Remember to claim that.

Listen.

You can hear it, can't you?

That's the sound of the mountain groaning, cracking, breaking, and shifting under the weight of that glacier…slowly but steadily being moved by heroes like you.

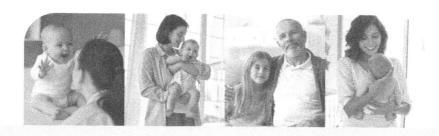

Expanding Your Primary Care Toolbox

Conversation Starters to Enhance Early Relational Health

Infancy (Birth–2 Years)

Questions That Promote Discussion of Resilience at This Age

- How are you feeling about this new role as a parent? *Or,* How is round 2 going for you?
- Who helps you with your baby? Who supports you?
- How do you perceive your child's temperament?
- It looks like your baby is on the move; how's that going?
- What do you do if you feel overwhelmed or stressed as a parent?
- How are you feeling about your relationship with your baby?
- What experiences did you have as a child that you want to replicate? How about any experiences you had that you're uncertain of or experiences that you don't want to duplicate?
- Do you want to raise your children how you were raised? Why or why not?

NOTICE: Watch for signs of postpartum depression, isolation from support systems, discord in the parent unit, or food/housing insecurities.

Early Childhood (2–5 Years)

Questions That Promote Discussion of Resilience at This Age

- What do you love about your child? *Or,* What do you appreciate about your child?
- We've all heard of "the terrible twos"; how's toddlerhood going?
- Does your child play with same-aged peers?
- How confident do you feel with discipline?
- What are your child's strengths?
- Who supports you?
- What are you noticing about your child's personality? Their character?
- How do you connect as a family?
- How are you doing mentally and emotionally?
- How are you coping lately?

NOTICE: Watch for discipline techniques and limit setting; notice awareness and insight in the parent about their child's behavior and their own needs as well as the need for support.

Middle Childhood (6–10 Years)

Questions That Promote Discussion of Resilience at This Age

- What's your family's schedule or routines? Do you carve out family time?
- What activities is your child involved in?
- Does your child have a best friend?
- Did you know your child can help out with family chores that are age appropriate?
- How does your family celebrate culture, faith, or community traditions?
- Do you have any concerns about your child feeling sad or worried or having low self-esteem?
- How did you feel about school when you were younger?
- Do you feel like you have tools for positive discipline?
- Do you find that you parent like you were raised? Differently? Tell me more.

NOTICE: Watch for signs of insight in the parent about their child's behavior and their own needs as well as the need for support.

Note: For early and late adolescence, there are conversation starters for both youth and parents/caregivers.

Early Adolescence (11–14 Years)

Questions That Promote Discussion of Resilience at This Age

FOR PARENTS/CAREGIVERS

- Who are in your children's circle of friends? Do you like them? How do they spend time together?
- Do you feel your child pulling away from you as they enter the teen years?
- What are your family's routines?
- Do you have any worries that your child feels sad or worried or has low self-esteem?
- Do you know how to help your child solve problems?
- Are you good at listening to your child?
- What are your child's strengths? What do you love about their character?
- How does your family celebrate accomplishments?
- What's your child's online behavior like? Have you had talks about this?

FOR PRETEENS/TEENS

- Have you witnessed or taken part in fights, either emotional or physical?
- What do you enjoy doing?
- Do you know how to handle conflict?
- Do you ever feel blue or worried so much that it interferes with your day or sleeping?
- Who are your best friends?
- Do you have a partner? If so, do they make you feel safe and loved?
- What are your strengths? What are you enjoying right now?

Late Adolescence (15–18 Years)

Questions That Promote Discussion of Resilience at This Age

FOR PARENTS/CAREGIVERS

- Are you monitoring texts and social media?
- Does your teen have close friends? What do you think about them?
- What are your teen's strengths?
- How do you talk about future goals?
- Do you know what natural consequences are for teens?
- What do you love about your teen right now?
- How do you spend time together?

FOR TEENS

- Who are your best friends? Who do you turn to if you're hurt or sad?
- What are your dreams?
- Do you have connections with the community?
- Do you have a partner? How do they make you feel?
- How's your mental health?
- How do you cope with bad days?
- How do you celebrate your accomplishments?
- Do you feel like you have someone to turn to if you're sad or overwhelmed?

GNOME Curriculum Planning Worksheet

Goals: What am I trying to accomplish with this training?

Needs: What information do I need to impart as a teacher/instructor? What gaps in skills/ knowledge do my learners need addressed?

Objectives: What do I want learners to know by the end of this training? What change in knowledge do I want to see? What skills do I want to have participants improve on? (You should have 2 or 3 clear objectives.)

By the end of this session, participants will be able to...

1.

2.

3.

Methods: What is the best instructional technique for this material? Didactic lecture, small group discussions, role-play, or something else?

Evaluation: How will I know that participants learned what I intended them to learn?

Baseball Analogy: A Resilience Pearl for Self-Care

Self-care is an important part of well-being, whether that be for the clinicians who take care of our patients or for the parents whom we care for, taking care of their families. First, individuals must recognize the importance of self-care and make time for it. All too often, we delay self-care or don't engage in it because we feel selfish or because other people or other responsibilities become a priority over self-care. Second, we have to prioritize caring for the other adults who take care of us as individuals and provide richness to our lives. These adults, whether they be a spouse or partner, a parent, or a great friend, provide us with a great sense of well-being, compassion, and empathy. They provide the emotional safety net we need when the rest of the world feels stressful. Finally, if we've taken care of ourselves and the people who support us (in that order), we can take care of our children and other dependents. In fact, if we do not engage in self-care as a priority, we will not be as effective in taking care of others. Here's an analogy Amy often uses with parents and colleagues around the issue of self-care.

Imagine yourself playing baseball and standing at home plate, waiting to hit the ball. On first base, you see self-care. On second base, you see care for your partner/spouse or other significant adults who bring you joy. On third base, you see your children or other dependents. If you want to hit a home run, where must you run first after you hit the ball? That's right: first base! But all too often, when it comes to making choices about how we spend our time, we run straight to third base and take care of our children (or jobs or other obligations) before we take care of ourselves. Parents are especially guilty of this delay in or lack of self-care because we are given the message to be selfless in parenting. However, it is important to remember that if we don't take care of ourselves, we cannot take care of children in our lives.

What does this mean? It means taking care of yourself first: run to first base! Take time for yourself. Focus on the triad of wellness: eating, sleeping, and physical movement. Even if you change just 1 or 2 unhealthy habits such as skipping breakfast, sleeping next to your phone, or being sedentary, you're on your way to healthier habits. Even 5 to 10 minutes a day of meditation can be positive self-care. *(Give lots of examples here to the parents you work with and permission for them to pursue these self-care activities.)*

After you've made progress in self-care, go ahead and run to second base. This means spending time with significant adults in your life who bring you joy (eg, your partner, your parent, a best friend, a book club). Making sure you have meaningful time in your life for this will decrease fatigue, burnout, and hopelessness. Plus, connected people are more resilient. Now, you have time and energy for kids—your own or those you work with daily.

Ever been to a Little League game? The cute little batter hits the ball and then takes off running to who knows where, on or off the diamond. They may even field their own ball! Or they may just watch it roll by. It's mayhem! Do not be a Little League player; plan your time with purpose and begin with self-care.

Play ball!

Basic Workflow Breakdown: Implementing Relational Health History Assessments in Practice

Every practice is a little different in terms of leadership, decision-making capacity, infrastructure, staffing, and resources available within both the practice and the community. These questions are designed to help you reflect on your own practice environment to help ensure the success of your assessment efforts.

Background Questions and Reflections

1. Do you have buy-in from your clinic leadership, clinicians, and staff? Whom do you need to inform, engage, and enlist in this project?

2. Who champions this work in your practice? Do you have a clinician champion(s) to continue to move this work forward? Do you have a quality improvement team for new projects in your office? Who would need to be involved in such a team (eg, clinician, nursing staff, mental health staff, administrative staff, parents and caregivers)?

3. Have you trained clinical and nonclinical staff in trauma-informed care? If no, how can this training be accomplished for your practice?

4. Do you have the ability to program or change your electronic health record? If no, what will you need to do or create to document results of a new screening protocol?

5. What has been your biggest challenge in implementing new projects in the past?

6. What has helped ensure success of new projects in the past?

_____

_____

_____

7. Does your clinic have a care coordinator? Can that person create a list of referral resources?

_____

_____

_____

8. What screenings or assessments do you need to implement first? Caregiver depression/ anxiety, social drivers of health, caregiver trauma, or social-emotional health? Do you have assessment tools for symptoms of trauma in children when it is indicated?

_____

_____

_____

9. What tool would be best for the assessment you've chosen for your setting?

_____

_____

_____

10. At what visits will you begin assessments? Well-child visits? Specific types of ill visits? All patients coming in? New patient/intake appointments?

_____

_____

_____

11. How often will you complete the assessment tool?

_____

_____

_____

12. Are there some visits where you will do screening and others where you will do surveillance?

_____

_____

_____

The Nuts and Bolts of a Screening Workflow

13. Who is responsible for ensuring that assessment tools are stocked in the office?

_____

_____

_____

14. Who will be responsible for handing out the assessment tool?

_____

_____

_____

15. Do you have any standardized language to explain the tool to the patient (either a cover letter or scripting for the staff member handing out the tool)? If no, who can develop this?

_____

_____

_____

a. Who is responsible for training staff on the scripting?

_____

_____

_____

b. Who helps communicate any workflow changes to staff members?

_____

_____

_____

16. Who collects the tool from the patient?

_____

_____

_____

a. Who helps recognize if a patient needs more time, encouragement, or a reminder to complete the tool?

_____

_____

_____

17. Who scores the tool?

_____

_____

_____

18. Who documents the results? Where is this documented in the record?

_____

_____

_____

19. Who discusses the results with the patient?

_____

_____

_____

20. Who discusses potential referrals with the patient?

_____

_____

_____

21. Does your practice have a centralized resource list? If so, where is this kept so it can be available for use during a visit?

_____

_____

_____

Screening Grid

Use this table to see which visits would be the easiest in which to implement relational health history tools. Fill in the tools you are already using, then decide where assessment tools would be least burdensome.

Newborn visit	2 weeks	2 months
4 months	6 months	9 months
12 months	15 months	18 months
24 months	30 months	36 months
4 years	5 years	6 years

Sample Caregiver Trauma Survey and Cover Letter

This is the tool that we have been using in The Children's Clinic to assess caregiver trauma, which we started doing in 2013. Although this tool includes the ACE questions—and we've covered all the controversies to this approach—it is included only for illustrative purposes. You can accomplish the same goals of approaching trauma in a caregiver by asking open-ended questions about their experiences from their childhood, such as how they were raised, what they'd like to repeat or have happen for their own children, and what they'd like to avoid. If you develop a tool for surveying caregivers about their trauma, remember a few important points:

1. Include a cover letter that explains why you are asking, with a message of caregiver autonomy (that they have choice in answering the questions); what you're going to do with the information; and how you intend to protect caregiver confidentiality.

2. Think beyond ACEs; as we've discussed, there are other traumas that are equally important. We've approached this in our tool with a section about "expanded ACEs" and an open-ended question.

3. Keep it balanced by asking about resiliencies or strengths. We've done this by asking about PCEs and by asking caregivers to reflect on what they want their child to experience.

4. We've included a list of resources at the end of our survey tool; this can be torn off and taken by caregivers if they choose. They can also take the resources even if they don't answer any of the questions—and that's OK. The tool is meant to introduce the concepts of trauma, resilience, and PCEs to parents and caregivers, so if all they want are some resources without doing any disclosures, that still accomplishes a critical educational goal.

5. Whatever method you use for assessing caregiver trauma, spend some time talking about the tool!

To the parents in my practice,

This survey asks questions about your past experiences as a child. While these questions are very personal, knowing about your experiences as a child can help us know how to help guide you through your parenting experiences over the lives of your children. You do NOT have to answer any questions if you don't want to.

What are adverse childhood experiences, and why are they important?

Adverse childhood experiences (ACEs) are stressful or frightening things that happen during childhood, such as abuse, neglect, or severe dysfunctions in the household. We know that people who experience a lot of ACEs may have more problems with their health and might also have a hard time making decisions about how to parent their children.

What is resilience?

Resilience is the ability to bounce back from stressful situations. Resilience can be learned, practiced, and improved on—and some studies have shown that good resilience skills help people avoid the health problems that come from ACEs. A lot of resilience comes from safe, supportive relationships that help us through difficult times.

Why does my pediatrician want to know this information?

Mostly because we care about you, and we care about your kids. Knowing what sorts of experiences you've been through will help us know how to guide you through your parenting decisions. That's all we're going to do with the information—to figure out how to best support you as a parent. Whatever you write on this form will be kept confidential.

THANK YOU for sharing this information. It may be hard to talk about these issues, but we are here to support you in your parenting journey.

Adapted with permission from The Children's Clinic.

ACE Questions

HOW MANY of these apply to you during the first 18 years of your life? You don't have to mark which specific statements apply to you. Write the total in the box:	

- Did a parent or other adult in the household often swear at you, insult you, put you down, or humiliate you OR act in a way that made you afraid you would be physically hurt?
- Did a parent or other adult in the household often push, grab, slap, or throw something at you OR ever hit you so hard that you had marks or were injured?
- Did an adult or person at least 5 years older than you ever touch or fondle you, or have you touch their body in a sexual way, OR attempt or actually have oral, anal, or vaginal intercourse with you?
- Did you often feel that no one in your family loved you or thought you were important or special OR your family didn't look out for each other, feel close to each other, or support each other?
- Did you often feel that you didn't have enough to eat, had to wear dirty clothes, and had no one to protect you OR your parents were too drunk or high to take care of you or take you to the doctor if you needed it?
- Were your parents ever separated or divorced?
- Was your mother or stepmother often pushed, grabbed, slapped, or had something thrown at her OR sometimes or often kicked, bitten, hit with a fist or with something hard?
- Did you ever live with anyone who was a problem drinker or alcoholic, or who used street drugs?
- Was a household member depressed or mentally ill, or did a household member attempt suicide?
- Did a household member go to prison?

HOW MANY of these apply to you during the first 18 years of your life? You don't have to mark which specific statements apply to you. Write the total in the box:	

- Did you experience repeated bullying as a child?
- Did you repeatedly experience discrimination based on ethnicity, skin color, or sexual orientation?
- Did you live in a neighborhood that experienced gang-related violence?
- Did you ever live in a foster home or group home?

Did anything else scary or upsetting happen to you as a child? Please describe that, if you feel comfortable: _____

_____

_____

_____

_____

_____

_____

_____

_____

_____

Adapted from ACES Too High. What ACEs/PCEs do you have? Accessed March 20, 2024. https://acestoohigh.com/got-your-ace-score.

Positive Childhood Experiences

For each of these questions, please answer yes or no.

Before the age of 18 years, I…

	YES	NO
Was able to talk with the family about my feelings		
Felt that my family stood by me during difficult times		
Enjoyed participating in community traditions		
Felt a sense of belonging in high school		
Felt supported by friends		
Had at least 2 nonparent adults who took a genuine interest in me		
Felt safe and protected by an adult in my home		

Adapted from Bethell C, Jones J, Gombojav N, Linkenbach J, Sege R. Positive childhood experiences and adult mental and relational health in a statewide sample: associations across adverse childhood experiences levels. *JAMA Pediatr.* 2019;173(11):e193007.

Which of these positive childhood experiences are you most excited to have happen for your child?

_____

_____

_____

How are you doing with making those experiences happen?
☐ I'm doing great.   ☐ I need some help with this.   ☐ I don't need to discuss it now.

Is there anything you think would be helpful for your pediatrician to provide right now?

_____

_____

_____

Other comments, questions, or concerns:

_____

_____

_____

This questionnaire was filled out by:
☐ Mom   ☐ Dad   ☐ Someone else (Please describe yourself: _____)

Have you filled this survey out before at The Children's Clinic—for example, with another child?
☐ Yes   ☐ No

How would you like to discuss this survey?
☐ During the visit   ☐ Afterward by phone   ☐ I don't want to discuss it

Resources You Might Find Helpful

Help Me Grow
1-833-868-4769
Email: helpmegrow@providence.org
Parent coaching, developmental supports, and connections to resources about parenting, normal child development, and other educational supports

211Info
Call 211 or text 898211.
Email: help@211info.org
Referrals and resources for community programs for financial and practical supports, like food, housing, parenting classes, and more

Baby Blues Connection
1-800-557-8375
www.babybluesconnection.org
Email: info@babybluesconnection.org
Support for parents experiencing depression or anxiety after birth. Includes a warm line, resources, support groups, and referrals to community mental health clinicians.

Websites With More Information

www.zerotothree.org: information about promoting your child's development

www.cdc.gov/ncbddd/childdevelopment/positiveparenting/index.html: tips about positive parenting and helping build your child's development

www.stresshealth.org: created by the Center for Youth Wellness, with ideas about managing stress and staying calm when faced with challenges

https://acestoohigh.com: dedicated to news and information about ACEs and what communities around the country are doing to combat the effects of childhood trauma

Books You Might Like

Parenting From the Inside Out by Dan Siegel, MD, and Mary Hartzell, MEd. Understanding how our own triggers may affect our parenting.

The Whole-Brain Child by Daniel Siegel, MD, and Tina Payne Bryson, PhD. Helping kids regulate big emotions, with practical tips for integrating their emotional and thinking brains.

The Deepest Well by Nadine Burke Harris, MD. Explores the effects of ACEs on health and wellness, describing Dr Burke Harris' journey into incorporating ACE knowledge into her pediatric practice.

What Happened to You? by Bruce Perry, MD, PhD, and Oprah Winfrey. Discusses ACEs, resilience, and healing among people who have experienced trauma.

The Happiest Baby on the Block and *The Happiest Toddler on the Block* by Harvey Karp, MD. Offers tips and techniques for helping your child calm and regulate themselves.

Building Resilience in Children and Teens: Giving Kids Roots and Wings by Kenneth R. Ginsburg, MD, MS Ed, FAAP, and Martha M. Jablow. Provides guidance on boosting children's confidence, fostering strength-based relationships, and helping children cope with stress.

Compassion-Informed Care

Inspired by concepts developed by the Substance Abuse and Mental Health Services Administration (SAMHSA) and Children's Health Alliance.

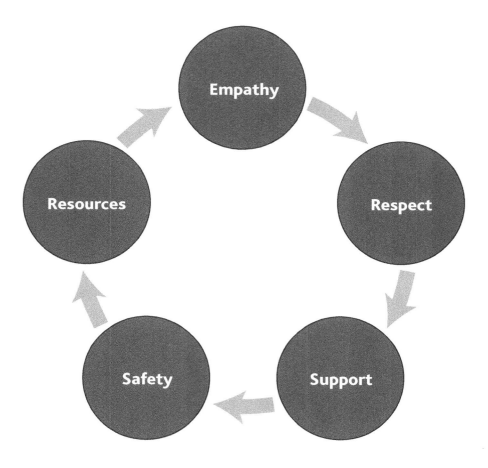

Compassion-informed care (adapted from SAMHSA's trauma-informed care) is a commitment

- To recognize trauma or chronic stress and know what it looks like
- To avoid triggering or increasing the trauma or chronic stress
- To restore safety, strength, and self-worth of the individual
- *To treat **all people** with compassionate and respectful care*

Restoring Compassionate Practices

Practice	How	Examples
Show empathy	For adults: Acknowledge that life has overwhelming moments, or that parenting is hard, or that being a provider for your family can be burdensome. For children: Let them know that you believe they're doing the best they can.	• Health problems • Behavioral problems • Sleep problems • Mental health problems • Addiction • Stress • Work-related problems • Marital issues • Chronic health problems
	Recognize that some people come from a background that hasn't prepared them for positive coping techniques.	• Lack of a positive parent role model • History of trauma or abuse themselves • Relationship issues that the practice may not be aware of
	Language example:	"I see that you are upset. I know you are not upset with me but at the situation. I will find a way to help you." "How has this experience been for you?"
Show respect	Acceptance and nonjudgment	• Have an open mind as you are speaking with patients and their families. • You may not know their full story/trauma.
	Acknowledge bias.	• Race • Religion • Socioeconomic status • Age of parents • Sexual orientation • Gender identity • Ability
	Build relationships.	• Between professionals and clients • Between professionals and staff • Between staff and families • Between colleagues
	Language example:	To a parent: "I remember that we talked about _____ last time. That's important to you, so let's revisit _____." To a staff member: "In our staff meeting yesterday, you seemed frustrated. That's not like you. Is something else going on? Can I help?"

Practice	How	Examples
Support the patient and family	Offer encouragement.	Let the person know they are not to blame when bad things happen that are out of their control.
	Give choices.	• Trauma = loss of control. • Balance patient needs and organizational needs.
	Know your resources.	Have a network of trauma-informed counselors and agencies for referrals.
	Focus on positivity and strengths.	Tell people what they *can* do, not what they *shouldn't* do.
	Communication	Make sure you are able to speak in the person's native language or provide a translator.
	Language example:	"This is a great opportunity for us to work as a team to develop a solution."
Provide safety	Physical safety	• Create calm and comfort. • Cast "warm eyes." • Be predictable. • Give choices. • Get down on the person's level. • No fast movements. • Allow a safe person to be present.
	Emotional safety	• Ask questions, and listen to the patient. • Be sensitive to trauma triggers. • It is OK to set limits on inappropriate behavior. • Be predictable. • Be trustworthy.
	Language example:	"We can talk about this together, or you can have a support person with you while you and I have a short discussion. What feels better for you?"

Case Study 1: Sara and Mia

Sara is late for her appointment with her 2-year-old, Mia. She arrives to the office visibly flustered, with tears in her eyes. Her last visit was a no-show. Records indicate that she has an unpaid bill with the clinic of about $70. When the front office staff indicates that it might be difficult for Sara to be seen today because she's late, she becomes angry and shouts at the front office staff, "Do you know how hard it was for me to get here today!"

Luckily, the pediatrician is able to see them. Mia is a healthy 2-year-old coming in for a well-child visit. Sara shares with the pediatrician that Mia has shown some behavioral changes over the past several weeks: disrupted sleep, increased clinginess, whining and resistance, and decreased appetite.

The pediatrician elicits a history that reveals that the changes correlate with Sara's recent separation from Mia's father.

Factors to Consider: Safety, Support, Empathy, Respect, and Resources

- Front office staff: What else might be going on for Sara? Is this typical for Sara and her family? Can you help decrease stress for Sara in other ways (eg, snack for Mia, reassurances, tissue, not overwhelming them with additional paperwork)?
- Nurse/MA: Notice changes in Sara and Mia's behavior. Check in with front office staff at transition: "Anything I should know?" Put off medical vitals until Sara and Mia are calmer. Provide reassurance and distraction. Point out what Sara is doing well.
- Pediatrician: Recognize that changes increase stress for children. Educate Sara on how stress shows up behaviorally. Provide support. Listen. Offer resources. You don't have to solve the problem to provide help.

Front office staff: Show empathy and compassion: "We're not sure how just yet, but we're going to try our best to see Mia today." If unable to fit Mia into the schedule, offer to call Sara later in the day to talk more about what is going on. Or perhaps see if a behavioral health consultant (BHC) can see Sara and Mia. Talk with back office staff about the situation. Share with the nurse/registered nurse that Sara came to the appointment visibly upset and provided an address change.

Nurse/MA: The nurse notices that Sara has indicated a change of address at check-in. Sara shares that she is currently residing at Mia's grandmother's house. Sara discloses to the nurse that she's worried about Mia's behavior. The nurse shares this information and the observations from the front office staff with the pediatrician.

Pediatrician: The pediatrician asks open-ended questions, uses neutral language, and shows empathy when Sara discloses details of her separation. They tell Sara that even 2-year-olds can pick up on changes in the home and in the relationship between their mom and dad. They ask if Sara would like a referral to a BHC.

Case Study 2: Tom and Taylor

Tom arrives for his son Taylor's adolescent checkup, phone and briefcase in hand as Taylor lags behind, also on his phone. Tom sighs, turns to Taylor, and says to the front office staff person, "We're here to get this guy fixed." Taylor turns crimson but smiles shyly. Usually, Taylor's mom brings him in for office visits.

Tom is a bit rude and inflexible with the medical assistant (MA) during the rooming process. He says to the MA, "I'm not sure what's going on with him. He's always on that thing [*pointing to Taylor's phone*], but his teacher says he seems different. My only worry is why he's failing 3 subjects. Maybe he needs Ritalin or something? I'll just wait out here." Then, Tom departs for the waiting room.

Alone with the MA, Taylor discloses that he's being severely bullied at school and on social media. Taylor says he *does not* want to talk about this with his dad, and when the MA asks about his mom, Taylor indicates, "She's really, really sick. I don't want to bother her."

Factors to Consider

Front office staff: Have we shown empathy and respect?

Nurse/MA: Have we provided safety, respect, and empathy?

Pediatrician: Have we provided resources and support?

Creating a Public Narrative: The Story of Me, The Story of Us, The Story of Now

Use this worksheet to create your public narrative: the 30-second elevator pitch that you'll use to motivate others in your practice to get on board with your quality improvement project. Test your narrative out on a colleague, and modify it as needed.

The Story of Me: Think of a clinical example that describes what personally motivates you to do trauma assessments or other components of the relational health history in practice. It's probably a patient whom you felt particularly challenged or moved by and who set you on your personal path toward trauma-informed care.

The Story of Us: How does this clinical example broaden to your (and your practice partners') personal day-to-day experiences? Use real data if you can—a simple statistic that illustrates the depth of the problem.

The Story of Now: How can you encapsulate the change that you want to make in practice related to trauma assessments? What tool or surveillance questions do you want to use? What will a clinician do if they identify trauma in their practice? How will they be helped to support patients and families?

Sample Shared Care Plan for Trauma

People involved in my care:

Primary care doctor:

Therapist/mental health clinician:

Care coordinator/peer navigator:

School counselor:

1. How will I know I need help? What behaviors, thoughts, or feelings tell me that I need to reach out to someone?

   _____

   _____

2. What coping strategies can I start with until I can reach out?

   _____

   _____

   Goals for self-care routines that will keep me well:

   _____

   _____

3. People I can reach out to for help (see Circles of Support on second page)

   _____

   _____

4. Resources (this page and the next):

Resource	Contact Information	Who Initiates Contact? (Patient, Clinician, Care Coordinator, or Other)
988 Suicide & Crisis Lifeline	Dial 988.	Patient (if needed in case of emergency)

Circles of Support

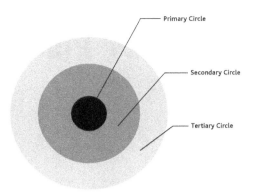

Circles of Support

Circles of Support

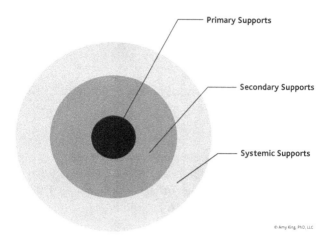

© Amy King, PhD, LLC

Primary supports: This circle usually comprises the core people in a person's life—the ones the person most trusts and goes to for support, advice, encouragement, and confidential listening. Most children and adults can identify 2 to 3 people within this circle.

> **Scripting:** *We all need go-to people in our lives. Who are the people you call, day or night, even at 2:00 am, if you're overwhelmed? If you're stressed, depressed, suicidal, scared, or in crisis, tell me 2 or 3 people you rely on who'll be there for you.*

Secondary supports: This circle comprises other supportive people in a person's life—the ones the person would turn to if the core group was not available to meet their needs. It's like the "second team" or "backup" helpers. Often, these are people within a system the person belongs to, such as work, school, neighborhoods, or other social groups. Most people can identify 3 to 5 people from their secondary circle.

> **Scripting:** *Now I want you to think of your backup people. Who might you call if someone from your primary circle isn't available? For instance, I see you have "X" in your primary circle. If they weren't available, who would you call or reach out to? Maybe these are people you wouldn't call right away at 2 in the morning, but these are definitely people you know would be there for you if you reached out.*

Systemic supports: This outer circle is usually systems that the person interacts with or people who are paid to be in that person's life. Pediatricians, teachers, and systems such as schools, religious organizations, and community centers may fall within this circle. Often, there are other systems the family *must* have in their lives, such as court-appointed therapy, human services, or case workers. Such systems can provide structure, oversight, and guidance. These are supportive people but not necessarily ones the person would go to for comfort or close relationships.

> **Scripting:** *OK, finally, I want you to think of other supportive people or groups in your life. People who provide you support or information or do helpful things for you or your family. Often, these are people whose job is to be in your life, such as me, your teachers, places of worship, etc. Who are these people?*

Secondary circle push: If the primary circle is empty or the individuals within it are unhealthy for or unavailable to that person, there must be an intervention. A *secondary circle push* happens by inviting people from the secondary circle into the primary circle. If you've identified that there are unhealthy people in a caregiver's or patient's primary circle, don't shame/blame the person or point that out; simply encourage more helpful people in that person's life.

> Scripting: *I noticed your primary circle doesn't have anyone within it. Or, I noticed that you could use some more supports outside your primary circle; we all can use more people. I wonder how it would feel to invite someone into your primary circle from your middle circle?*

Note: Most people feel nervous or uneasy about burdening others or feeling rejected. Be sure to address this fear with reassurance.

> Scripting: *I know asking for help can be hard. Do you have "X's" phone number? Have you thought of asking them for help? We could even create a little script together about how to ask. Or, I could sit with you while you call. Or, I can call with/for you. What I know is that most people want to help and don't even know when others are struggling. I'm sure that's the same for "X." I'm sure they would want to help you. Let's try together.*

Remember, although "systems" is the label for the tertiary circle of support, systems may be on any level of the circles and are often critical supports to have in place. Don't forget to encourage a push for systems as well. Food boxes, suicide helplines, utility companies, domestic violence shelters, and counseling centers are examples of systems you can add to a person's circle.

Becoming a Baby Observer

For Clinicians

While in office, point out to parents how and when they attune to their baby. Greater attunement promotes attachment, which ultimately prevents poor health outcomes. However, most parents don't know that these interactions are so critical. Some parents do them without effort, whereas others need quite a bit of guidance. Here are some interactions to look for and observe during visits. Pointing out these critical moments between babies/toddlers and caregivers promotes Competency, Connection, and Confidence (3 of the 7 Cs) in parents.

Following are some things you can say:

- Look at how she is smiling at you.
- Wow, he was crying and you knew just what he needed!
- Look at those eyes; she's really tracking your voice.
- I really like how you're holding him. He's facing you, and that helps him feel safe.
- What have you noticed lately about your baby's sleep patterns?
- Did you know you can hold/nurse/rock your baby while we give vaccines? This will help comfort your baby.
- What does your baby/toddler really love doing with you?
- I notice that your toddler really watches you. She's really interested in your emotional state (your feelings). That's great!

For Parents

Being a baby observer—watching, paying attention to, recognizing, and responding to your baby's cues—helps promote greater connection, which leads to healthy attachment with your baby. Being a baby observer or an attuned caregiver is critically important for you and your baby. Greater attunement promotes attachment, which prevents poor health outcomes. If you're like most parents, you may not realize how straightforward yet important being attuned can be for your baby. Some parents do it without effort, whereas others need quite a bit of guidance. Here are some ways you can become an expert baby observer.

What seems to interest your baby? What overwhelms them?

Watch your baby's face: How are they feeling? Can you mirror that feeling?

If your baby gets upset or starts crying, what works to comfort your baby?

Watch how your baby responds to your voice and your touch. What soothes?

What feelings do you notice in your baby? Can you narrate those feelings out loud?

What makes your baby giggle?

What happens if you play peekaboo?

What happens if you make new sounds your baby has never heard?

Be curious about what your baby notices, what they like and dislike, what startles them, and what soothes them. Observers are curious detectives about baby cues.

Have you watched yourself dance with your baby?

Mimic sounds your baby makes, and watch your baby's face in the mirror.

Think about the 5 senses (sight, touch, smell, taste, and sound): try out soothing or stimulating your baby/toddler with different senses. Watch what happens.

The more you observe your baby/toddler and they observe you, the more attuned you'll become to their needs. Babies and caregivers who are attuned experience less disruptive behavior later on. It's as if you've told your child, "I understand you." This builds resilience in your baby/toddler and promotes attachment!

Yolky Feelings

Sometimes, processing feelings is difficult for children because they lack the proper terminology to sort through the complex feelings they have inside. Also, children (like adults) mistake secondary feelings as primary feelings, which often leaves them feeling misunderstood or corrected or lands them on the receiving end of discipline.

Primary feelings: Primary feelings are just that: the core feeling of what's going on inside of us. They best exemplify what is happening and, if labeled properly, most often lead to help.

Sadness, worry, and confusion are 3 primary feelings; they may also be called by synonyms (eg, *blue, anxious, misunderstood*). Other feelings children often list include boredom, disappointment, and loneliness. But for the purpose of the exercise, we try to stick with primary feelings.

Secondary feelings: Secondary feelings are still *very real* feelings, but they often mask our primary feelings. Examples of secondary feelings include anger, upset, annoyance, jealousy, "being mad," and contempt. Secondary feelings often lead to fights, discipline, and defensiveness. They rarely get us the help we need.

The Yolky Feelings exercise is meant to help children sort through their emotions and identify primary feelings so they can get the help they desire. Here's the script we utilize while drawing a picture of an egg, cracked open.

> "Sometimes, when you're sad or worried or confused, it comes out as anger. *(Give an example here of when this has happened to you or the child.)* When your feelings come out as yelling, screaming, or pushing, it's hard for you to get the help you need. In fact, I bet sometimes you might even get anger in return, or, worse yet, punishment for your behavior.
>
> You see, the inside of this egg [*pointing to the yolk*]—the squishy, yolky part—is what contains our 'yolky feelings.' These feelings are *sad, worried,* and *confused.* The outside of the egg and the part surrounding the yolk contain protective feelings—just like the egg whites protect the yolk from getting broken. Our 'egg white feelings' protect our yolky feelings. These feelings are *anger* and *mad (or any synonym for those).*
>
>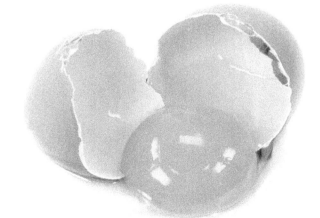
>
> When we express anger, the helpers in our lives can't lend us the support we need. If I'm screaming or yelling, many people will scream or yell back at me, right? But if instead, I think about my yolky feeling and identify how I felt on the inside, I will get more help. Let's try it."

Sample Script

Pediatrician: Remember when your mom mentioned that you'd crumpled up your homework and thrown it at her? How were you feeling then?

Child: Mad!

Pediatrician: I bet you were. And I wonder if you were feeling any of these other yolky feelings as well?

Child: Well, I was really confused because I didn't understand my homework.

Pediatrician: Sure, I get confused too.

Child: And I was worried because my teacher said if we don't get our homework done, we have to stay in from recess and I don't want to miss recess.

Pediatrician: Ah, I see. What would it be like if you had told your mom about feeling confused and worried? Do you think she would have helped you?

Child: Yes, but instead I got sent to my room because I was mad.

Pediatrician: Right. I want you to get the help you need. And yolky feelings help adults know 2 important things: how you're feeling on the inside and how to help. Way to go!

Flipping Your Lid

Let's face it: everyone loses it at times. But it's important to understand why it happens and how to respond. Flipping Your Lid is a model and guide to understanding triggers and survival behavior that is based on the work of Dan Siegel, MD.

First, watch the video on Flipping Your Lid (https://youtu.be/dAgzqaqWKkQ?si = xdRLU7KEf7r82hnq)

or a similar one by Dr Siegel (https://youtu.be/G0T_2NNoC68?si = qjvbSSKkrrn7q1LH).

These videos have wonderful insight and a model to follow.

Second, it's important to understand the difference between being in a "flipped-lid" state and a calm, regulated state. When we're calm and regulated, we can think, make decisions, weigh pros and cons, consider our responses, and stay open and curious. When we're in a flipped-lid state, we're in a fight-or-flight state. Our number one goal in this state is survival. We don't have access to more complex thinking. No learning happens when we've flipped our lid, and all rational thinking is absent.

Next, determine if you or your child is in a calm, regulated space or a flipped-lid space.

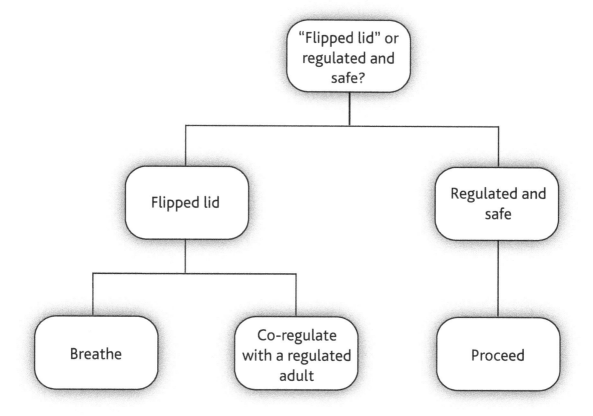

If your child is in a flipped-lid state, the only goal should be to get them to a space that feels calm and safe. Only then can your child access the ability to think, be rational, and make healthy decisions. If your child is in a calm and regulated space, wonderful! You can proceed with reassurance that your child has the ability to learn and stay curious.

Finally, you might explore triggers that lead to flipped-lid states and exercises that help your child get to a calm and regulated state.

Remember: as adults, we get triggered and flip our lids as well.

Following are examples of triggers for children:

- Hungry
- Tired
- Lonely
- Worried
- Scared
- Confused
- Disappointed

Following are examples of triggers for adults:

- Tired
- Running late
- Worried
- Multitasking
- Confused
- Helpless

Discussions about triggers, flipping your lid, and ways to restore safety and calm are excellent family conversations. When we talk about topics like this early and often, we create an environment that says we're open to talking about feelings. That creates resilience for your child!

Special Time

Derived from Matheson RC. DIR floortime therapy. *J LC Spec Educ.* 2016;12(1):2; and Greenspan SI, Wieder S. *Engaging Autism: Using the Floortime Approach to Help Children Relate, Communicate, and Think.* Da Capo Lifelong Books; 2006.

General Guidelines

✔ 10 to 15 minutes per day

✔ 3 to 4 times per week

✔ Time with a loving, caring adult (eg, mom, dad, grandparent, foster parent)

✔ Distractions turned off

✔ Child-led activity

✔ No games with rules

✔ No screens

✔ "Parent hat" (or "teacher hat," etc) taken off

Remember, unless there's a safety issue, the child leads the time together. It doesn't have to be deep conversations, just hanging out together. When possible, point out feelings your child is having, express curiosity, and remind the child that you enjoy this time.

Scripts

For young children: I would love to play with you. Will you play with me? We can play anything you would like to. This will be our special time! I'm going to set a timer for about 10 minutes, and when the timer goes off, I have to do some other things, but we'll play again soon!

For school-aged children: What are you up to? Would you like to hang out? What would you like to do? I've got about 15 minutes, and you have all my attention. Let's do something fun; it's up to you!

Or: Hey, what would you like to do if you had all my attention for the next 15 minutes or so? Anything at all? I would love to spend some time with you doing whatever you want, and I promise, I won't talk about *(fill in whatever your kid would like to avoid talking about)* and we'll just hang out. How's that sound?

For teens: Have a you got a few minutes? Can I hang out with you? *Or,* Would you like to go for a drive? *Or,* Can I sit with you for a bit? I'm interested in what you're doing.

Ideas for Special Time

Babies and Toddlers

✔ Bath time

✔ Singing

✔ Dancing

✔ Reading

✔ Mirror play

✔ Playing on the floor with toys

School-Aged Children

See all the above, plus the following:

✔ Baking

✔ Crafts

✔ Walks/hikes

✔ Building

✔ Creating structures

✔ Taking apart electronics

✔ Listening to music

Young Children

See all the above, plus the following:

✔ Baking

✔ Reading together

✔ Art/crafts

✔ Walking around outside

Teens

See all the above, plus the following:

✔ Going for drives

✔ Sitting next to you during homework

✔ Journaling

✔ Gardening

✔ Teen DJ

Beginning Discipline: Full Text

After introducing the subject, I start with drawing a 4-quadrant graph on the exam room paper, and I fill in the parenting styles as I describe them.

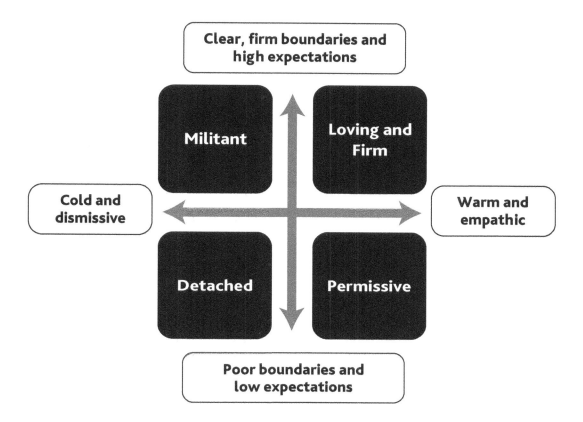

Here's the script.

"There are 4 basic parenting styles, based on expectations (the rules, regulations, and boundaries for the child) and empathy (the love, affection, and warmth we show our kids). Low expectations and low empathy—in other words, 'We don't care about our kid, and we don't care what they do'—make up what I call 'detached,' or neglectful, parenting. Obviously, this isn't a good place to be, since kids need love and guidance from us. A lot of people grow up in families where there were a lot of rules but not a lot of love and affection; this was certainly the dominant parenting style in the generations before I was born. These are militant households—with a kind of 'kids should be seen but not heard' mentality or 'do as I say, not as I do' type of caregiving. These households are very clear about boundaries, but they don't always feel warm and loving, so growing up in a cold household like that may make it harder to build loving relationships later in life, and kids may later act out because they have not internalized problem-solving skills but simply do as they're told. People who grew up in households like that often want to do something different, so they go the other direction on the empathy spectrum, as they should, but drop the expectations. This is permissive parenting. It turns out, though, that kids need rules and regulations to feel safe and secure; they need to know someone is in control. Without that, they might start feeling anxious. The other unfortunate outcome of permissive parenting is that kids tend to have poor social skills and can be self-focused. Obviously, what I want you to be is the loving and firm type of parent, a balance of the two.

That's because supportive parenting comes down to 3 basic ideas:

1. Kids raise or lower themselves to whatever expectations we set for them, so don't be afraid to have high expectations. Your kids will want to try to get your approval, so having clear and consistent rules will lead to better behavior.

2. Love your child, even if you dislike behavior. Kids need and deserve unconditional love from us.

3. Kids learn more from what they see us do than what they hear us say. This means that when you're enforcing rules, yelling at a child to get them to calm down is confusing. So is hitting or spanking; it teaches them more about the use of force than the behavior you're trying to teach. It also means that we have to model the behaviors that we most want to see in our kids.

Now, you're going to have some days when you're in each of these different parenting modes, and that's OK. Some days, you'll be here or here or even here *(I point to each of the different quadrants in turn, usually ending with 'Detached')*. It's where you are most of the time that matters."

Yes, it's a long script…but I think it's an important one. If you're familiar with parenting literature, the actual names for the parenting styles are *neglectful, authoritarian, permissive,* and *authoritative.*[1,2] *Authoritarian* and *authoritative* are such similar words to me that I avoid them for clarity's sake; they are less relatable, whereas *loving and firm* is clear and relatable. I always follow up with "What questions does this bring up for you?" If you have time, you can consider having parents and caregivers reflect on the parenting style they grew up with and what they might want to do similarly or differently. You might also ask caregivers whom and where they turn to for messages and advice about parenting.

From Amy: A few considerations when talking with parents about parenting styles and discipline: First, as R.J. points out, normalize that caregivers learn from their models and they're doing the best they can based on their family of origin, cultural message, and trial and error. Often, when there are 2 caregivers in a household and one of them is on an end of the continuum that feels overly harsh (militant) or overly permissive, the second caregiver likely will try to compensate for that behavior. I encourage caregivers to move toward each other on the continuum instead of trying to move in the opposite direction for balance. It helps kids feel like discipline is more consistent. Second, remind parents that *discipline* means "to teach" and that we want to model behavior and promote the outcome we're looking for. So, I'll often ask parents when they're exasperated with a behavior, "What do you want your child to learn?" and that helps refocus them toward engaging in a lesson that helps their child get to that goal or outcome. For instance, if your toddler is melting down when being asked to pick up toys and you either yell at them to pick them up right away and threaten to throw them out (militant) or do it for them in an effort to stop crying (permissive), you'll lose the opportunity to teach your child the goal: when we make a mess, we pick up after ourselves. So, I encourage the caregiver to find that happy medium, being loving and firm: "Oh, it looks like you've made a mess with all these toys. Looks like we need to pick them up before we can go outside to play." When the child refuses and begins to cry, the caregiver can say, "I can see you're sad *(loving and empathic),* but we can't go on with our day until these are put away *(firm and clear).*" Third, I want parents to give themselves grace and patience. As R.J. points out, it's normal to move on these continuums depending on your day or energy level. We simply want to land in the space of being loving AND firm, kind AND clear, and warm AND boundaryed as much as possible. A final note is to regard cultural humility when it comes to parenting styles. It is clear that parenting style affects outcomes for children, but be sure to focus conversations on approach and fluidity versus the "best" approach. Parenting styles are also a reflection of the society parents belong to, which transmits values, expectations, behavior patterns, belief systems, and guidelines about optimal and deficient parenting.[3] Stay curious about parenting styles and you're likely to have engaging conversations with incredible people doing the best they can based on what they've learned.

References

1. Baumrind D. Current patterns of parental authority. *Dev Psychol*. 1971;4(1, pt 2):1–130
2. Kuppens S, Ceulemans E. Parenting styles: a closer look at a well-known concept. *J Child Fam Stud*. 2019;28(1):168–181 PMID: 30679898 doi: 10.1007/s10826-018-1242-x
3. Checa P, Abundis-Gutiérrez A. Parenting styles, academic achievement and the influence of culture. *Psychol Psychother Res Study*. 2018;1(4):pprs.2018.01.000518

Finding Calm to Prevent Overwhelm

My WHY: _____   My THEME SONG: _____

Goal for Today

Priorities

Self:

Relationships:

Job:

Daily Check-In

☐ I created a boundary around my workflow today.

☐ I said yes to help when offered.

☐ I stretched, walked, and moved between patients.

☐ I ate lunch and snacks and drank water.

☐ I took 90 seconds to breathe.

☐ I left work at work.

☐ I delegated a task to someone else.

One Boundary

One Piece of Joy

Appendix S

PDSA Cycle Worksheet

SMART aim statement (**S**pecific, **M**easurable, **A**ttainable, **R**ealistic, and **T**imely or time-specific):

Plan: What change will I implement to achieve my SMART aim statement?

Do: How will I make this change happen?

Study: How will I measure whether the change is successful?

Act: What are my next steps? If my initial PDSA cycle was successful, do I need to expand the test to a larger group of patients or clinicians? If not successful, what changes can I make?

Creating Boundaries

✔ Boundaries let people know what's OK and what's not OK.

✔ Boundaries assume that we want to stay *in* a relationship with a person or an organization, *not* that we want to depart.

✔ To create a script around boundaries, take the following steps (an example script follows):

1. Reflect on what's going wrong (use the table below).
2. State what's going on objectively with just the facts: who, what, when, and how.
3. Think about how it could be different or what outcome you would like to see.
4. Make a specific request to address the situation.
5. Finish by focusing on your overarching goal: to stay in a relationship with a person or an organization.

WHAT'S OK	WHAT'S NOT OK	MY DESIRED OUTCOME

Example Script for Creating Boundaries as a Medical Professional

[Fill in name and organization],

I truly enjoy working here. I enjoy my patients and love my colleagues. And I'm committed to exceptional patient care. I'm feeling burned out [or *overwhelmed, overscheduled,* or a more specific example, such as *I'm not being able to take my lunch*]. It has really gotten in the way of how I want to show up. To that end, I would like to advocate for [fill in the blank, such as *blocking out 15 minutes before my lunch hour so I can catch up* or *not having scheduled meetings during my Monday lunch hour*].

Please let me know when we can talk about creating this change so I can continue to show up as an incredible physician committed to my patients and our organization.

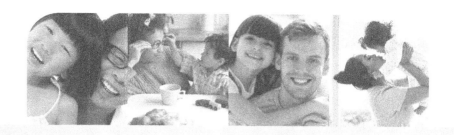

Index

Index

Page numbers followed by *f* indicate a figure; by *t*, a table; and by *b*, a box.

A

AAP. *See* American Academy of Pediatrics (AAP)
A-B-C of behavior, 123
Accountability, 206
ACE. *See* Adverse childhood experiences (ACEs)
Addressing Mental Health Concerns in Pediatrics, 30
Administration/clinic leadership, motivating, 193–194
Adverse childhood experiences (ACEs), 1, 3, 6, 11, 13–14. *See also* Screening and assessments
 debate about screening for, 14–16
 driving health disparities, 21
 in parents and caregivers, 101–104
Advocacy, 213–214
Ages & Stages Questionnaire, 88
American Academy of Pediatrics (AAP), 4
 Addressing Mental Health Concerns in Pediatrics, 30
 Bright Futures, 28, 151, 153–154*t*, 190
 on building resilience, 68
 conference series by, on being trauma informed, 210
 National Resource Center for Patient/Family-Centered Medical Home, 140
 on parents and caregivers as coaches, 76
 on peripartum mood disorders, 84, 96
 on positive parenting, 122
 on preventing childhood toxic stress, 75
 on public health threats from ACEs, 59
 Screen and Intervene toolkit, 99
 Screening Technical Assistance and Resource Center, 89, 99
 on trauma-informed care (TIC), 42
Anda, Robert F., 14, 28
Angelou, Maya, 39
Anticipatory guidance, 109–111, 144–145
 on exercise and getting out in nature, 119–120
 on good caregiver mental health, 121–122
 on healthy relationships, 111–113
 on mindfulness, 120–121
 on nutrition, 117–118
 on positive parenting, 122–127, 126*b*
 on resilience, 64
 roadmap for, 152–154, 153–154*t*, 191–192*t*
 on sleep and caregiver self-care, 116–117
 on trauma education, 113–116
Ask Suicide Questions (ASQ), 146
Assessments. *See* Screening and assessments
Atkins, Sue, 95
Augsburger, David, 159
Aunt Bertha, resource clearinghouse, 34, 201, 212
Autonomy, health care ethics principle, 16*t*, 19–20
Awareness of trauma, 43

B

Baby observers, becoming, 136, 151, 255–256
Baby Pediatric Symptom Checklist, 88
Baggage, trauma as, 17, 18, 43–44
Barriers, 25–26
 caregiver acceptance of trauma and SDOH questionnaires, 34–36
 clinician confidence, 29–30
 dysregulation, 31–33
 lack of resources, 33–34
 to resilience education in pediatric settings, 66–68
 responding to trauma-informed care (TIC) adoption, 49–52
 time, 26–28
Baseball analogy for self-care, 170–171, 227
Bedtime routines, 116
Being fully human, 172–175
Belly breathing, 121
Benevolence, health care ethics principle, 16*t*, 18–19
Beyond the ACE Score, 166
Big Brothers/Big Sisters, 34
Block, Robert, 59
Blue Zone Communities, 204
Bodies, listening with our whole, 162
Born for Love, 83
Boundaries, creation of, 271
Boynton-Jarrett, R., 50, 113
Boys & Girls Clubs, 34
Brain responses to trauma, 53–55
Breathing exercises, 120–121, 144
Bright Futures, 28, 151, 153–154*t*, 190
Brown, Brené, 83
Building Relationships: Framing Early Relational Health, 90
Building Resilience in Children and Teens, 65, 239
Bullock, L.M., 61
Burnout, 177, 179–180
 finding community and connection to mitigate, 183–184

C

Care coordinators, 147–148
Caregivers. *See* Parents and caregivers
Care plans, shared, 141–147, 251–252
Center on the Developing Child, Harvard, 39, 55, 66, 210
Childhood Trauma and Resilience: A Practical Guide, 21, 42, 85, 201
Children's Health Alliance (CHA), 39
Choices, giving, 162
CICT. *See* Compassion-informed care training (CICT)
Circle of Friends, 133
Circles of Support, 133–136, 133*f*, 164, 251–254
Clinical skills, 157
Clinical staff, motivating, 194
Clinical systems monitoring, 204–209